# Creating Nursing's Future

Issues, Opportunities, and Challenges

# Creating Nursing's Future

## Issues, Opportunities, and Challenges

**Eleanor J. Sullivan, RN, PhD, FAAN**
Professor
School of Nursing
University of Kansas
Kansas City, Kansas

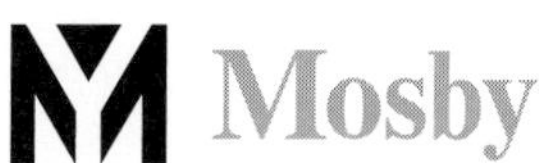

St. Louis Baltimore Boston Carlsbad Chicago Minneapolis New York Philadelphia Portland
London Milan Sydney Tokyo Toronto

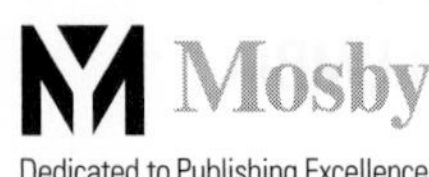

Dedicated to Publishing Excellence

A Times Mirror Company

*Publisher:* Sally Schrefer
*Editor:* Michael S. Ledbetter
*Developmental Editor:* Lisa P. Newton
*Project Manager:* John Rogers
*Senior Production Editor:* Cheryl A. Abbott
*Designer:* Bill Drone
*Manufacturing Manager:* Don Carlisle
*Cover Designer:* E. Rohne Rudder



Composition by Clarinda Company
Printing/binding by R. R. Donnelley & Sons Company

Mosby, Inc.
11830 Westline Industrial Drive
St. Louis, Missouri 63146

**Library of Congress Cataloging in Publication Data**

Sullivan, Eleanor J., 1938-
Creating nursing's future : issues, opportunities, and challenges / Eleanor J. Sullivan.
p. cm.
Includes bibliographical references and index.
ISBN 0-323-00239-0
1. Nursing—United States—Forecasting. 2. Medical Care—United States—Forecasting. 3. Twenty-first century—Forecasts. I. Title.
RT42 .S84 1999
610.73'01'12—dc21

98-46292
CIP

99 00 01 02 03 / 9 8 7 6 5 4 3 2 1

*To the nurses upon whose work we stand today*
*and to the nurses who will follow us.*
*We wish you the best.*

*Time keeps on slippin', slippin', slippin' into the future.*

**Dave Barry quoting the Steve Miller Band**

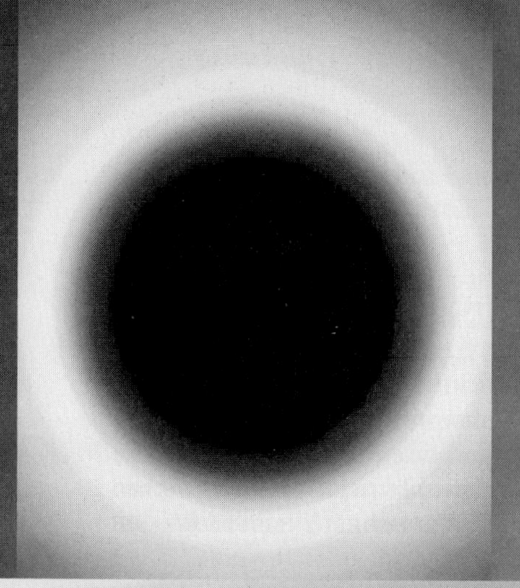

# Contributors

**Lea Acord, PhD, RN**
Dean and Professor, College of Nursing
Montana State University
Bozeman, Montana

**Carole A. Anderson, PhD, RN, FAAN**
Dean and Professor
College of Nursing
The Ohio State University
Columbus, Ohio

**Janis P. Bellack, PhD, RN, FAAN**
Associate Provost for Education and Professor of Nursing
Medical University of South Carolina
Charleston, South Carolina

**Akiko M. Berkman, MPAHA, MPH**
Project Coordinator
Healthy Communities
Portland, Oregon

**Marjorie Beyers, RN, PhD, FAAN**
Executive Director
American Organization of Nurse Executives
Chicago, Illinois

**Clement Bezold, PhD**
Executive Director
Institute for Alternative Futures
Alexandria, Virginia

**Rachel Z. Booth, PhD, RN**
Dean and Professor, School of Nursing
University of Alabama at Birmingham
Birmingham, Alabama

**Jennifer Bosma, PhD**
Executive Director
National Council of State Boards of Nursing
Chicago, Illinois

**Fay L. Bower, DNSc, FAAN**
Past President, Clarkson College
Omaha, Nebraska
Past President, Sigma Theta Tau International
Consultant, Nursing, Health, and Higher Education
Clayton, California

**Ann Marie T. Brooks, RN, DNSc, MBA, FACHE, FAAN**
Chief of Nursing Affairs
King Faisal Specialist Hospital and Research Centre
Riyadh, Kingdom of Saudi Arabia

**Roger J. Bulger, MD**
President and CEO
Association of Academic Health Centers
Washington, D.C.

**Myra J. Christopher**
President and CEO
Midwest Bioethics Center
Kansas City, Missouri

**Jacqueline F. Clinton, RN, PhD, FAAN**
Professor and Director
Center for Nursing Cultural Awareness and Sensitivity
University of Wisconsin
Milwaukee, Wisconsin

**Helen R. Connors, RN, PhD**
Associate Professor and Associate Dean for Academic Affairs
School of Nursing
University of Kansas
Kansas City, Kansas

**Linda L. Davies, PhD**
Director of Academic Support
University of Kansas
Medical Center A.R. Dykes Library
Kansas City, Kansas

**Sue K. Donaldson, PhD, RN, FAAN**
Dean and Professor, School of Nursing
Professor of Physiology, School of Medicine
The Johns Hopkins University
Baltimore, Maryland

**Joyce J. Fitzpatrick, PhD, MBA, RN, FAAN**
Elizabeth Brooks Ford Professor and Former Dean
Frances Payne Bolton School of Nursing
Case Western Reserve University
Cleveland, Ohio

**Maryann F. Fralic, RN, DrPH, FAAN**
Professor and Director
Corporate and Foundation Relations
School of Nursing
The Johns Hopkins University
Baltimore, Maryland

**Susan C. Fry, MEd, RN, CNAA**
Vice President, Patient Operations
Via Christi Regional Medical Center
Wichita, Kansas

**Sherril B. Gelmon, DrPH, FACHE**
Coordinator, Oregon MPH Program
Associate Professor of Public Health
School of Government and School of Community Health
College of Urban and Public Affairs
Portland State University
Portland, Oregon

**Suzanne Gordon**
Journalist and author
Arlington, Massachusetts

**Patricia A. Grady, PhD, RN, FAAN**
Director, National Institute of Nursing Research
National Institutes of Health
Bethesda, Maryland

**Trevor Hancock, MD**
Health Promotion Consultant
Kleinburg, Ontario
Canada

**Ada Sue Hinshaw, PhD, RN**
Dean and Professor, School of Nursing
University of Michigan
Ann Arbor, Michigan

**Karen Kelly, EdD, RN, CNAA**
Director, Behavioral Healthcare/Social Services
St. Elizabeth's Hospital
Belleville, Illinois

**Karlene Kerfoot, PhD, RN, CNAA, FAAN**
Vice President of Patient Care and Organizational Development
Memorial Hermann Healthcare System
Houston, Texas

**Diane K. Kjervik, JD, RN, BSN, MSN, FAAN**
Professor and Associate Dean for Outreach and Practice
School of Nursing
University of North Carolina–Chapel Hill
Chapel Hill, North Carolina

**Alice Kuramoto, PhD, RN, C, FAAN**
Professor and Director of Continuing Education and Outreach
School of Nursing
University of Wisconsin–Milwaukee
Milwaukee, Wisconsin

**Victoria J. Larson, RN, BSN**
Founder/Past President Ackley Nursing Services, Inc. and Ackley Home Health, Inc.
San Diego, California

**Andrea R. Lindell, DNSc, RN**
Dean and Professor, College of Nursing
Interim Dean, College of Allied Health
Associate Senior Vice President for Interdisciplinary Education
University of Cincinnati
Cincinnati, Ohio

**Karen L. Miller, RN, PhD, FAAN**
Dean and Professor, School of Nursing
Dean, School of Allied Health
University of Kansas
Kansas City, Kansas

**Virginia L. Morse, RN, MN, CEN, CCRN, CS**
Clinical Nurse Specialist/Program Director
Trauma Services
Truman Medical Center
Kansas City, Missouri

**Jane S. Norbeck, RN, DNSc, FAAN**
Dean and Professor, School of Nursing
University of California–San Francisco
San Francisco, California

**Nancy Rainville Oliver, PhD, RN, HNC**
Associate Professor, Department of Nursing
California State University–Long Beach
Long Beach, California

**Daniel J. Pesut, PhD, RN, CS, FAAN**
Professor and Chair, Department of Environments for Health
School of Nursing
Indiana University
Indianapolis, Indiana

**Tim Porter-O'Grady, EdD, PhD, FAAN**
Senior Partner
Tim Porter-O'Grady Associates, Inc.
Atlanta, Georgia

**Marla E. Salmon, ScD, RN, FAAN**
Professor and Dean, Graduate Program
University of Pennsylvania
Philadelphia, Pennsylvania

**Toni Smith, RN, EdD**
Director, Nursing Methods, Procedures and Quality Control and Recruitment and Marketing
Strong Memorial Hospital;
Associate Professor of Clinical Nursing
School of Nursing
University of Rochester
Rochester, New York

**MaryCarroll Sullivan, RN, MTS, JD**
Vice President and Chief Operating Officer
Midwest Bioethics Center
Kansas City, Missouri

**Diana L. Taylor, RN, PhD, FAAN**
Associate Professor
Department of Family Health Care Nursing
School of Nursing
University of California–San Francisco
San Francisco, California

**Virginia P. Tilden, DNSc, RN, FAAN**
Professor and Associate Dean for Research
School of Nursing
Director, Program of Research on Ethics and End of Life Care, Center of Ethics
Associate Director, Center for Ethics in Health Care
Oregon Health Sciences University
Portland, Oregon

**Patricia A. Trangenstein, RN, PhD**
Associate Professor
Coordinator of User Support
Center for Academic Technologies and Educational Resources
College of Nursing
University of Cincinnati
Cincinnati, Ohio

**Connie Vance, RN, EdD, FAAN**
Dean and Professor
School of Nursing
College of New Rochelle
New Rochelle, New York

**Mary Wakefield, PhD, RN, FAAN**
Director, Center for Health Policy
College of Nursing and Health Science
George Mason University
Fairfax, Virginia

**Betsy E. Weiner, RN, PhD**
Professor of Nursing
College of Nursing
Director, Center for Academic Technologies
Acting Associate Director
Academic Information Technology Services
University of Cincinnati
Cincinnati, Ohio

**Eileen Zungolo, EdD, RN**
Dean, College of Nursing
Northeastern University
Boston, Massachusetts

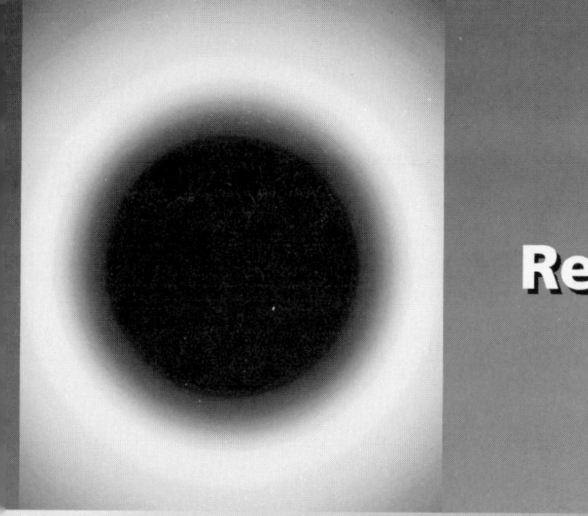

# Reviewers

**Joy Brands, MPH, CNM**
Assistant Professor of Nursing, Retired
Bellarmine College
2001 Newburg Road
Louisville, Kentucky

**Jean Bohomey, MS, RN, CS**
Assistant Professor of Clinical Nursing
University of Rochester
School of Nursing
601 Elmwood Avenue
Rochester, New York

**Carla L. Mueller, MS, RN**
Assistant Professor
University of Saint Francis
Department of Nursing
2701 Spring Street
Fort Wayne, Indiana

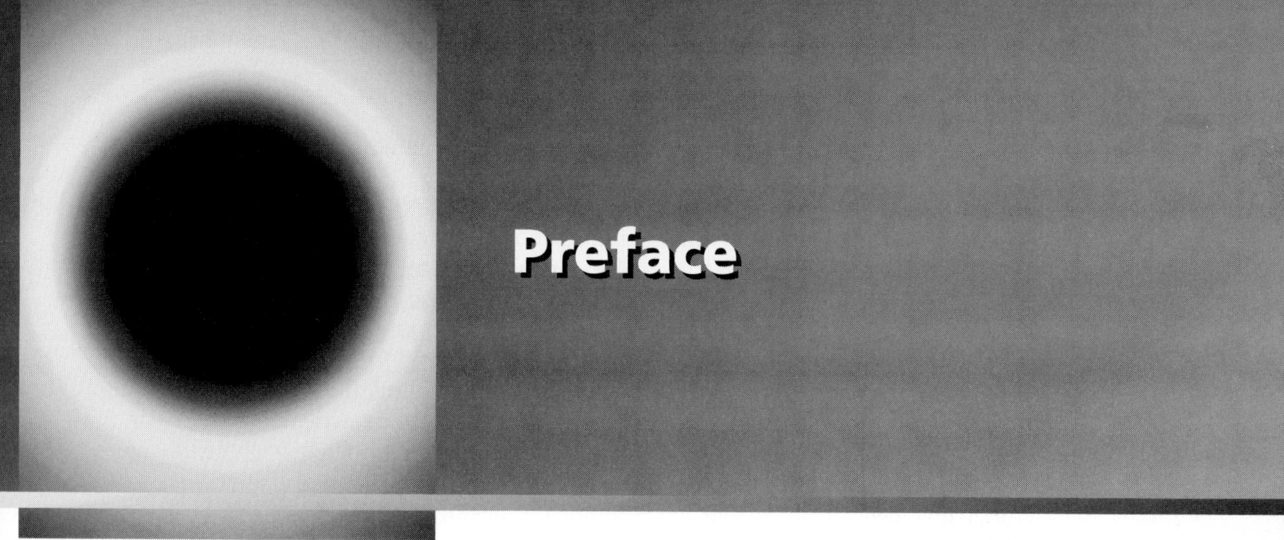

# Preface

The future is unknown. Therefore any book about the future is necessarily speculative. What is recognized clearly, however, is that we affect the future by what we do or fail to do today. That's what this book is about. It is designed to help nurses and others create a preferred future for nursing. Its purpose is to bring attention to the issues affecting nurses, explore the opportunities inherent in the future, and use challenges as stepping stones to creating a desired future.

*Creating Nursing's Future: Issues, Opportunities, and Challenges* is like no other text on nursing issues or nursing's future. Its strength is its conceptual framework, based on the work of futurists Trevor Hancock and Clement Bezold, that proposes comparing the probable future (if current trends continue) with a preferred future (the one we'd like to see happen), which enables us to design strategies to achieve the future desired.

Another strength of the book is the expertise of its chapter authors, including leading figures in nursing, health care, bioethics, law, and journalism. Their sections build on Hancock and Bezold's framework and draw from the authors' extensive experiences as leaders and scholars. The result is a one-of-a-kind textbook in nursing that covers the issues of nursing and health care—a snapshot of the present and a vision of the future.

Today's health care world is continually shifting and adapting to changing economic, scientific, and clinical demands. Nurses, like other health care professionals, often wonder what their future will bring. Examining possibilities and ways to achieve a desired future gives nurses the tools to create a better tomorrow for themselves, the profession, and their patients.

Each chapter includes Discussion Exercises for readers to complete on their own. These are designed to help readers recall relevant situations in which they might now, having read the text, understand or respond differently. Some are designed for readers to imagine themselves in hypothetical situations with real-life problems to solve. All are intended to evoke creative, contemplative solutions to problems and set a pattern of innovative thinking about possibilities for the future.

The book is arranged in six parts. Part I, **Nursing in Society,** examines nursing from a futurist perspective, explores the future of the health care system and nursing's role in transforming that system, includes nursing's role in health care policy and in the public domain, and concludes with a chapter on enhancing nursing's public image.

Part II, **The Future of Practice and Education,** considers nursing practice of the future and how to prepare nurses for that practice in both beginning and advanced practice roles, envisions creative settings for clinical teaching, discusses scientific discoveries and technology, explains how information technology can be used in practice and teaching, suggests innovative faculty practice models, explores continuing education and staff development of the future, and spells out the challenges facing nursing in higher education now and in the future.

Part III, **Administration in the Future,** describes how to organize, plan, and manage in tomorrow's health care system; discusses collective bargaining in the future; and explores management of academic nursing programs.

Part IV, **Accountability, Quality, and Control,** answers many questions about the future of accountability, quality, licensure, and accreditation and considers the ethical and legal issues of the future.

Part V, **Nursing's Scientific Future,** includes information about the future of nursing research, the expansion of collaborative and interdisciplinary research, the preparation of nurse researchers for the future, and the career trajectory of a nurse scientist.

Part VI, **Expanding the Boundaries,** is designed to stretch the imagination from *what is* to *what is possible.* Alternative health care, interdisciplinary practice and education, growing multiculturalism, entrepreneurship, globalization, and the role of professional organizations explore contemporary ideas and innovations. Scenarios of health care's future complete the text.

The appendixes are an especially valuable addition to this book. Contents include listings of international resources, current and proposed doctoral programs in nursing, and a directory of nursing organizations in the United States.

The future is a wide-open vista, a blank canvas on which to transform our vision into reality. There is no inextricable mystery here—we simply pose the questions: what is best for our clients, the patients? What is best for our profession? What can I do to make a difference? What works? What doesn't work? In a perfect world, how would nursing and health care be configured?

Generations of nurses and their patients are relying on our imagination, intellect, and daring. By examining the issues, seizing the opportunities, and accepting the challenges, nursing is poised to create a vision for the future into the years to come. The future of nursing depends on it. And on you.

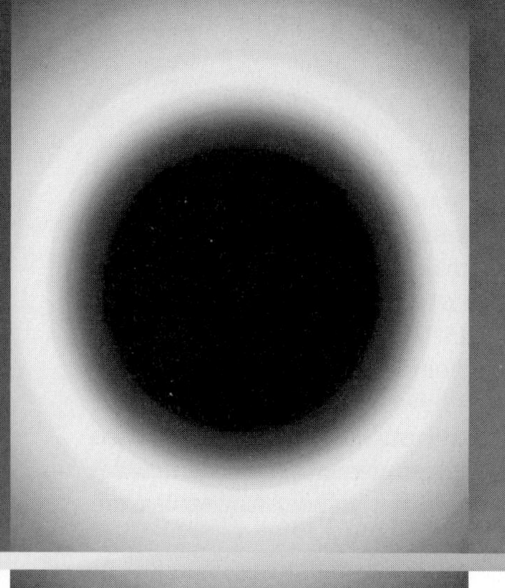

# Acknowledgments

The quality of this book and the potential it has to help create nursing's future is largely due to the contributions of the chapter authors. Without them this book would not exist. Nursing leaders in practice, education, administration, technology, policy, ethics, law, nursing science, entrepreneurship, and professional organizations all offered their best thinking on the possibilities in nursing's future. The contributions of futurists Trevor Hancock and Clement Bezold to the conceptual framework and as chapter authors were invaluable and greatly appreciated. Physician Roger Bulger, journalist Suzanne Gordon, academician Sherril Gelmon, and bioethicist Myra Christopher all made essential and exemplary contributions in their respective chapters.

The support of the School of Nursing at the University of Kansas is appreciated. Rita Clifford, Barbara Langner, and Susan Fry all shared their wisdom, expertise, and advice.

Carole Anderson and Polly Bednash kindly recommended contributing authors. Connie Lacker and Marcia Pressly provided accurate and swift typing services.

At Mosby Lisa Newton coordinated manuscript preparation, secured permissions, and kept in constant contact throughout the development phase of the book. Jeff Burnham and Michael Ledbetter were, successively, Mosby's editors on the project and guided the book from conception to completion. Cheryl Abbott did an outstanding job as production editor.

Reviewers are always invaluable in creation of a new book, and Joy Brands, Jean Bohomey, and Carla Mueller offered valuable comments and suggestions.

To everyone who contributed to the fine quality of this book, I thank you.

**Eleanor J. Sullivan**

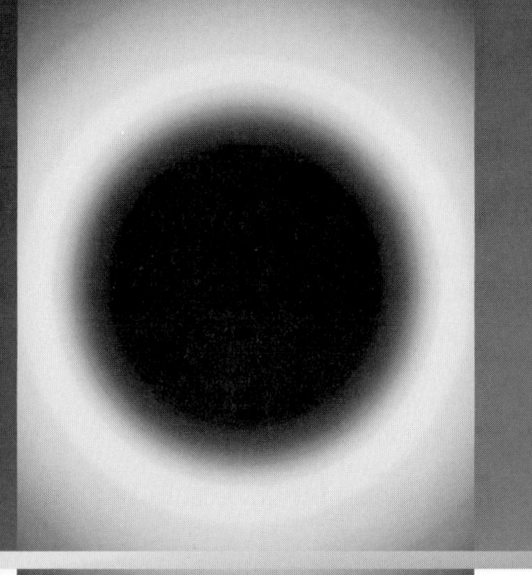

# Contents

## PART I
## NURSING IN SOCIETY

# I

# Nursing in Society

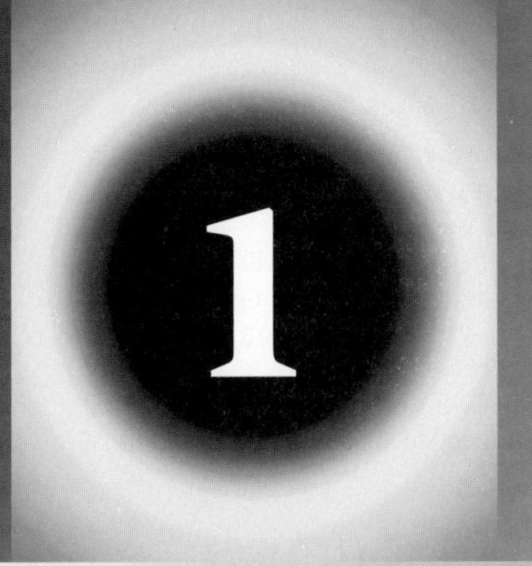

# 1 Examining Nursing From a Futures Perspective*

**Clement Bezold**
**Trevor Hancock**
**Eleanor J. Sullivan**

*Thinking about the future is only useful and interesting if it affects what we do and how we live today.*

**James Robertson**
British expert on alternative futures

Since the beginning of time, we have tried to predict the future. Changes in the solar system, natural phenomena, or animal behavior, among others, have been suggested as signs of pending events. Fortune telling has enjoyed continuous success in spite of scientific evidence of its fallibility. End-of-the-world predictions have failed to materialize, but the world's demise continues to be prophesied. Myths guided beliefs about the past and foretold the future (Box 1-1).

Two beliefs characterized predicting the future: the future would repeat the past, for example, a person could count on the seasons to change, crops to grow, babies to be born, the old to die, and life generally to stay the same; and that if and when there was change, it was caused by an external force such as a supernatural power or more powerful people or governments. Individuals had little or no ability to affect their future or the world.

As the twentieth century marched on, social, economic, and political changes occurred more rapidly. That rate and magnitude of change continue to increase. Demographics, including birth rates and migration, are altering the face of specific locales and will affect the future of places that experience population losses, gains, or changes. Education, literacy, governments, agriculture, and social conditions are shifting, changing constantly. Mapmakers struggle to keep world maps current and are challenged by constantly changing regional borders and names.

The growth of technology, especially communication technology, is unprecedented. As people live longer, they see revolutionary changes occur over the course of their lives. There

---

*Parts of this chapter are modified from Bezold and Hancock (1996) and Hancock and Bezold (1994).

**Box 1-1**

It was 1982—a boom time for hospital growth. In the average U.S. community, inpatient care had peaked at 1134 days per thousand. When the planning shop of a major hospital chain asked a futurist firm to explore the outlook for inpatient care and the implications for hospital strategies, they worked together and reached an estimate: by 2010 inpatient care would be reduced by 50% to 60%. By 1990 this forecast was proving accurate: inpatient demand had dropped to 607 days per thousand—down nearly 50% from its 1982 level. Unfortunately, the organization failed to respond to that early warning; it was at odds with the dominant acute-care paradigm of the time. And 5 years later the system's CEO was painfully acknowledging that they had missed a major shift.

From Hancock T, Bezold C: Possible futures, preferable futures, *Healthcare Forum J* 37(2):23, 1994.

are people in today's technologic world who can remember life without cars, planes, or telephones. The world has shrunk to a global village connected by transportation, communication, business, and government; what occurs in one part of the world has the potential to affect widely diverse areas.

Environmental change also has the potential to affect the lives of millions of people all over the world. Global warming will increase the range of malaria and other insect-borne diseases, alter climate patterns and food production, increase the severity and frequency of storms, and create millions of "eco-refugees." Depletion of forests, fisheries, fossil fuels, and other resources; pollution and impaired ecosystem health; and the fraying of the web of life all have dramatic health effects, both locally and globally (McMichael, 1995).

Social change, however, is slower in coming. Technologic advances are forcing decisions that heretofore were unimagined except in science fiction. Decisions about cloning, genetic research, and assisted suicide challenge long-held notions of right and wrong. The best thinking of right-minded people is needed to envision a future committed to the health and well-being of the world's citizens, succeeding generations, and the environment.

The study of the future has never been more imperative. Nursing has never had a greater need to understand the future, to envision a preferred future, and to develop strategies to create the preferred future than it does today. Vision and commitment are needed more than ever before.

## WHY STUDY THE FUTURE?

Although many people think that it is the job of futurists to predict the future, the task is better left to fortune tellers. Truly effective futures work engages people who are not futurists in thinking more effectively and creatively about the future and in applying that thinking to their present activities. As a result they may be better able to define the future they prefer and to work to create it while avoiding the future they fear.

Health futures work must be both imaginative and plausible, but it also has to confront the will to act. To be helpful, it has to influence learning, encourage commitment to action, and inspire those involved to question their sacred assumptions.

Health futures work does more than identify what might happen; it enables individuals and organizations to find or enhance the leadership necessary to move in desired directions. This means that good futures work includes both futures research and vision. These in turn contribute to strategic management by aiding in anticipation, setting direction, and securing commitment.

## SHAPING THE FUTURE

Failure to understand these points leads some people to assume that the future is fixed and is approaching with an awesome inevitability—that there is nothing we can do about it. Such a passive way of thinking inevitably results in apathy and a feeling of impotence and lack of control, a not uncommon experience in nursing.

Futurists by and large take a proactive stance with regard to the future. There is no certainty in studying the future, because it does not yet exist. Rather, futurists study ideas about the future and often believe that the future is plastic and can be shaped. If they are not actively involved in seeking to create change themselves, futurists are certainly aware that their presentations and predictions will form the basis for others who seek to create change.

Futurism is, to use a phrase coined by Alvin Toffler, author of *Future Shock* (1970) and *The Third Wave* (1980), a form of "anticipatory democracy," helping people to decide what sort of future they want and how they might go about achieving it (Bezold, 1978). In the case of health futures, such thinking should not be confined simply to the health care system but should encompass health in the broader sense. Although health care futurists are chiefly concerned with issues of human biology, disease treatment, services and technologies, the role and scope of practice of health care professionals, and the funding of health care, health futurists are mainly focused on the environmental, social, economic, political, cultural, behavioral, biologic, and health care determinants of health. It is not enough to create a vision of a preferred twenty-first century health care system; we need a vision of a healthier future for all (Hancock and Garrett, 1995).

## Assumptions About the Future

Two relevant assumptions about the future can be made. First, the future is uncertain. There is no single, certain forecast for the future of health and health care. Although we would like to eliminate this uncertainty, we must be able to live with it effectively and creatively. Understanding key trends and alternative futures for health conditions, for health care, for our organizations, for our profession, and for our communities can enhance our effectiveness and creativity. Second, we choose and create major aspects of the future by what we do or fail to do. Although the future is uncertain and much of the future is beyond our control, there are large aspects of the future we can influence. Visions and strategies linked to a clear sense of trends and scenarios make us better able to shape the future we prefer.

## Four Futures

Canadian futurist Norman Henchey (1978) proposes four ways of thinking about the future.

The *possible future*—what may happen—encompasses everything we can possibly imagine, no matter how unlikely, including "science fiction" futures that transgress presently accepted laws of science. For example, one possible future is that we will learn how spiritual healing works and will be able to treat people by using the energy aura of the healer.

The possible future includes "wildcards," those dramatic and seemingly implausible changes that can occur very swiftly. Wildcards are typically low-probability but high-impact events such as the fall of the Berlin Wall, the transformation of the Soviet Union, or the bombing of the federal building in Oklahoma City. We need to be flexible enough to deal with surprises when they occur, so having a sense of what type of wildcards might arise is useful. However, most planning efforts do well to focus on dealing with more plausible futures.

The *plausible future*—what could happen—represents a narrower scope, emphasizing those possible futures that seem to make sense given what we know today. Plausible futures can be discrete forecasts of individual trends or a set of scenarios, each combining differing trends and together describing a range of alternative futures.

Examples of common plausible futures are a high-technology growth scenario; a "green" or sustainable society scenario; a scenario of environmental, economic, and social decline and/or a more controlled society; and a "high spirit" or transformation scenario. For each of these we can describe a quite detailed societal scenario, including a description of health status and of the health care system. The health care system will reflect the society of which it is a part, not the other way around, which is why we need to consider the societal scenario first.

The alternative futures approach enables us to compare a range of quite plausible future options and to choose among them. In making that choice, we make explicit the values we hold, individually and collectively (see Bezold and others, 1997, for an example of this approach applied to health promotion).

The *probable future*—what will likely happen—is based on our examination of our present situation and our appraisal of likely trends and future developments. It is one of the plausible futures and is sometimes referred to as "business as usual" or the "official" future.

Most people see the future as an extension of the present with little significant change. Likewise, most government and business planning assumes that the probable future will be a straightforward extrapolation of the present.

Until very recently, the probable future of the health care system was seen to be hospital based, physician dominated, and high tech. Today, that assumption, or some aspects of it, has already changed (health care is no longer hospital based) and other aspects of it seem less certain. Ironically, history shows that this image of the most likely future often turns out to be the least likely to occur. Descriptive forecasts based solely on recent trends can preclude futures that are different; they also often turn out to be the future we don't want! As University of Hawaii futurist James Dator (1993) has remarked, "Trends can take us with unerring accuracy to where we don't want to be!"

The *preferable future*—what we want to have happen—is sometimes called *prescriptive futurism* or *normative forecasting*. Preferable futures are visions that generally begin by identifying and trying to create a future that does not yet exist. Vision moves reality beyond the present toward the best that can be.

Figure 1-1 illustrates how these four futures relate to one another and shows that all of these futures start from where we are today but then diverge. From our up-close vantage point in the present it is hard to tell them apart, but clearly, choices made now can have dramatic effects over time.

Creating a shared vision of the preferred future health care system or of a healthy com-

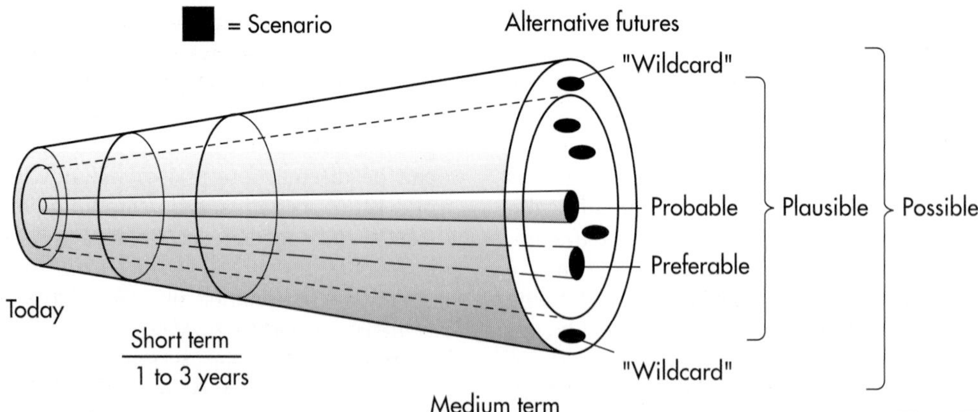


**Figure 1-1** Types of futures. (From Hancock T, Bezold C: Possible futures, preferable futures, *Healthcare Forum J* 37(2):25, 1994.)

munity can be a powerful technique for mobilizing an organization, a community, or a profession around a common purpose.

### Liberating the Future

A marked difference between the future we think is likely to happen and the one we would prefer to have happen often exists. Examining both can be very liberating.

Too often our image of the future is the scenario we think will most likely happen. If we don't like the way we think things are going, this may bring with it an awful sense that the light at the end of the tunnel is a train bearing down on us. The probable future is something that seems to be done to us, something over which we have little or no control, and often something we don't like very much.

If the field of health futures focuses too much on the probable, which it has a tendency to do (planners, be they politicians, civil servants, or private business persons, like to know what to plan for, as do ordinary people), then it runs the risk, perhaps inadvertently, of disempowering people and denying them choice. If people are told "this is the probable future," then the only choices left for them are how to prepare for it, how to brace for it, and how to deal with it when it arrives.

The preferable future, on the other hand, is a liberating and empowering future, especially when it touches our more creative capacities. It not only enables but also encourages people to say, "This is the future that we value and that we want to create." The energy and creativity released in a preferable futures process can be quite astonishing.

## HEALTH VERSUS HEALTH CARE FUTURES

It is extremely unfortunate that we have come to use the words *health care* almost synonymously with the word *health*, thus confusing two very separate concepts: health and health care (or more accurately, sick care). Thinking about the future of health is not the same thing as thinking about the future of health care. The field of health futures is concerned with the future of our state of health, which is dominated by environmental, social, economic, and political determinants and to a lesser extent by biophysiologic, genetic, and health care factors. Will we be more healthy or less healthy in the future? What will be the major influences on health? What values will we attach to health, and what role will health play in our decision making? What will be the relationship between health and health care?

A great deal of health futures thinking is concerned with societal futures in general, particularly those aspects of societal futures that affect health and well-being. This includes such issues as wealth and poverty, living and working conditions, the sustainability of our environment, the state of social networks and social support, the extent of participation and empowerment, and a whole host of other issues that affect personal and collective health and well-being. Health futures also considers the subject of health/public policy, or the health impacts of public policy in nonhealth sectors. What future policies might be developed if health and well-being were prime determinants of public policy? (Hancock, 1982)

Health care futures, on the other hand, is a subset of health futures and deal with a comparatively minor determinant of future health. It is concerned with the future of the institutions and professions of the medical/sick/health care system. Such issues as the size, structure, and financing of health care services; the role of physicians, nurses, and other health care professionals; future technologies and therapies; and the impact that health care services may have on overall health and well-being are also concerns of health care futures. Although forecasts and visions for the future of the health professions and health care delivery are essential, it is important to avoid becoming overly concerned with health care futures and losing sight of the primary objective: health (see Hancock and Garrett, 1995).

## The Influence of Medical Care

Until recently, the concentrated wealth of the medical sector usually meant that in any discussion of health, including any discussion of the future of health, medical care and medical futures predominated. This occurred in part because many people who work in the medical care system continue to believe that medical care played a major role in improving health during the past 100 years.

However, major improvements in health in the nineteenth and twentieth centuries resulted primarily from improved food supply, better hygiene and sanitation, and reduced family size resulting from economic development and the education of women and their participation in the workforce (McKeown, 1979). MeKeown's work shows that although vaccines and antibiotics had some effect (mostly after 1935), much of the decline in mortality for many of the major infectious diseases occurred before effective vaccines and antibiotics were available. Similarly, much of the decline in cardiovascular disease mortality in the United States in the past 20 years has been attributed not to medical treatment but to changes in lifestyle related to smoking, diet, and exercise (see Evans and others, 1994; Hancock and Garrett, 1995; and Sagan, 1987 for broad overview of the determinants of health).

At the global level the World Bank's *World Development Report: Investing in Health* (1993) has emphasized the importance for future health status of measures to increase the income of those in poverty; to improve education, especially for girls; and to promote the rights and status of women. In the future, as in the past, it is likely that these environmental, social, and economic factors will continue to be of greater importance in determining health status than medical care. This is why it is necessary to begin futures work with an environmental scan that scopes out the future shape of society then projects what health status and health care would be like in such a society. Nursing can then see where its skills and talents fit into the need for health and health care. Of course, in designing our preferred future, we need to understand the major forces that will likely be affecting health and health care in the future.

# NURSING'S FUTURE

Nursing's future is inextricably, and rightly so, bound to society's future and the future of health care. The value placed on health (or not), the willingness of a society to expend its resources to improve or maintain health, societal beliefs that all citizens are entitled to health care, and the commitment to improve and maintain public health all determine the role and scope of health care in a society. Nursing, then, complements the components of health activities that the society values and participates in offering services that society values.

A variety of futures for nursing can be surmised for the following scenarios. A *possible*—though not very likely—future for nursing might include a radical change in the structure of health care systems in which nurses act as the primary managers of care and physicians and all other health care providers report to nurses. A more *plausible*—slightly more likely—future could envision an expanded role for nurses in which holistic nursing care becomes the predominant value in the health care system. A *probable*—more likely—future might suggest that the current invisibility of nurses will continue; that nurses will lack power, vision, and cohesiveness; that the health care system will continue to disempower nurses; and that nursing care will decline as a societal value. The *preferable*—and one we would like to see happen—future for nursing might predict that the holistic care delivered by nurses will be recognized as integral to the health care system and that nurses will serve as the first line of care in promoting healthy communities and will be recognized as integral to the health care team (Sigma Theta Tau International, 1996).

The focus of this book is on nursing's preferable future, with predictions about the probable futures—what will happen if current trends con-

**Box 1-2**
***How Far Away Is the Future?***

Most futurists share the belief that the future will be shaped by human decisions and actions. The immediate future (1 to 5 years) is largely shaped by decisions previously taken (of course, "discontinuities" such as the 1989 fall of the Berlin Wall or the 1991 Iraqi invasion of Kuwait can dramatically and swiftly alter the future). But the medium-term future (5 to 20 years) and the long-term future (20 to 50 years) are substantially shaped by the decisions we make today and in the years ahead.

Beyond 50 years, the future is so far removed that thinking about it is extremely difficult. How much of what we accept as commonplace today could have been anticipated in 1930? How little of what was commonplace in 1930—most of the mechanical and electrical equipment of the twentieth century—would have been anticipated in 1880? This does not make thinking 50 years out irrelevant, but it does free us to make use of science fiction literature, which can be very helpful even in thinking about dramatic changes that could surprise us in the next decade.

Modified from Hancock T, Bezold C: Possible futures, preferable futures, *Healthcare Forum J* 37(2):23, 1994.

tinue—used for comparison. Sometimes, the two are the same; that is, what one expects to happen is what one prefers to happen. Often, this is not the case, and—to the extent that the probable and preferable futures differ—this difference is the target for new visions and strategic planning action (Box 1-2).

## COMPONENTS OF HEALTH FUTURES

Trends, scenarios, visions, and strategies are four components of health futures work. Trends and scenarios explore what might happen. Visions clarify what we want to create. Strategies link plausible and preferred futures to action (Bezold and Hancock, 1996).

### Trends

A trend is a pattern of change over time. Trends typically focus on discrete topics, for example, health care costs, disease prevalence, and therapeutic advances. They generally involve plausible forecasts, usually extrapolated from recent or past experience (though at times those who monitor trends or their clients inappropriately confuse what they think is plausible with what they prefer). There are a variety of quantitative and qualitative methods for developing trends, including environmental scanning with various degrees of quantification, Delphi and other surveys, and expert judgment.

It is important to understand how trends evolve and how to spot a trend in its early stages. As trends grow in visibility and importance, they often become issues—changes or problems on which we take action. Figure 1-2 illustrates this emergence of a trend into an issue.

Once an issue has emerged, it is easier to observe by scanning the mass media. Many trends, however, can be spotted years in advance in trade or scientific media. Even before that, artistic or visionary thinkers will explore the ideas or forces that will make up the trend. Victor Hugo's *Les Miserables* depicted the plight of the poor in France and foretold future societal attention on these problems, which may have been instrumental in improving conditions. In the early 1960s pollution was seldom thought to be a serious problem in the United States, and environmental concerns were relatively low. Rachel Carson had a different opinion of trends in environmental conditions and wrote *Silent Spring* (1962), which hastened today's concern about the environment. More recently, Suzanne Gordon's book, *Life Support* (1997), which chronicles the work of three nurses and illustrates nurses' essential role in health care, has been hailed by the *Washington Post* (Benderly, 1997). The *Post* states that *Life Support* "belongs in the august company of Rachel Carson's *Silent Spring* . . . and other pivotal works with the power to shift the nation's consciousness." This is remarkable praise for a book about nursing that was written for the general

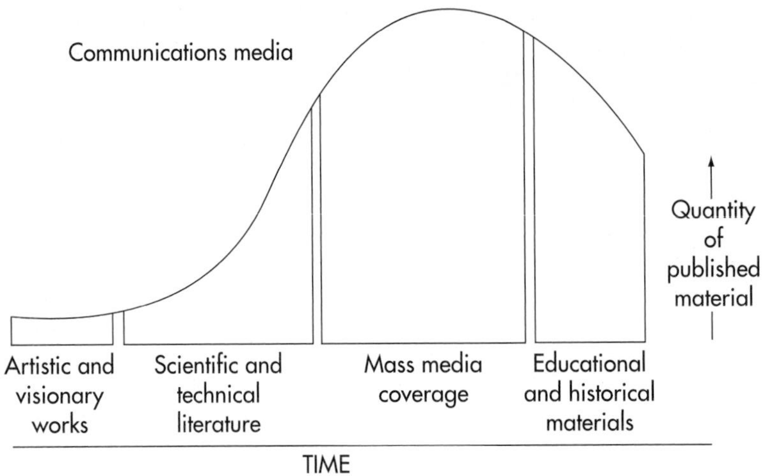


**Figure 1-2** Emergence of a trend into an issue. (From Bezold C, Hancock T: Health futures: tools for wiser decision making. In Bezold C, Mayer E, editors: *Future care: responding to the demand for change,* New York, 1996, Faulkner & Gray.)

population, and the future will tell if the *Post's* predictions come true.

In most areas of health care, trends are found at these various stages of development. The earlier a trend is spotted, the greater flexibility an organization has to respond to it. Some organizations and most governments wait until trends become issues, often waiting for the issue to reach a crisis state before taking action. When a trend is at a crisis state and is getting significant attention in the media (the top of the curve in Figure 1-2), the decision costs for policy makers are higher and the range of options for solving the crisis becomes narrower.

Attempting to look farther into the future is important to alert us to threats and opportunities. Positive change can be accelerated to the extent that we look ahead at what should be changed.

## Scenarios

Trends focus on change in certain specific topics over time, for example, poverty, acquired immunodeficiency syndrome (AIDS), therapeutic breakthroughs, and health care finance. However, trends often move in conflicting directions. Scenarios are powerful tools that were developed for considering how interacting sets of trends might lead to a range of conditions in the future. Scenarios are compilations of trends into differing images of the future. These images of the future allow their users to consider a broad range of possibilities. As the cone in Figure 1-1 indicates, scenarios "bound the uncertainty" of the future by defining what is plausible and what becomes possible if wildcards were to emerge. The use of scenarios grew significantly in the 1980s in both corporate and community planning, particularly in the United States and Europe.

Scenarios can be developed in a variety of ways and in varying degrees of detail, yet a set of scenarios should be both plausible and challenging. Scenarios provide a powerful opportunity to learn both about the future and about our current thinking, including the assumptions and paradigms to which we have become blind.

The Institute of Alternative Futures (Bezold and Hancock, 1996) often uses a set of archetypes including a "best guess" extrapolation of current trends—the official future or "business as usual" scenario (e.g., managed care continues to expand). Next, a "hard times" scenario is explored that asks "What could go wrong?" (e.g., quality of care declines). Participants are then invited to create two very different scenarios to portray more visionary possibilities (e.g., new low-tech, noninvasive therapeutic techniques are proven effective; healthy lifestyles are common). This approach has recently been used by the World Health Organization to generate a set of global scenarios as a basis for exploring the future of health promotion. It was concluded that one scenario leads to "health for many," one to "health for a few," and one to "health for all." The implication for health promotion strategies and actions today can then be explored (Bezold and others, 1997).

Scenarios are simplifications of complex current realities extended into the future. The future that actually occurs is likely to be a mixture of scenarios, somewhat like a mosaic, but one in which one future predominates, just like one color can predominate in a mosaic.

Scenarios invite us to think about the relative likelihood and relative preference of the different futures. Interestingly, the scenarios thought to be most likely often turn out to be far less preferred than the more visionary ones. However, many organizations focus their planning on reacting to the more likely futures, reinforcing them and preventing the more desirable ones from occurring. Although organizations can identify more creative, productive futures that they would prefer, their planning and decision-making processes often do not allow them to take the steps necessary to realize their preferred future. As a result they focus too much on what is and ignore what could be and what ought to be. This leads to the next type of futures tool: vision.

## Vision

Scenarios are "futures for the head." They provide intelligence, identifying threats and opportunities and stretching our imagination. Visions are "futures for the heart." They touch and move us.

Scenarios deal with plausible futures, yet futures thinking should be used to lead us to wiser action. Action is often strongest when it comes from our deep commitments—from our heart. Vision is a statement of our values projected into the future we want to create. Visions define the best that can be—something that those who subscribe to the vision will commit to creating.

Thus a vision is a compelling, inspiring statement of the preferred future that the authors and those who subscribe to the vision are committed to creating. The critical dimension of a vision is not the statement itself but the commitment and behavior that the vision draws out of those who pursue it.

Examples of vision can be found in both the public and private sectors. In its Health for All campaign, the World Health Organization offered a positive vision of the future. The Reinventing Government initiative, headed by Vice President Al Gore, is another example. In their book, *In Search of Excellence* (1982), Tom Peters and Robert Waterman report that companies that authentically communicated a strategic vision to their employees could tap a higher level of productivity from employees because the vision touched their hearts.

In *The Fifth Discipline* (1990), Peter Senge emphasizes that for a vision statement to effect positive change, two conditions must be met. First, the vision must be a shared vision to which members of the organization are committed. They will stretch themselves and the organization to make it happen, creating the conditions necessary. Second, the members of the organization must believe that they can make it happen; "vision becomes a living force only when people truly believe they can shape their future." This is why it is vital that the crafting of a vision be undertaken in a way that is as broad based and participatory as possible, whether it is a vision of a health community (Hancock, 1993), a health care system, a hospital, or any other setting or organization.

**Box 1-3**
***Comparison of Strategic Plan With Visions***

| Strategic Plans | Visions |
|---|---|
| Directional | End-state oriented |
| Linear | Holistic view—a snapshot |
| React to trends and competition | Desire to create in the world |
| Work forward to the future | Work backward from the future |
| Have to know how to get there | Unclear how to get there |
| Completed plan | Dynamically incomplete—a process |
| Plan language | Vision language |
| Cool | Hot |
| Rational | Heart/spirit |
| Mind focused | Intuitive |
| Bureaucratic | Poetic |
| Secret | Public |

From Doyle M: Quest for vision, *Assoc Manage,* p 29, September, 1990.

## Strategies

Strategies and visions are both important for moving forward, but they are not the same. An organization could have a marvelous vision of where it wanted to go but could have no plans for getting there. Likewise, an excellent strategic plan might be developed but not be based on a preferred vision of the future. As American futurist John Naisbitt noted in his book, *Megatrends* (1984): "A strategic plan is worthless without a strategic vision." Both are essential to move an organization, a community, or a profession toward its preferred future. Box 1-3 compares strategic plans with visions.

Although we have not been short of strategic plans, there has been a comparative dearth of strategic vision. From a futures point of view, however, what is important is the combination of strategic vision and strategic planning.

Vision is influenced by the threats and opportunities of the external environment best summarized in scenarios. Vision is also guided by factors internal to the organization, community, or profession, including its strengths and weaknesses and its competitive position. Once we have a vision, strategies are needed to focus our efforts on achieving the vision. Strategies are high-level, integrated sets of actions we will take to make our vision a reality.

# CONCLUSION

Futures thinking is a tool for wiser action that stimulates the imagination, encourages creativity, identifies threats and opportunities, and allows us to relate possible future choices and consequences to our values. The challenges for planners, policy makers, and health care and nursing leaders seeking to use health futures are three-fold as follows:

- To integrate more visionary and scenario-based futures methods with the more standard, near-term (often within the old paradigm) planning approaches
- To consider the roles of health care providers within the wider role of the determinants of health (e.g., where are the greatest points of leverage, and in that context, what is the appropriate role for health care providers?)
- To involve the whole range of customers and the entire community in designing the health and health care system that the community wants

The value of thinking about health futures is that it requires us to look beyond our preoccupation with the health care delivery system to examine the real determinants of health and health status. It serves to focus our attention on the human and ecologic ends rather than the economic and technologic means that are so often the preoccupation of health care futurism. Thinking about the future in this way should lead us to examine more closely what we do and how we live today and to ask what it takes to create a healthier future for all.

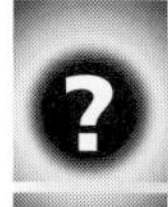

## *Discussion Exercises*

1. Identify reasons why studying the future is important to nursing.
2. Select an aspect of nursing (e.g., practice, education, research) and create four scenarios (possible, plausible, probable, preferable) of nursing's future.
3. Explain how trends, scenarios, visions, and strategies intersect in achieving a preferred future. Use nursing as an example.

## References


Benderly BL: Cure for an epidemic: a compelling cry to put patients first in health care, *Washington Post,* May 26, 1997.

Bezold C, editor: *Anticipatory democracy,* New York, 1978, Random House.

Bezold C, Hancock T: Health futures: tools for wiser decision making. In Bezold C, Mayer E, editors: *Future care: responding to the demand for change,* New York 1996, Faulkner & Gray.

Bezold C, and others: *World health 2020: global scenarios for health promotion* (conference working paper, 4th International Conference on Health Promotion, Jakarta, Indonesia, July, 1997), Geneva, 1997, World Health Organization.

Carson R: *Silent spring,* Boston, 1962, Houghton Mifflin.

Dator J: Health futures symposium, Geneva, 1993, World Health Organization.

Doyle M: Quest for vision, *Assoc Manage,* p 29, September, 1990.

Evans R and others, editors: Why are some people healthy and others not? In *The determinants of the health of populations,* New York, 1994, Aldine deGruyter.

Gordon S: *Life support: three nurses on the front lines,* Boston, 1997, Little, Brown.

Hancock T: Beyond health care, *Futurist* 16(4):4, 1982.

Hancock T: Seeing the vision: defining your role, *Healthcare Forum 36*(3):30, 1993.

Hancock T, Bezold C: Possible futures, preferable futures, *Healthcare Forum 37*(2):23, 1994.

Hancock T, Garrett M: Beyond medicine: health challenges and strategies in the 21st century, *Futures 27*(9/10):935, 1995.

Henchley N: Making sense of the future, *Alternatives, 7*:24, 1978.

McKeown T: *The role of medicine: dream, mirage or nemesis?* Oxford, 1979, Blackwell.

McMichael AJ: *Planetary overload,* Oxford, 1995, Oxford University.

Naisbitt J: *Megatrends,* New York, 1984, Warner Books.

Peters T, Waterman R: *In search of excellence,* New York, 1982, Random House.

Sagan L: *The health of nations,* New York, 1987, Basic Books.

Senge PM: *The fifth discipline: the art and practice of the learning organization,* New York, 1990, Doubleday.

Sigma Theta Tau International: *Nursing leadership in the 21st century: a report of ARISTA II,* Indianapolis, 1996, Center Nursing Press.

Toffler A: *Future shock,* New York, 1970, Random House.

Toffler A: *The third wave,* New York, 1980, Random House.

World Bank: *World development report: investing in health,* Washington, DC, 1993, World Bank.

# 2 What Will Health Care Look Like in the Future?

**Roger J. Bulger**

*We have the best sick-care system in the world. The problem is we don't have good health care.*

**Jocelyn Elders**
Former Surgeon General of the United States

In the first chapter of this book, we learned that futurism's value for the profession of nursing is not so much to predict the future accurately, which of course no one can accomplish, but to provide as rational a basis as possible for proactive efforts to deal with and possibly to affect that future in positive ways. This same statement can be made with regard to attempting to anticipate what health care will be like in the next century. If one thinks back to what health care was like at the beginning of the twentieth century and compares that with health care today, it is clear that very little could have been accurately prognosticated. Even the most superficial of analyses would quickly demonstrate that perhaps technologic advances, unexpected and unimaginable 100 years ago, played the major role in what has transpired over the last century, along with changing social, demographic, political, and philosophic realities and beliefs. We probably cannot safely say more than that about what health care will be like in the year 3000.

Having thus disposed of planning for the next millenium, it seems prudent to consider possible scenarios for the next 20 to 25 years. First, we should consider the social background of our current environment and the major transformational forces currently confronting the health professions and the health care delivery world; second, some current forces, issues, models, and trends in health care delivery; and third, two contrasting scenarios for the future, one probable as an extension of existing trends and the other preferable, as an example of the best possible realistic outcome based on the values, ideals, and aspirations of our society with relation to health care. Finally, a proposal by which health professionals can link their foundational values to the evolving delivery system and the implications of these scenarios for health professional education in general is discussed.

## ENVIRONMENTAL SCAN AND TRANSFORMATIONAL FORCES

We now live in the postmodern era. Postmodernism initially referred to architecture. Its roots, however, lie in the philosophic questioning of the intellectual foundations of modernism, that is, the belief in science, rationality, deductive reasoning, objective observation, and unending progress through industrialization, capitalism, and materialism. Postmodernism suggests that modernism was not enough, that rationality and science are insufficient to bring meaning and happiness to individuals, and that credence must be given to other ways of knowing than those that flowed from the Renaissance and Enlightenment. Postmodernism refers to an era after modernism and before whatever will come next.

We are in an uncertain, ambiguous period of change between the incredible successes and disappointing failures of modernism and the next era, which we may think of as the "post–postmodern era" to begin we know not when and to be determined by people possibly as yet unborn and by events and concepts as yet unimagined. If the whole society is between reigning cultural paradigms, we should not be too surprised that the health care world is in some disarray as well. Thus we in health care are not being selectively targeted by some evil genie; we are instead experiencing our part of a general social condition.

In such a transition, would it not be wise to wait and buy time? Perhaps, but this transition, certainly as we are experiencing it in health care, is full of change and flux. Realistically, we cannot wait. Those in health care must participate and work to guide potentially major and even massive change out of the values we most trust, struggling all the while with our philosophic, professional, and personal priorities and with the diversity increasingly characteristic of our society.

### Movement Toward Patient-Centeredness

#### Nursing

Nursing's professional star is rising; political power and prestige are growing; scope of practice is expanding into areas once reserved for physicians; the general population increasingly expresses enhanced trust in nurses and increasingly loses confidence in physicians as true advocates. The temptation is real for organized nursing (and for other health professions) to move through this period thinking primarily about how to preserve, consolidate, and enhance their profession's status and power. This, based on any reasonably objective history of our various professions' behaviors and anticipating a tendency toward professional unionization, is what one might identify as a likely scenario for the next few decades until the shakeout to something more stable in health care is finalized. However, such an approach fails to take into account one of the transformational forces with which we must all contend and which may help the whole industry to pull together instead of apart: the new and growing sense of "patient-centeredness."

#### Patient-Centeredness

This concept is expressed most prominently in the United States because our tradition of individual liberty and self-determination is so strong. We have moved to "patient as decision maker" and have been the first Western society to significantly deviate from the paternalistic, authoritarian, physician-dominated mode to a more participatory and active role for patients in deciding their futures. Patient-centeredness is expressed almost as dramatically in the movement to patient outcomes as the dominant benchmarking techniques for quality and effectiveness of care.

#### Interprofessional Practice

In terms of interprofessional relations and professional goals, placing patient-centeredness at the head of the list of professional values will lead the major professions to relate to each other in those terms. Thus if it is best for the patient that care be provided by nurse midwives, then so be it; if data make it clear that patients in other situations should be cared for by obstetricians, then so be it. If circumstances are ambiguous, then trials should determine if a judgment should be made that favors one or the other. In this construct the professions each seek to support the practices that are best for specific patients in specific situations and would therefore recognize that there may well be appropriate ongoing shifting of task assignments from one profession to another. This is also true regarding the legitimate overlap of services. The patient-centered approach reduces the likelihood of interprofessional turf wars and supports a seamless web of highly competent, collaborating health professionals who serve patients.

## Expanding Definition of Health Care

The second new force in health care is the expanding definition of health care. For the past four decades, the wonders of reductionism, biomolecular science, and medicine have held us all in thrall. *Medical care* meant a sophisticated operation or a precise therapeutic agent determined by advanced technologic diagnostic tests. It seemed that not a week went by without a new miracle intervention or cure being announced and celebrated. The genetic revolution, which is only now beginning to unfold around us, promises even more striking interventions in the future, when diseases will be treated before they make people ill. Genetic manipulations may be preemptive strikes to reduce the risk in genetically predisposed individuals. Such discoveries have given way to a broader understanding of health care and an insistence that it include prevention of disease and promotion of healthful behavior, as well as an increased attention to those suffering from diseases we can neither prevent nor cure.

The treatment of those suffering from chronic disease is to help the afflicted cope with new life situations and with incurable debility. Whereas one used to worry that the borders of medical care were being expanded unnecessarily because of the excessive medicalization of diseases or conditions that may have had social or other causes, we now are faced with the borders of health care moving to include much more comprehensive programs in prevention and chronic care. Long-term implications of this change are stupendous.

## Demography

The third major driver of our efforts during the next century is demography. Our population is growing inexorably older and dramatically more ethnically diverse. The women's health movement has raised gender bias to an increased level of awareness. Clinical practice is beginning to adjust to awareness of women's issues and the biases that have sometimes clouded the clinical thinking of a male-dominated medical profession. Perhaps the best example of this (and one of the earliest) was the observation that women experience the first signs of an impending heart attack differently than do men, and that subsequently the diagnosis was missed by clinicians who placed too much emphasis on the pain radiating down the arm, a symptom much less often experienced by women having a heart attack than by men.

When AIDS burst on the scene in the early 1980s, it was perceived essentially as a disease of the male homosexual community because early studies show a prominent incidence among sexually promiscuous gay men and drug users. It is possible that the AIDS epidemic will eventually become identified with the other forces that have raised the consciousness of our society to various subgroups and their particular plight in our culture.

Finally, the burgeoning elderly population will clearly place great strain on our health care resources, especially if we try to practice good clinical prevention practices, provide good health promotion and disease avoidance services, and also expand our services to the elderly with chronic disease and debility. No one profession can do it all; organized delivery systems of one sort or another may have a chance if they can creatively involve all health professionals in a coordinated effort on behalf of the patient.

## The Technologic Imperative

Technology has been a forceful driver in American life generally for almost 200 years; it has been a major factor in our health care for the past 50 years. Historian Daniel Boorstin (1989), who has called the United States "the Republic of Technology," believes that our optimistic faith in material progress and our capacity for technologic achievement and know-how have kept us relatively free from demagoguery and the domination of any of the narrow belief systems that have seemingly overtaken other nations. As Boorstin explains it, we look less to the next great dictator, leader, or grand philosophy to bring us to the next level than we look to the next great technologic advance. Of course, we have received those advances, one after another, either from the genius of our own citizens or from that of those starting elsewhere and who come to the United States where their ideas and inventions have a better chance of becoming reality.

One could argue that the postmodern era recognizes that technologic success has failed to bring us happiness and that the meaning of postmodernism lies in a turning away from technology and that we should see this as a key to the future. Although the inhumanity of pure technology is undesirable and technology by itself does not bring happiness, there is little evidence that shows that we are turning away from our fascination with new technologies in most spheres of people's daily lives, especially in the health arena.

Several points illustrate this. First, through the 1980s and early 1990s the United States dominated the new and emerging biotechnology industry largely because of enlightened policies at the federal government and university levels. These policies encouraged faculty scientists to turn new discoveries into viable products, which continue to flow from the basic science laboratory to the applied science laboratory and then to the patient. Second, the much-hyped Human Genome Project has become a major public symbol for its expectation that genetic advances will be so voluminous and effective in the decades just ahead that they will reconfigure completely much of medical interventionism from treating people after they become ill to treating them for the reversal of their genetic risk factors while they are healthy. Third, engineering advances such as robotics, imaging, organ replacement with prosthetics, and xenotransplantation continue to occupy the public mind, and such scientific and technical advances are highly prized by the citizenry. Fourth, the inexorable advance of the computer and informatics applied to health care and the health sciences continues at an ever quickening pace.

In indicators such as these, there are considerable concerns about the unfettered use of new advances. This is especially true in the areas of informatics, the electronic medical record, and the genetics revolution. The potential placed before us by the electronic medical record has been well articulated and includes the capacity to conduct important population-based health services research on the incidence of disease, the effectiveness of treatments, and the quality of the care provided; however, there is public doubt that sufficient security can be provided through the computer to prevent inappropriate disclosure of personal information. These concerns must be addressed before the full potential of either the genetics or the informatics revolution can be realized.

## Cost Control and Rationing

The prevailing mandate for health care in the United States is to control costs. The rapid movement from fee-for-service to managed and even capitated care has produced major shifts in financial incentives for providers, even where the sweep to managed care is not fully realized. In California, experts believe that once capitated or "tightly managed" care covers about half of the population, the whole system will react to the cost control and price measures (Felt and others, 1995). In the current health care structures, the fat in the system is being rapidly squeezed out. Soon there will be no more excesses to eliminate, and further decreases will lead to the loss or rationing of effective interventions from the menu of services offered to patients.

"Rationing" is a bad word in the United States; it means limits applied to individuals, most often by someone else (Bulger, 1996). Those of us in the health care world appreciate that the allocation of scarce resources in a rational manner, *rationing,* has been routinely carried out within the daily practices of caregivers, probably since the health care enterprise began. Now, however, we can see the time coming when our love of new technology conflicts directly with our financial ability to access all of these technologies. Clearly, the convergence of these two forces will create still greater pressure for us to conduct the proper studies to determine what works and what does not so that we can enjoy the outcomes of as many truly effective technologies as possible.

It is useful to ask some basic questions about rationing: "What is rationed?" and "Who rations?" Three things are rationed: technology, time, and people. It might be well to emphasize once again the intrinsic importance of technology to Americans' sense of progress and hope for the individual's capacity to get up from the sickbed and have another chance at life, in essence, to the optimism and hope of Americans that they live in a supportive, responsive, and generous nation.

The prospective payment, capitated system creates the circumstances through which the rationing of time becomes either a blunt instrument or a fine art. The central issue in the rationing of time lies hidden in the results of an experiment done at Princeton University more than 25 years ago (Darley and Batson, 1973). The lessons of that experiment are timeless and are cogent to our considerations here. The subjects in the experiment, students in their last year at Princeton Theological Seminary, knew only that they were participating in a study on religious education and vocations but did not know exactly to what end. Each completed a personality questionnaire, then had a scheduled one-on-one session with a faculty member, at which the student was asked by an assistant to prepare for a 3- to 5-minute talk on either the parable of the Good Samaritan or the jobs in which seminary students would be most effective.

The assistant returned after a few minutes to indicate that the student's appointment would be in an office in the next building and to provide directions. The assistant also had one of three different messages for the student with respect to time: (1) the student was expected a few minutes ago and should hurry over ("high hurry"); (2) the student should please go right over ("intermediate hurry"); or (3) the student would be expected in a few minutes but could go over and wait there briefly ("low hurry"). As students walked or rushed through the alley to the next building, they passed a motionless man, slumped in a doorway, groaning and coughing like the sufferer might have done in the parable of the Good Samaritan. However, this was no real sufferer but was instead a trained observer who noted which students stopped and what they did when they stopped.

The only factor that correlated with whether a student stopped to help was how much time the student had. This result seemingly implied that character meant nothing in human affairs, a depressing thought. On further reflection, however, one conclusion from the experiment can be that no matter how well prepared, even the best of people may be incapable in certain circumstances of expressing their compassion to other suffering human beings because they need time in order to actually provide the needed services. Thus we ration time at our peril. It should be noted that other factors, such as a person's instincts or beliefs, must have had some effect because about 25% of the students did not stop even when they had the time, whereas 10% stopped even when they had no time and were in the "high-hurry" state. The implications of this study for tightly managed organized delivery systems are dramatically obvious.

Michael Ashley-Miller (1996) reported an incident that illustrates an extreme of the tendency for managers to cut costs by cutting personnel. In considering the financial plight of a British hospital, a consulting group recommended to the hospital management that its financial problems could be solved by a reduction in the nursing force of 350 full-time equivalents. The consultants went on to say that the remainder of the nursing work force could accomplish all the relevant work including what the departed 350 would have done if they simply stopped talking to the patients.

Who rations? There are five options: the health professional (typically the physician), the politician, the patient, the manager, or some combination thereof. For many years in the modern era, the answer lay somewhere between physicians and politicians and neither group wanted the mantle of "rationer-in-chief." Physicians knew that they could allocate scarce resources and did so virtually every day as long as they were asked to distribute those resources according to medical need. A good example of this sort of allocation is in the assignment of patients to beds in the intensive care unit; the sickest and most medically needy patients are typically given entry. However, physicians in the United States are much less willing than their counterparts in the United Kingdom, for example, to withhold expensive and complex treatments from elderly patients (who would otherwise benefit from the intervention) just because they are older (Aaron and Schwartz, 1984).

Politicians, on the other hand, have been loath to accept the responsibility for rationing. Increasingly, as the paternalistic, physician-dominated model of health care has given way to a patient-control model, it has seemed to some that the patient would gain greater influence and perhaps even control over the provision of personal services and that an enlightened patient would, in fact, not want unnecessary or ultimately futile treatments. With the collapse of the Clinton health care reform plan, the private-dominated, managed competition model for the delivery of health care has taken hold across the country and managers of organized delivery systems have in effect taken over, and threaten to dominate, the allocation of resource decisions. The answer to the question of "Who rations?" is still unclear and is, in fact, muddled; it should most certainly be kept very much on the radar screen of all concerned about health care in our society.

## HEALTH CARE PARADIGMS

Three intellectual paradigms govern modern health care. Even though it may well be an important force affecting health care in the twenty-first century, the extension of routine health care services to include prevention and chronic and rehabilitative care in addition to curative medical care is nevertheless based on three quite distinct paradigms rooted in modern science and the Enlightenment (Bulger, 1998). These are the biomedical, the biopsychosocial, and the epidemiologic. Traditional faculty in medical schools are generally locked into the biomedical, reductionist, molecular paradigm, which seeks the molecular causes of individual diseases and the molecular treatments to cure them.

Nursing, on the other hand, is very much involved with the patient or client as a person and think in terms of the biopsychosocial paradigm, aiming to enhance the patient's response to illness, trauma, or treatment. In addition, nurses use their interpersonal skills to further enhance positive patient outcomes.

Public health faculty are traditionally locked into the population-based, epidemiologically driven paradigm, which seeks to understand and enhance the health status of the population as a whole. The environment is likely to interest them more than particular diseases, except when the focus is on how to prevent those diseases from occurring and how to take effective steps to alter behavior toward a more health-promoting mode.

Of course, it has always been true that each of these three major health professions finds meaningful advocates and significant expression within all three paradigms. Dentistry, pharmacy, and other allied health professions have also tended to move beyond their immediate intellectual frame of reference in efforts to be more effective, more tolerant, and more understanding across the spectrum of health care delivery as we now envision it for the twenty-first century.

## WHO AND WHAT IS A HEALER?

The concept of personal development and enhancing one's own personal competencies may be more fully developed in the nursing literature than in medicine—excluding, perhaps, the psychiatric literature. Carol Taylor (1995) of Georgetown University School of Nursing argues that moral competence should be added as a fourth nursing competency to the traditional triad of intellectual, interpersonal, and technical skills. Taylor asserts, "An increasing tendency to focus primarily on the intellectual and technical competence of nurses is radically redefining nursing and threatening nursing's ability to respond to human need." She describes some practical strategies for developing and maintaining interpersonal competencies among nurses and in effect shows how this can be incorporated into total quality improvement efforts.

In his 1983 book, *The Physician's Covenant*, William May describes five images of the physician as healer (Box 2-1). It is not entirely clear whether May thinks that any one healer might adopt any or all of these images at one time or another or whether he thinks that most physicians tend to fall into one of the image categories. Furthermore, it is not certain that he sees the fifth image, the physician as teacher, as the final step to maturity as a healer.

In Box 2-2, the elements of the evolution of the mature physician, nurse, dentist, or other healer are listed. Against a background of scientific competence, the healer must learn about the richness of human suffering; such awareness will elicit the felt need to communicate more effectively with patients and to better understand the nature of their personal circumstances and their sense of their pain. Clinical experience soon brings a growing awareness of the need to confront the prospect of one's own death before having to face it firsthand. All of this attunes the clinician to the subtleties of the placebo effect and the human role in the optimization of the beneficial effects of treatment.

One of the most extraordinary examples of the therapeutic effect of a human interaction connected with a professional intervention is described by physician-author Fitzhugh Mullan in his autobiographic work, *Vital Signs: A Young Doctor's Struggle with Cancer* (1975). As Dr. Mullan tells it, after an almost unbelievable hospital stay of several months' duration during which he, his family, and his caregivers endured a dramatic

### Box 2-1
### *Images of the Healer*

*Fighter:* Makes war on death and disease
*Parent:* Demonstrates compassion and benevolence
*Technician:* Believes technical performance is ultimate
*Covenanter:* Values responsibility, service, and fidelity
*Teacher:* Assists patient in coping with incurability

Modified from May W: *The physician's covenant: images of the healer in medical ethics,* Philadelphia, 1983, Westminster Press.

### Box 2-2
### *Characteristics of the Healer*

1. Scientific and technical competence
2. Understanding suffering
3. Ability to communicate
4. Knowledge of the placebo effect and its role in scientific medicine
5. Coming to terms with death
6. Expanded roles and three paradigms
7. Commitment and loyalty

Bulger RJ: *The quest for compassion: the forgotten ingredient in health care reform,* Charlottsville, Va, 1998, Carden Jennings series of clinical ups and downs, he was at last ready to go home. On the morning of his planned discharge, he suddenly became frightened and overwhelmed with a desire to kill himself, a feeling he had never known before. Feeling himself on the verge of jumping out of the window, he informed the nurse of his situation and asked for help. She contacted the psychiatrist on call.

The psychiatrist who responded was unknown to Dr. Mullan but appeared to be approximately the same age and level of seniority. The psychiatrist listened carefully to Dr. Mullan's words, and then asked just one question: "Do you want me to hold you?" Dr. Mullan broke down. One leaves the scene with the picture of two people holding onto one another, the vulnerable one gaining the strength necessary to go on to the next stage of recovery from the other, stronger and healthy person who somehow knew enough to use the right seven words. The encounter empowered Dr. Mullan to overcome his panic, to go home, and to undertake successfully the rest of his long and laborious return to the full health he now enjoys.

## ALTERNATIVE HEALTH CARE

The expansion of alternative (complementary) health care and the increasing proportion of the population using such care, in addition to startling estimates of the extent of our collective investment in nontraditional medical care, is finally getting some attention from the health care establishment (Majino, 1987). There are even many traditionalists whose minds are open to the unknown and who are willing to study and consider the potential value of such unusual interventions. Beneath this renewed interest is a clear message that our usual model of care is not providing what people seem to want. Thinking about this missing element has led to a reconsideration of the importance of cost and efficiency and to a reexploration of the healing relationship, the placebo effect, and the nature of the trust between patient and professional, between patient and professional team, and possibly even between patient and the institution or organized delivery system.

> The placebo effect: a pill or operation, a healing person, an institution . . . or all of the above?

Lain Entralgo (1970) identified the seminal importance of Hippocrates' cleavage of the science and practice of medicine from the intervention of words and the incantations of the shamans who practiced their art at the time. According to Lain Entralgo, Hippocrates created the tradition of medicine as the silent art, which led to the separation of medicine from psychiatry, which from then on developed along a separate track. Freud and Jung and their various followers evolved the practice of using words in therapy in ever more arcane and separate venues from the traditional activities of scientific medicine, which in turn had become more closely associated with the reductionist, biomolecular paradigm, which seeks answers in our molecules and genes to medicine's questions. However, recent developments in the neurosciences (e.g., neuroendocrinology and neuropharmacology) have seemed to draw the two areas together (Kiecolt-Glaser and Glaser, 1986). As the molecular biology of emotion gets addressed more effectively by traditional science, we can understand how emotions and beliefs can influence the incredible pharmacy we carry in our own brains. As it becomes clearer in more and more specific situations how neuroendocrinologic or neuropharmacologic response may change under different environmental circumstances, it becomes easier in principle to conceive of the nature of the well-known phenomenon we call "the placebo effect."

The placebo effect is defined as any effect occurring in association with an intervention but not resulting from any known physiologic function of the intervention. In fact, placebo effects are not always beneficial; major skin rashes and other reactions have been demonstrated to come from nonallergenic placebos in a small percentage of subjects. Because Americans have been enamored of technology virtually since our nation's inception and because our medical profession is known worldwide to be highly interventionistic in its utilization of the many new drugs and other techniques constantly being made available, patients in the United States are presented more often than patients in other countries with new instruments of hope and new venues through which to profit from the combination of the intrinsic effectiveness of the therapy and its associated placebo effect.

In days gone by, physicians were essentially bereft of effective therapies and were left with only the placebo's benefits (Bulger, 1991). Thus one of France's greatest early nineteenth-century clinicians was quoted as advising the use of all new medicines as often as possible before they ceased to become effective. Oliver Wendell Holmes echoed these sentiments when he postulated in the midnineteenth century that if all of the medicines in the world were tossed into the sea, it would be good for the people and bad for the fish. Finally, in Flexnarian times, L.J. Henderson (Bulger, 1991), the famous twentieth-century biochemist said, "Sometime between 1910 and 1912, it became true that for the first time in history, a random patient visiting a random doctor would have had a greater than fifty-fifty chance of profiting from the encounter." Because the placebo effect generally is believed to be in the range of 30% to 50%, Henderson can be interpreted as saying that, finally in the twentieth century, physicians had the tools to improve on the placebo effects of their interventions.

Most of us in modern health care practice tend to minimize the placebo effect and in fact study it all too infrequently. For example, we have no idea about individual variation in providers' abilities to elicit the placebo effect from patients, although Benson declares that the elicitation of such benefits depends on the degree of trust in the relationship between the provider and the patient (Benson and Epstein, 1975). It is the conventional wisdom of many experts that the most pervasive and intense placebo effects are elicited when both the patient and therapist believe that the intervention will work and that the benefit is less marked when one or the other doesn't really believe the therapy may work. This point was made in the 1950s when, based on convincing evidence in experimental animals, a well-known surgeon concluded that tying off the internal mammary artery in patients with compromised coronary artery blood flow would increase the blood flow through the impaired coronaries such that those with severe angina and cardiac dysfunction might experience symptomatic improvement. He performed surgery on a series of the most severely ill coronary patients and got highly gratifying results, with 85% of his patients experiencing dramatic improvement and some even returning to work pain free. As word spread around the country, others performed the surgical procedure with only half to two thirds of patients experiencing improvement, thus justifying a randomized controlled trial in which every other patient had a sham surgical procedure. When it became apparent that the sham surgery produced results comparable with those from the real surgery (Cobb and others, 1959, Beecher, 1961), the trial was stopped and the surgical procedure was never performed again. It has been said, however, that many of the original patients continued to stand behind the validity of their surgery and of the improvement they enjoyed from it.

One of the most powerful, scientifically sound experiments to demonstrate the power of the placebo effect was performed by Stewart Wolf (1950), a respected gastroenterologic physiologist who undertook a study of the nausea associated with pregnancy. Each pregnant volunteer subject agreed to have a tube placed in her stomach through which Dr. Wolf could record intragastric pressures. Thus he recorded the reverse peristalsis in the stomachs of the pregnant women when they reported feeling a wave of nausea. When their stomachs were quiet, he dropped in some ipecac and measured the immediate and expected reverse peristaltic response, along with the reporting of the subjective feeling of being nauseated. Dr. Wolf then told each of them that he was about to deliver a medicine through the tube into their stomach that he believed would stop their nausea. He waited until the subjects were experiencing the nausea, and then he delivered his medicine, which invariably did stop the nausea and reverse the antiperistaltic movements. The striking fact is that the medicine he delivered was ipecac, which has exactly the opposite pharmacologic effect. Dr. Wolf interpreted these results as showing that the patient's trust in him led them to believe that the medicine would work and that their belief caused the in vivo secretion of some blocking agent, which prevented the action of ipecac, as well as of whatever molecule caused the naturally occurring nausea of pregnancy. He concluded, "Placebo effects which modify the pharmacologic action of drugs or endow inert agents with potency are not imaginary, but may be associated with measurable changes at the end organs. These effects are at times more potent than the pharmacologic action customarily attributed to the agent."

The previously scientifically tenuous connections between our minds and our bodies are being more fully explicated and explored by a talented array of modern investigators and clinicians (Benson and McCallie, 1979; Pert and others, 1985; Kiecolt-Glaser and Glaser, 1986; Institute of Medicine, 1989). The holistic movement in general speaks to treatment of individual patients by individual therapists. However, can we think of beneficial effects occurring to patients on the basis of the trust relationship with groups of people or with institutions? Nurses are well aware of the studies that purport to show that mortality rates in an intensive care unit are lower when the level of communication between doctors and nurses is high rather than low. A most telling illustration of a kind of institutional placebo may be found in a report of a randomized controlled trial involving 616 primiparous women and the care they received during delivery at a Houston hospital (Kennell and others, 1991). All patients were cared for by the same team of nurses and doctors, who applied the same logic and practice standards to each patient throughout the study. In the control group, 18% required a cesarean section and 55% had epidural anesthesia. One of the two experimental groups had only one added feature to the control treatment and environment: a woman who stood in the corner of the delivery room in a white coat with a clipboard and who neither introduced herself nor spoke to anyone during the birthing process. In this group the rate of cesarean sections dropped to 13%.

The second experimental group differed from the control group only by the presence of a doula, that is, a woman who introduced herself by name to the patient; who told the patient that she had no expertise in obstetric care, except for having had a baby herself; and who further told the patient that she would stand by her side, hold her hand, and be available to talk or answer questions for the patient as needed. In this third group the cesarean section rate fell to 8% and the use of epidural anesthesia dropped to 7.8%. There were analogous progressive improvements in administration of pain medication, neonatal problems, and length of hospital stay for mother and child. These results have been substantiated in subsequent studies in other settings.

In the Houston hospital the hiring of the doula proved to be cost effective. The importance of studying such interventions by caring figures in different clinical settings has been more recently demonstrated by the Robert Wood Johnson Foundation–financed study of terminal hospital care, in which the addition of a trained nurse to the care team was evaluated. (SUPPORT Principal Investigators, 1995). The function of the nurse was (1) to facilitate physician–patient interaction, (2) to develop patient directives and thereby shorten the period during which terminal patients are on mechanical life support, and (3) ultimately to reduce the total cost of terminal hospitalizations for seriously ill older patients.

In this randomized trial of patients determined in advance to have a life expectancy of 6 months or less, a quarter of the patients presenting to the hospital died in the hospital; one third of those who died spent their savings and/or those of their family to pay for the terminal hospitalization. It was believed that the intervention of a trained nurse would lead to a breaking of the communication logjam and a reduction of all of the worst statistics. To everyone's surprise, the trial proved otherwise, showing that the nurse had a positive effect on only the patients' families' view of the terminal event. Thus the addition of a person to facilitate communication and caring in this instance produced no measurable benefits sufficient to justify the expenditure of funds necessary to do the job. (See Chapter 31 for more on alternative care.)

## COMPETING MODELS OF THE HEALTH PROFESSIONAL AND PATIENT RELATIONSHIP

Medical sociologist Charles Bosk (1997) believes that two models of physician–patient interaction are vying for dominance in our rapidly changing health care environment: (1) the professional service model, which is characterized (or caricatured) as the physician-governed, paternalistic, "doctor-knows-best" model in which the patient plays a passive, subordinate, and compliant role and whose path to a cure is to follow the doctor's orders steadfastly; and (2) the patient-choice model, in which the patient is active in choosing diagnostic approaches and therapies, takes an active role in the healing process, and for whom the altruism of health care personnel can no longer be taken for granted.

In the patient-choice model, the physician is in a far more passive role, which often creates tension between professional competence and expertise and patient autonomy and the ability of patients through informed consent to decide their options effectively and to take control of their fate. Bosk prophesies that the emergence of advanced informatics tilts the pendulum farther away from the first and older model toward the second and newer model. For example, if patients with certain diseases form a community using electronic communication to share information and to develop other venues of mutual support, they may come to rely on one another to achieve the therapeutic support once provided by a sympathetic physician. In fact, Brennan and others (1995) report on such a model of support for caregivers of Alzheimer's patients. This model is similar to the philosophic foundation of self-help groups (e.g., Alcoholics Anonymous) in widespread use today that use nonprofessional volunteer members as leaders.

Anticipating that doctors and patients in the managed care world are in danger of missing the chance to "overcome" the dominance of the clinical algorithm in the individual case, Bosk acknowledges that this trend to "algorithm-driven" practices could drive doctors and patients closer together. However, he worries that, instead of uniting in the face of being overrun by an army of managers, physicians and patients will seek to defend their own turf and to extend it, with both sides fighting for the remaining crumbs of autonomy. Bosk foresees the gradual loss of the "therapeutic person" as professional time, talk, and touch are eroded. He implies, but does not assert, that the most hopeful path for the health care enterprise would be for the patients and their doctors to join hands in their insistence on high-quality care.

Bosk's analyses certainly seem plausible, but there is another way to envision the situation and our opportunities fruitfully. This vision recognizes that until recently a technology-poor medical world was dominated by medical care in which a physician brought succor and a limited set of technologies to bear upon a given patient's ills. The fee-for-service system prospered in association with the proliferation of specialties and the technologies that scientific progress made available until out-of-control costs brought the trend to capitated, population-based financial plans. The financial system that heretofore had buttressed the patient's hopes for a personal physician advocate with strong monetary incentives to provide the patient with the best care available has been turned upside down, such that a majority of patients find themselves in health care plans that reward the providers for providing less costly care.

Physicians who worry that these changes will erode the trust upon which much of their status and respect and placebo-based therapeutic capacity has been built are correct, because this is exactly what has happened. One could argue that it is now too late to worry about that loss of trust, because it has already been lost. Now is the time to figure out what to do in the face of that erosion or loss. It is well to remember that the collective status of physicians in the public's view has historically always been in flux, with deep nadirs and high peaks if one looks back for even only a few centuries.

At the same time, as scientific discovery brings the neuroendocrine and neuroimmunologic worlds into greater consonance with our emotions and enhances our understanding of some placebo-based successful therapeutic results, polls and focus groups reveal that patients and public alike have lost faith in hospitals and in physicians to be their true advocates. Consumers understand that if they are willing to switch doctors for a monthly reduction in fees, surely their doctors are not likely to give up too much of their own financial well-being just to provide patients with the very best treatment available. Such is the price for the move from less than 15% of the population in capitated plans to more than half.

As the final excesses of cost are wrung from the system, the public will resist further shrinkage. Partnerships between professionals and patients are emerging to counter unfettered cost cutting by overzealous managers, and one can expect a heightened sensitivity on the public's part to the rationing of health care.

Polls and focus groups tell us that the public trusts the nurse. The nurse, it is believed, will still advocate for patients and advise them sympathetically and patiently. People believe that nurses will remain true, sympathetic caregivers, a belief and trust that is increasingly being shown to enhance patient outcomes and improve results quantitatively as long as somewhere on the team or in the caregiving apparatus that compassion is dispensed. Increasingly, more respected clinicians are accepting of the expanded definition of the placebo effect, popularized by Herb Benson, that identifies the placebo effect outcomes with any treatment not explainable by the known physiologic or pharmacologic effects of the intervention.

Effective collaboration between physicians and nurses who form recognized delivery teams will lie at the core of the twenty-first-century approach to sustaining the benefits of the patient's trust in caregivers. Furthermore, such leadership by doctors and nurses will serve to bring other health professionals onto the team. We can, in effect, turn this potential problem of erosion of trust into an advantage.

Another change that influences the multiprofessional team approach is the new, more expansive view of the nature of health care. As previously discussed, the new definition includes not only prevention and curing of disease but also the care of the chronically ill whose diseases have not been prevented or cured. No single profession can do all that, yet any responsible system of health care would seek to accomplish the full spectrum of preventing, curing, and caring in an integrated multiprofessional manner. Finally, the new "patient-centeredness" rhetoric has been matched by a new emphasis on the evaluation of health care outcomes, an emphasis that in effect validates "placebo-based improvements."

Doctors, nurses, and other health professionals continue to fight over turf instead of collaborating for the benefit of their patients. In the simplest of terms physicians need to recognize that health care can no longer be delivered solely by doctors and that even the best doctors and nurses can have their finest efforts thwarted by the incompetencies of others on their team. Hippocrates seemed to include under his plane tree at Cos all who would follow him in the learning and practice of scientific medicine. Today, if Hippocrates considered that prevention and chronic care belonged in his purview, he would include a wide variety of health professionals under his learning tree and he might insist that, as his followers develop their set of covenants, they should refer to *all* scientifically based health professionals. He might insist on the goal of developing for patients a seamless web of scientifically based health professionals. He would insist on the goal of a team of highly competent professionals being deployed in the patients' interests, and he would recognize that the patients were joining the team, sometimes as the leaders. He would tell us to meld Bosk's professional service and patient-choice models, and he would ask physicians and nurses to lead the other health professionals in yielding, if need be, some professional autonomy in the interests of restoring the trust and confidence of the more autonomous patients. If the placebo effect can be recognized as resulting from the efforts of individual healers and can be validated as being associated with health professional teams' interventions, we must consider extending the effort to whole institutions and organized systems of care.

Hippocrates would encourage us to embrace the patient-centeredness concept as the way to bring the health team together, and in considering his own Hippocratic Oath, he would advocate that we add "collaboration" to the centuries-old trio of "competence, commitment, and compassion." Furthermore, he would advocate that language similar to the following be added to every health profession's covenantal statement:

> As a health professional dedicated to enhancing the health care status and well-being of individuals and communities, I pledge collaboration with all of my health professional colleagues similarly committed and promise, should tensions or conflicts of interest arise, to place patient and public interest above the perceived self-interests of my individual profession.

## TWO POSSIBLE SCENARIOS FOR THE FUTURE

### Most Likely Model

The most likely scenario is based on the U.S. tradition of creeping incrementalism. We have too many vested interests on both sides of almost any issue, too many checks and balances within our governmental processes, and too much of a capacity to use the media to instill fear or to create it over the unknown in any dramatic alteration of the status quo to justify predicting that anything else but creeping incrementalism will be true of the health care enterprise over the next few decades. In addition, market mentality and managed competitiveness have brought a halt to the upward escalation of health care costs.

Economist Uwe Reinhardt (1996) suggests that we are now aimed at the perpetuation of a three-class system in health care. Assuming that Medicare and Medicaid continue to move toward a capitated mode, their participants, along with most of the working class, will receive prepaid care via Health Maintenance Organizations, (HMOs) or point-of-service plans that offer comprehensive services at a capitated level; this will be the predominant mode of service delivery for most of the population.

The second mode will be a more traditional indemnity insurance program that allows free choice of physician and hospital, which will appeal to 10% to 20% of the higher-income population. The third mode will be whatever is made available through the community to serve those who have no plan or who lack insurance. Depending on what steps society takes, this population will include the working poor, those who elect not to have any insurance, illegal aliens, and all others who cannot qualify for the other avenues of health care.

What is done about quality control, accessibility, and technologic innovation in health care in a price-driven market will depend largely on state and federal initiatives and reactions to circumstances. One would expect a plethora of legislative attempts to solve problems that the public cannot support for one reason or another, such as the legislation of an extended hospital stay for normal delivery, or the passage of a law that requires physicians and other caregivers to tell patients all of the options theoretically open to them even if some of the options may not be available through their plans, or the recent passage of a law in Texas that allows HMOs to be sued for malpractice for undertreating patients.

The most likely scenario will suffer from major deficits in each of the three foundational areas of access, quality, and cost. We now have more than 40 million people who have no insurance or other mechanism to finance their health care, and in the year 2010 we will still be the only Western democratic society that has not found a way to provide health care for all of its people. Quality standards, regulation, and oversight will remain largely in state hands and will be spotty, uneven, and grossly deficient. Because so many people will be outside of the main system, cost cannot be capped and the system will be exploited. Costs will continue to rise, perhaps faster than in the majority of our Western-nation colleagues.

## Ideal Model

The ideal model would be similar to the Canadian system. It would be established according to federal guidelines, mandates, and standards as follows:

1. Everyone will be covered.
2. Coverage will be portable from state to state.
3. Quality-of-care standards will be developed at the national level but will be implemented at the state level.
4. Costs will be monitored and evaluated in terms of total costs: costs of prevention, costs of caring for the chronically ill, and the costs of curative acute care.

Research on the outcomes and quality-of-health services will be carried out on a dramatically increased level so that proper evaluation can inform allocation decision makers. In this more perfect world, we shall be paying for significantly fewer ineffective interventions and will not have to forgo supporting many useful interventions.

This more perfect model will value the healing clinician and the time necessary for that intervention. It will value and evaluate the contributions of all health professionals. It will explicitly value patient-centeredness and in this regard will focus on the patient as decision maker and will rely heavily on patient outcomes as an evaluative tool. This ideal system will place a high priority on raising the health status of the entire population and will invest more heavily in the treatment of those whose illnesses cannot be cured.

The ideal (but less likely) scenario will promote efforts to address the realities of our changing demography and will underscore the value of all contributing health care team professionals. On the other hand, the ideal scenario will properly support technical advancement and innovation. In the best of our brave new worlds, the best available safeguards on computer-based medical record security will be established and data sharing for research and quality-improvement efforts will continue to evolve. Advances in informatics and genetics will be welcomed through publicly accountable processes. The issue of "rationing" in all its permutations will be a subject of important public dialogue, and professional time and technologies will be supported.

The publicly perceived excesses of market competitiveness will be modulated by legislation and regulation so as to foster a patient-centered approach by organizations and by the system overall. Social policy will promote the development of a functional teaming of patients with health professionals as an important countervailing force to the singular drive of managers toward cost control and profit. Quality and value will be the subject of debate and explicit public education.

Finally, the ideal health care system will have aligned its incentives to encourage the health professions to come together to provide the seamless web of competent care that patients and the public expect and deserve.

## Strategies to Achieve an Ideal Health Care System

How can those of us who are concerned about health services for the next century have an impact on what emerges? Many of us who work in the field and who have university roots see the future of our society as a whole tied to our basic values and our aspiration for a true learning society made possible by the interaction of the new informatics and our best values as Americans. Thus what emerges for health care must, in the end, be the product of an intersection of our basic societal values, the professional values of the major health professions, and the university's values, expressed through a more businesslike management culture in the context of patient-centeredness and public health concerns.

We should test each and every incremental step, forward, backward, or sideways, that someone proposes for our future health care delivery system against (1) the societal values for health care of justice, autonomy, hope, and mercy; (2) the professional values of competence, commitment, caring, and collaboration with other professionals in a patient-centered and public-focused effort; and (3) the university values of learning from experience, developing new knowledge, and storing and disseminating what is known for the benefit of the community as a whole. To the extent that we can infuse our strategies with these values, our nation could in fact form a more perfect system of health care even as it seeks to expand services to include more prevention and chronic care within a business ethic; the fully developed iteration of the system must be turned more toward the creation of value in preventive and therapeutic services (for the sick and for the enhancement of the health status of the population at large) and less toward the creation of wealth (for stockholders and providers).

It is far less important for any so-called experts to proclaim what they believe and foresee than it is for them to advocate for a process that people in health care at every level (local, regional, state, or national) can use to establish their goals and strategies and to define the benchmarks and outcomes they will utilize to assess their progress toward their goals. It may be useful to illustrate the sort of process by which we can interact with market and social forces to influence the outcome of the evolution of our health care system as we move into the next millennium.

Table 2-1 summarizes the move from an identified list of foundational values in a health care delivery system to an analogous list of missions and goals, thence to a list of guideposts along the way; from such a list of guideposts, it should be relatively easy to determine what benchmarks and outcome measures will circumscribe any ongoing assessment efforts. As can be seen in Figures 2-1 and 2-2, one should be able to evaluate the delivery of health care according to our basic and foundational values; if we actively interact with those assessments to effect improvements and alterations, we will move our system or our part of the system into closer consonance with what we want as health professionals and as citizens and potential patients.

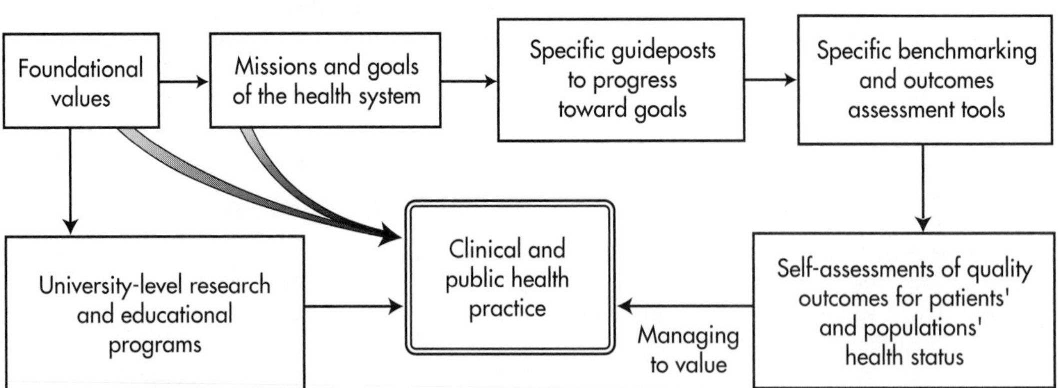


**Figure 2-1** Process for preserving our values throughout time of rapid evolution.

**TABLE 2-1 Sample Progression From Foundational Values to Assessment Tools**

| Fundamental Values | Missions and Goals of Health Care Organizations and Systems | Guideposts Open to Assessment | Identification and Use of Specific Benchmarking and Outcomes Assessment Tools |
|---|---|---|---|
| Justice<br>Autonomy<br>Hope<br>Mercy<br>Competence<br>Commitment<br>Caring/compassion<br>Collaboration<br>Learning<br>Basic research<br>Applied research<br>Education<br>Professionals<br>Public<br>Health care service<br>Patient-centered<br>Public-centered | Increase access<br>Increase patient and public consultation<br>Effective technology<br>Efficient/cost-effective services<br>Increase quality<br>Increase health status of population<br>Decrease mortality and morbidity<br>Increase years of quality living<br>Enhance research efforts<br>Increase quality<br>Decrease cost<br>Increase public education<br>Effective expansion of HPDP* and chronic care, including care of the dying | Demography<br>Special populations<br>Cultural and ethnicity<br>Cost control/resources allocation<br>Patient-centeredness<br>Professional service vs. patient-choice models<br>TQI†, patient outcomes, and HSR‡<br>The evolution/ development of new teams of caregivers<br>Alignment of financial and other incentives with goals<br>Patient/clinician balance with management and financial concerns<br>Healing clinicians and the placebo effect<br>The healing institution<br>Technologic intervention and transformational inventions<br>HPDP<br>Curative service<br>Chronic and end-of-life care | Relevant population<br>Selected financial data<br>Patient satisfaction<br>Survey-outcomes<br>Patient and profession survey<br>Selected data<br>Collection/analysis<br>Listing of specific new teams and measures of performance<br>Presentation and analysis of incentives plans and effects<br>Value-oriented, data-patient, and profession survey usage<br>New surveys<br>Time-management data<br>Patient and profession survey<br>Professions, management, and patient survey<br>New developments and collect/analyze data on efficiency and effectiveness<br>Population health-status data<br>Patient disease-specific data<br>Patient quality-of-life-oriented data<br>Family survey<br>End-of-life care |

*HPDP = Health promotion and disease prevention
†TQI = Total quality improvement
‡HSR = Health services research

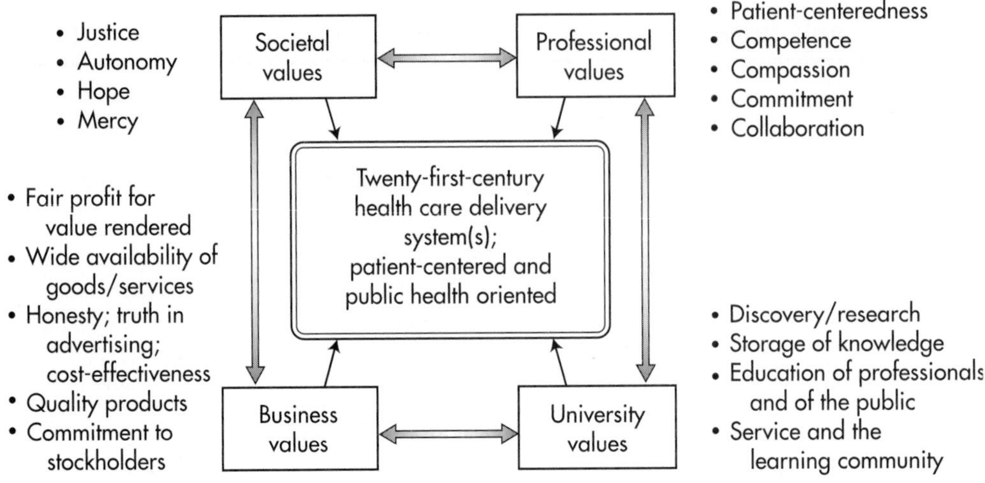


**Figure 2-2** The interplay of various sets of values (sample lists for illustration purposes only) on the emerging health system in the United States.

Figure 2-1 diagrams the process by which we can work to preserve our societal, professional, and university values as we develop our new care models in a business-oriented environment. Figure 2-2 illustrates the interplay of values from all four sectors, suggesting that societal, professional, university, and business values all serve not only to influence the health care delivery system but also to influence each other.

## CONCLUSION

It is useful to keep four major points in mind as we consider our health care future. First, science and technology will shape the future more than we can possibly imagine. Second, the effectiveness and efficiency with which we adapt to the breadth of the new demands being placed on the system will be determined by the effectiveness of new health teams and multiprofessional collaborations that must be devised to cope with the new environment. Third, much will depend on our collective ability to educate individual healers and therapeutic teams of health professionals who are capable of empowering patients to summon their own energies for self-healing. Fourth, as health professionals we should adopt a slogan (e.g., "By their outcomes ye shall know them!") to remind us constantly that we must look daily to clinical, evaluative, and other health services research to provide self-corrective data for our practices.

Obviously, all of this places a tremendous responsibility on us as health professionals to explore more fully our understanding of our societal and professional values so that we can effectively lead or influence the policy decisions that will be made every day by institutions; organized delivery systems; employers; and local, state, and federal government entities, which taken together will shape and determine the ultimate expression of health care in the United States in the twenty-first century.

## *Discussion Exercises*

1. Discuss potential conflicts between the movement toward patient-centered care and characteristics of the health care system, such as cost control, rationing, use of technology,

patient/provider relationships, and structure of health care organizations.

2. How likely is the ideal health care system proposed in this chapter? Explain your rationale.
3. Do you agree that the reductionist, biomolecular, scientific model of medicine will change in the near future? Discuss the forces that could promote an expanding view of health care and those forces that might constrain it.

## References


Aaron HJ, Schwartz WB: *The painful prescription,* Washington, DC, 1984, Brookings Institution.

Ashley-Miller M: *United Kingdom issues.* Paper presented at the Annual Meeting of the Association of Academic Health Centers, September 2, 1996.

Beecher HK: Surgery as placebo: a quantitative study of bias, *JAMA 196:*1102, 1961.

Benson H, Epstein MD: The placebo effect: a neglected asset in the care of patients, *JAMA* 232:1225, 1975.

Benson H, McCallie DP: Angina pectoris and the placebo effect, *New England J Med* 300:1424, 1979.

Brennan PF and others: The effects of a special computer network on caregivers of persons with Alzheimer's disease, *Nurs Res 44*(3):166, 1995.

Boorstin D: The republic of technology and the limits of prophecy. In Boorstin D: *Hidden history,* New York, 1989, Vintage Books.

Bosk CS: The transformation of the therapeutic relationship. In Holmes DE, editor: *The digital decade: promise and peril for the academic health center,* Washington, DC, 1997, Association of Academic Health Centers.

Bulger RJ: The demise of the placebo effect in the practice of scientific medicine: a natural progression or an undesirable aberration? *Trans Am Clin Climatol Assoc* CII:285, 1991.

Bulger RJ: Old wine in new bottles. *J Prof Nurs* 12(6):338, 1996.

Bulger RJ: *The quest for mercy: the forgotten ingredient in health care reform,* Charlottsville, Va, 1998, Carden Jennings.

Cobb and others: An evaluation of internal mammary artery ligation by double-blind technic, New England J Med 260:1115, 1959.

Darley JM, Batson CD: From Jerusalem to Jericho: a study of situational and dispositional variables in helping behavior, *J Pers Soc Psychol* p 100, 1973.

Felt S and others: *How academic health centers are changing in response to the market,* Washington, DC, 1995, U.S. Department of Health and Human Services.

Institute of Medicine: *A research briefing: behavioral influences on the endocrine and immune systems,* Washington, DC, 1989, National Academy Press.

Kennell J and others: Continuous emotional support during labor in a U.S. hospital, *JAMA* 265:197, 1991.

Kiecolt-Glaser JK, Glaser R: Psychological influences on immunity, *Psychosomatics 27:* 621, 1986.

Lain Entralgo P: *The therapy of the word in classical antiquity,* New Haven, Conn, 1970, Yale University Press.

Majino G: The lost secret of ancient medicine: the essence of healing rediscovered. In Bulger RJ, editor: *In search of the modern Hippocrates,* Iowa City, Iowa, 1987, University of Iowa Press.

May WF: *The physician's covenant,* Philadelphia, 1983, Westminster Press.

Mullan F: *Vital signs: a young doctor's struggle with cancer,* New York, 1975, Farrar, Strauss, Giroux.

Pert CB and others: Neuropeptides and their receptors: a psychosomatic network, *J Immunol* 135(suppl):820s, 1985.

Reinhart U: Personal communication, 1996.

Support Principal Investigators: A controlled trial to improve care for seriously ill hospitalized patients, *JAMA* 374:1591, 1995.

Taylor C: Rethinking nursing's basic competencies, *J Nurs Care Qual* 9:1, 1995.

Wolf S: Effects of suggestion and conditioning on the action of chemical agents in human subjects: the pharmacology of placebos, *J Clin Invest* 29:100, 1950.

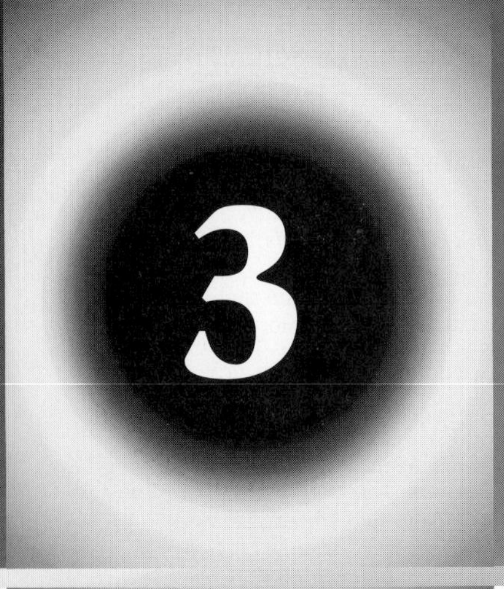

# 3 Nursing's Role in Transforming the Health Care System

**Tim Porter-O'Grady**

*Adventures don't begin until you get into the forest.*

**Mickey Hart**
Grateful Dead drummer

Much is happening in health care that is changing its face forever. The burgeoning of technology has had perhaps the greatest impact on the growth and changes in health care services (Berman, 1989). The times are quickly moving the health system in the United States in new directions, not all of them perceived as desirable. Nonetheless, these transformations bode well for a challenging and intriguing time for the health care system and those who work in it (Beckham, 1996).

Whether the changes now confronting health care will have a positive impact on the practice of nursing depends on two questions:

1. How early can the key change points in health care be identified and strategies be enumerated to respond quickly?
2. How desirable will those changes appear to nurses, and how willing will they be to embrace them and give the future form?

Nursing has a jagged history in terms of its positioning for success and for making a difference (Porter-O'Grady, 1995). In times of war and great crisis, nurses have been able to respond in an exemplary manner, often with great bravery and significant contribution. However, in times of routine changes nurses have been more circumspect. Sometimes nurses have been perceived as genuinely inert. The truth of nursing's response to change lies somewhere in between the two extremes.

Current conditions call for a relatively quick response. The changes in both design and function in the health care system are challenging health professionals to make significant strides toward addressing their implications and responding in kind (Argyris, 1993). The nature of this response is critical to the ability of the professional bodies to make clearly effective and appropriate responses. The onset of managed care, capitated systems, mergers and systems integration, point-of-service delivery models, interdisciplinary teams, case management, continuum of service, and a host of related circumstances have changed health service forever. The ability to thrive now requires hospitals to become health systems and to integrate service around capitated populations in a wide variety of forms and arrangements (Lowe, 1996).

Nurses are plunged into this reality precipitously and without much preparation. It often appears as if the changes came as a thief in the night, changing nurses' reality forever and challenging nurses to respond to a world into which they never asked to be thrust. Just as quickly, nurses have been asked, indeed demanded, to adjust and to accept the conditions for this change regardless of its appropriateness or value. Often those who have led systems, in their enthusiasm to respond and position the organization well in the marketplace, have never fully considered the impact of adjusting the service framework without more forethought and care. Nevertheless, the times are upon health care that demand response and require a sustainable framework for the future (Shortell and others, 1996).

## KEY FACTORS

Several circumstances will have a sustaining influence on health care for the foreseeable future:

- Health care is becoming increasingly subscriber based, with providers knowing their patients before they provide service to them.
- Payment for service is being made in advance of service at a capitated rate.
- Physicians are moving from privilege to partnership in their relationships in the health service structure. Most will be in some model of partnership or employment relationship.
- Consumer/population-driven service structures will predominate, thus creating the need for constructing and supporting a comprehensive continuum of linked services.
- The new architecture for the future of health service is an information infrastructure that creates the conditions that no longer require institutional approaches to the planning and delivery of clinical services.

These five new realities are challenging and changing the conditions for health service forever and affecting the professions in a dramatic and significant way. They also offer an opportunity to redesign health services in a much more functional way, leading to a better level of health and a more positive relationship between providers and with patients (Beckham, 1994). These demands create a real opportunity to build community, population-based, linked, and early engagement health services. Insight, wisdom, creativity, and good timing will be critical factors in making this happen.

As a result there are two scenarios for nurses that can play out in the emerging paradigm. One reflects nurses' current level of response; the other mirrors an ideal outcome that reflects a different sort of engagement on the part of nurses and their profession. Which one of these will predominate depends on the congruence between the profession's actions and the demand for response.

## REACTING TO A NEW REALITY

Without much change in the current strategy of the professional leadership of nursing in their response to the reality shift in health care, one can safely anticipate some specific results. At present, much of the action of nurses has been reactive, rather than proactive, to change. Some of the following are the most visible nursing responses to the changes thus far in health care:

- Voicing strong concerns about the move to integrate the disciplines around the patient and diminish or eliminate nursing as a separate department
- Indicating that changes in staffing levels threaten patient safety
- Enumerating that cross training and using assistive clinical personnel threaten the safety of patient care.
- Indicating that downsizing the hospital threatens nurses' jobs and jeopardizes the delivery of patient care
- Proclaiming that shortening the length of hospital stay threatens patients' safety and creates the conditions that make patients sicker and increase readmissions
- Stating that downsizing the number of nurses in the system creates a reduction in the standard of care and threatens the safety of increasingly sicker patients

In spite of nurses' pronouncements, there is no evidence that any of the above conditions are true or even substantiated in any valid manner. Although there are a host of anecdotal stories to support the threatening claims, there is precious little evidence to validate them.

This is not to suggest that there are not serious issues at hand in the retooling of patient care services for the future. Some decisions made by less than insightful leadership are creating havoc in a number of settings across the country and putting both organizations and patients at risk. Although real, these scenarios are fortunately less common than many would have the public believe.

A script is unfolding for a preferred future for health care. The key question is whether nurses are at the table proactively writing the script or at the door lamenting the need to write it. The call of the times is to perceive and conceive a desirable approach to health service that is truly value driven and cost effective. Whatever is decided, the product will be radically different from the one we have become accustomed to over the past 50 years (Coile, 1997).

## A PROBABLE SCENARIO FOR NURSING AND HEALTH CARE

In this depressing scenario the health care system continues to develop outside the institutional framework. The move to capitated systems requires professionals to move to various locations along the system's continuum of service. Without too much creativity one can assume that some shifting of the locus of control will create key changes in the system over the next decade:

- Capitation will continue to expand its influence and will include all services, both public and private, across the service landscape.
- Costs will level off for the short term and then will escalate, moving toward the rate of growth that accrued in the 1980s.
- Tight control over the payment of services will continue to increase payer scrutiny of doctor and hospital charges, requiring justification for all medical-related activities.
- Managed care administrators, buyers (e.g., employers), and payers will continue to squeeze providers until a standard of performance or algorithm for clinical activity emerges that more clearly ties cost and service together.
- Tightening service activities and blending functions to produce specific outcomes will require that professionals have a template from which they operate in rendering specified patient care services.
- Hospitals and health systems will still tend to emphasize illness services at the expense of creating real health-based service in conjunction with the plan's subscribers.

These key elements are embedded in current responses to the vagaries of health care in much of the United States today. Controls on the part of payers and managed care companies are creating a sense of defensiveness and a minimalist approach to service provision. Although a minimalist approach to service provision is nonsustainable, it does provide the foundation on which most providers will live for the foreseeable future.

## Nursing and Medicine in the Probable Scenario

For nurses the probable scenario centers around some specific responses. In this probable scenario nursing will frequently be positioned to play a functional role in the delivery of point-of-service care. Much of the planning and direction for that service will continue to come from policy makers who are not service providers and who have established an economic and financial relationship with physicians.

Nurses, in this scenario, will continue to respond to demands within the parameters of their own profession, directing most of their conversations to each other rather than to other partners in health planning from other disciplines and health care service structures. Furthermore, nurses will still seek entré into the policy forums where health system planning unfolds. Nurses, with the exception of a precious few, will be generally excluded or, more accurately, simply not included in high-level health business and service planning.

Physicians will maintain control of the clinical and practice arenas of health care and will control the practices of all other health providers. The economic balance favoring the clinical work of advanced practice nurses will continue to be ignored and under-researched because of the power relationship among physicians, health business leadership, and politicians. Nurses will continue the effort to be heard and to share evidence of their viability in the clinical and financial arena, but little progress will be made and little attention to nurses' value will be generated.

Although physicians will attempt to maintain control of practice, the demand for primary care advanced practice nurses will continue to accelerate. Group practices and a wide variety of health plans will hire advanced practice nurses as employees to do much of the routine medical and primary clinical work that physicians neither value nor have time for. They will continue to be paid and to benefit as other employees, sharing little of the decisions that govern the practice, policy, finances, and business activities of the practice. Nurses will generally not share in the equity of the practice or the health system.

Nurses will continue to move out of hospitals and other institutions, as health care becomes increasingly continuum driven and noninstitutional in design. The growth of outpatient services will continue at an accelerating rate, and there will be a corresponding decline in inpatient beds. As these beds are no longer used, staffing will continue to decline in bed-related activities until about 50% of the beds are gone. The nurses displaced in this reconfiguration will either be unemployable or, after seeking retraining, will be used in non–bed-based clinical activity.

Several change factors will continue to operate and unfold in our scenario, further affecting the role and position of the nurse in varying capacities:

- Departments of nursing will fold, leaving no organizational structure for the articulation and definition of nursing practice in health systems.
- Nurse managers will continue to be eliminated, removing the nurse from key management roles throughout the system.
- The nurse executive will cease to function in that capacity, which will be eliminated as a key role in the organization's leadership.
- Increased use of case management will require a higher level of education than most nurses currently have, thus allowing diverse graduate-school practitioners (e.g., social workers and health educators) to function as case managers.

- The influx of more physicians into positions of leadership and management in many health systems will create supervisory relationships with nurses and others in clinical practice.
- Payment and remuneration processes will slow the growth in nurses' salaries, which will remain at the lower midline in health care salaries and will be consistent with salaries for functional rather than professional roles.
- Preparing too many nurses for a compressing marketplace will create for the first time in a century an overflow of the number of nurses. These nurses will not find work and will be unemployed for a considerable period.

### Impact of the Probable Scenario

This scenario described does not look particularly different from the current status of nursing in the marketplace today. With little proactive and assertive response to the changes going on all around the health system and with the current rate of change, it is easy to see how nurses can be dramatically and immediately affected.

Many of the forces necessary to create this probable scenario are already underway in the health care system (Blouin and Brent, 1996). Nurses are reeling and reacting to changes affecting their current understanding and practices and how health services are provided and how they should be offered. At present, there is a tremendous loss of place and of value in the current delivery of health services. With the loss of a center point or power location in the system, nursing has no sense of itself. Nurses are finding it difficult to cope with the magnitude and trauma associated with the demand for the radical reshifting elements of the health service structure. Nursing has positioned itself frequently to be viewed as the protector of all that is stable, historic, and right, through pleas of patient endangerment to the loss of good standards of care. Much of this positioning is causing the conditions for this probable scenario of the ebb and flow of faddish nonsustainable service approaches that simply cannot be well designed when a key player in the process is missing from the table where these processes are conceived and engineered.

As a result, nurses are perceived as dragging their feet rather than proactively acting as planners and as players in designing a more cost-effective, value-driven health care system. This lack of nursing participation in health care planning causes health care leadership to impose changes that may not be well thought out and are defensive rather than proactive. Nurses need to participate in leadership roles to positively affect changes in locus of control, service, and structure in health care. Otherwise, nurses will continue to service changes that are made without nursing input. Without leadership and participation in decision making, nurses will continue to be spectators.

## CONSTRUCTING THE PREFERRED SCENARIO FOR NURSING

Many of the changes occurring within the health care system are long overdue. Many of the intentions driving much of the change are responses to variables that now lie outside the control of most of the players. The health care system must respond to the demand for value if it is to be sustained and healthy enough to provide good service for all of its subscribers.

The introduction of value as an important component in the equation to balance health care choices has changed the rules for everyone in our preferred scenario. The best choices can no longer guide every decision. Value to patient and community, as well as good service within a set of acceptable financial imperatives, becomes the ethical leader's obligation.

There is an entire frame of reference that guides the understanding identified in newer point-of-service designs in this preferred scenario. These models remove much of the hierarchy and move most of the decisions into the point of service where many of the key values are located and the key providers are configured. This change demands a shift in both locus of control and the behaviors necessary to thrive in the new environment. The challenge for nurses is to be able to identify the signposts of change early enough and then to engage in the efforts to affect positive outcomes in the process and continuously throughout the health system. Indeed, nurses anticipated their specific responses to the new environment, out of which they developed a viable format for the delivery of cost-effective nursing and health services for the foreseeable future.

The desirable health system of the future will have three major elements, which are currently in place and will be driving its construction for the next two decades:

- Continuing development of a subscriber-based health system
- Fixing prices for services in advance of providing service
- Building a progression of linked services across the continuum of care

All of the elements necessary to create this scenario are already in progress and are generating the circumstances that will drive health care services for the next two decades. Everything about the change is providing a firm and positive baseline for the future of nursing practice to reach a potential only dreamed of in past generations of nursing service.

In our preferred scenario, late engagement health service (sickness care) gives way to early engagement health service (health care). This shift is driven by the structure of prepayment, which shifts the focus away from high-intensity health intervention to high-intensity health prescription. The health system has successfully made the transition to population-based services and has finally accommodated advanced pricing strategies that by now have become standard approaches to setting prices for defined health services across the continuum of care. Health systems are beginning to participate in setting regional standards of service to provide a comprehensive range of services.

In our preferred scenario many positive forces that were previously at the periphery of health services have moved toward the center of the health care system:

- Physicians have been mostly repositioned into group practice arrangements and into new partnership in the health system that has a full range of providers.
- A primary care approach has laid the foundation for a more integrated approach to health service, building stronger patient-driven service structures within the health system.
- New partnerships with the business community have moved the locus of control and service more toward employer-based health services, creating service partnerships between provider organizations and employers.
- The burgeoning growth of technology has further limited high intervention and invasive strategies, creating a more decentralized service environment.
- Technology has furthered portability of service, making it much easier to bring services to consumers in their homes, clinics, community centers, and mobile units in rural and inner city settings.

## Role of the Nurse

This scenario has created a nutrient foundation for the growth of nursing practice. It became clear to the policy makers early in the move to primary care that broad-based, cost-effective providers were needed at the point of service to ensure that access to primary services could be obtained in a wide variety of urban and rural settings across the country. Preparation of an adequate number of primary and family practice physicians was a long way off, and the demand for primary services was growing at an accelerated rate. Through extensive education and lobbying of members of Congress, sufficient education dollars were made available for the preparation of a growing number of advanced practice nurses. In conjunction with the emphasis at the federal level for adequate primary care providers was the passage of the "Advanced Nurse Practice Equity Act," which constrained states from passing restrictive practice laws limiting the full practice of nursing, including nurse prescriptive privileges. These measures went far to create equity-based clinical partnership arrangements between physicians and nurses.

As the health care system became increasingly decentralized, the role of the nurse changed radically. Decreasing market demand caused considerable reduction in the number of nurses who have associate degrees and diplomas. A concomitant increase occurred in the number of nurses who have baccalaureate and masters degrees. As a result the role and function of the nurse changed considerably in the health care organization:

- Case management of patients grew from 20% to nearly 60% as institutions became centers of intensive intervention with a strong need to refer patients back to a continuum of services to manage reintegration into the social mainstream.
- Nurses developed a more mobile skill set, creating increased flexibility in their utility across the continuum of services and facilitating the continued expansion of nursing services in noninstitutional settings.
- Nurses became the integrating and coordinating members of clinical teams, providing a role that focused on the linkage and integration of the work of the clinical team and ensuring that expectations for service and outcomes were consistently achieved.
- Nurses provided the majority of consumer-based education and development for professionals to assist subscribers to handle their life processes, to reduce late cycle demand for high-intensity service, and to facilitate patient self-management of chronic health concerns.
- Nurses identified their influence on sustainable health care outcomes measured by quality monitoring and the advancement of clinical pathways through the synthesis of the processes of care.
- Systems leadership required an increase in the number of nurses more than ever before because of their skill in linking and integrating the various components of the system and their ability to focus the structure and resources of the system on facilitating decision making at the point of service. More nurses than at any time in nursing's history have moved into CEO roles in a variety of service structures in the continuum of services.
- More nurses than ever before have moved into alternative locations for the delivery of health services. As more service configurations have emerged because of the focus on health, new service constituents have been added to the array of health services in the system. As evidence of their impact on health becomes increasingly clear, nurses have positioned themselves to provide a broad range of services from life management processes to nutritional therapy and healing processes across the health continuum.

## System Leadership

The organization of health services has also changed considerably. As health service is driven more directly from the point of service, the system's leadership is devoted mostly to providing resource and decision support services. The focus of systems leadership is to predominantly ensure that the right information is available to decision makers in a form they can use when they need it. Furthermore, system leadership provides the tools of information management to the provider in a format that makes their use both easy and routine. The information infrastructure now drives the health care system by producing integrated clinical and financial outcomes data that provide immediate feedback on choice and performance to both leader and provider (Box 3-1).

### Box 3-1
### *Point-of-Service Team Work*

Sandy Cannon, RN, has been the multidisciplinary team leader in the Women's Health Center for 7 months. The Health Center has moved completely to population-based service design, which places all consumers at the center of the organization and decentralizes the system around the specific service populations. Women's services are a major initiative of the Health Center, and transdisciplinary clinical teams are constructed around specified patient activities. The medical staff organization is redesigned to parallel the patient service structure to improve the relationship and increase interaction between physicians and the other clinical staff. A strong clinical partnership developed between the advanced practice nurses and the physicians. Service protocols were developed by the various teams and placed into the computers so that all team members could practice within their parameters. Best practice guidelines for each team member are included in the protocols. They contain the financial profile, expected outcomes and the evaluative criteria for each critical path (protocol).

Sandy worked closely with the team to develop its skills in team process. Getting the team to work together and to understand the contribution of each member was challenging. Giving up nonintegrating behavior and determining how each role would support the achievement of aggregated outcomes was difficult at first. The team had grown significantly over the past few months and the physicians, nurses, and clinical staff had begun to build a strong relationship around the patient protocols they had developed together. Sandy found that her time and efforts were less focused in the arena of making decisions for the staff. Instead, she spent much of her time mentoring and facilitating their development of skills in problem solving, decision making, and solution seeking. Much of her time is now spent in seeking and applying resources to the teams and in obtaining information necessary to support their work. Sandy is now able to say to herself that the chances of building a sustainable team-based and point-of-service system is looking stronger every day. Even physicians are happier with getting involved and problem solving and believe that they can make a difference and get real results. Patient care appears more coordinated, and patients are responding well.

## CONCLUSION

The basic shift in our preferred scenario is the creation of structure and process that support the principles of a new age for work: partnership, equity, accountability, and ownership (Porter-O'Grady and Krueger-Wilson, 1995). These principles drive sustainability of systems in the new era for health care. As nurses and others configure their practices around these principles, they create the conditions for strong clinical relationships and the foundations for good health service. The difference between the probable scenario and the preferred scenario is the generalized commitment of every member of the health team to these principles. The preferred scenario is certainly not outrageous nor even outside the realm of possibility. Whether it unfolds depends on the insight and energy of nurses and organized nursing. There will certainly be a role for nurses in the unfolding health system. How vital and central nursing is to what the health care system is becoming depends entirely on the willingness of nurses to engage the change process early and to do the work necessary to make the desired change possible. The ability of nurses to thrive depends entirely on the capacity of nurses to create a tightness-of-fit between what the changing health care system needs and what nurses have to offer. This is nothing short of a revolutionary mandate for the profession. Time will tell how well nurses answer the call.

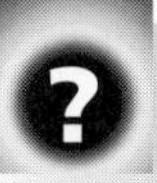

## *Discussion Exercises*

1. Major differences between the probable and preferable scenarios are described in the chapter. Discuss strategies that nurses can undertake to create the preferable scenario.
2. The chapter suggests that nursing responses to changes in health care have been reactive rather than proactive. Do you agree? How can nursing respond proactively?

3. Do you think nurses will "answer the call" as described in the chapter? Explain your reasons.

## References

Argyris C: *Knowledge for action,* San Francisco, 1993, Jossey-Bass.

Beckham D: The power of primary care, *Healthcare Forum J* 37(1):68, 1994.

Beckham D: Hearing the tidal wave, *Healthcare Forum J* 39(2):68, 1996.

Berman M: *The reenchantment of the world,* New York, 1989, Bantam Books.

Blouin A, Brent N: California Nurses Association et al *v* Alta Bates et al: possible implications for restructuring, *J Nurs Adm* 26(2):10, 1996.

Coile R: *Five stages of managed care,* Chicago, 1997, Health Administration Press.

Lowe A: Reducing variation in patient care: nursing responds to capitation, *J Nurs Adm* 26(1):14, 1996.

Porter-O'Grady T: Managing along the continuum: a new paradigm for the clinical manager, *Nurs Adm Q* 19(3):1, 1995.

Porter-O'Grady T, Krueger-Wilson C: *The leadership revolution in healthcare: altering systems, changing behavior,* Gaithersburg, Md, 1995, Aspen.

Shortell S and others: *Remaking health care in america,* San Francisco, 1996, Jossey-Bass.

# 4 Nursing's Future in Health Care Policy

**Mary Wakefield**

*We must not, in trying to think about how we can make a big difference, ignore the small daily difference we can make which, over time, add up to big differences that we often cannot foresee*

**Marian Wright Edelman**
Children's advocate

Poised on the verge of a new millennium, health care delivery in the United States and in countries around the world is undergoing unprecedented change; it transcends not only state borders but also international borders, with providers, health care delivery systems, and managed care organizations increasingly serving populations around the globe. The geohealth landscape, ranging from where and how services are delivered to the expected competencies of providers, is rapidly reconfiguring. Much of this change, from local to international levels, is contingent on the action or inaction of governments.

## RECENT HEALTH POLICY EFFORTS

With the 1994 demise of efforts to overhaul our nation's health care system through President Clinton's Health Security Act, state governments and the private sector moved rapidly to design their own substantive changes in health care. Although the full aftermath of these transitions is yet to be played out, fundamental shifts have already resulted in a major reallocation of power and decision making from providers and health care facilities to managed care organizations and purchasers of health care. Wilensky (1997) identifies one significant component of this power shift, noting that "the erosion of professional authority . . . has diminished the role that health care professionals might otherwise have taken in ensuring quality in the new world of managed care." This trend alone, that is, shifts in the locus of decision making, should prompt the nursing community to actively engage in the policy dialogue. Concomitant with shifts in power, insecurity in the American psyche is increasing, with public concerns voiced regarding issues as basic as whether providers have the interest of the patient or the payer of care as their first priority.

Policy makers at all levels of government evaluate and, through public policy initiatives, often respond to significant changes in health care. Public policies are "authoritative decisions made in the legislative, executive, or judicial branches of government that are intended to direct or influence the actions, behaviors, or decisions of others" (Longest, 1996). As such, public health policy is a vehicle for creating an environment that maximizes the health of individuals and communities. Directly and indirectly, policy affects the practice of every provider. Through the enactment of public policy then, governments are pivotal players in the health care arena.

Worldwide, nurses increasingly recognize the significance that public health policy and political activity have on their practice and the health of their patients. Acknowledging these critical linkages, Affara and Styles (1992) assert that all health professions have the responsibility to participate in prioritizing and formulating policy. Specific to organized nursing, they state that "a system of governance for the profession must provide for . . . participation of the profession in the development of public policy." To fully participate in the policy-making process, nurses need to be cognizant of the overarching health care issues that have driven and will continue to drive public policy for the foreseeable future. From local to national levels, the major policy discussions revolve around *health care costs, inadequate access to care,* and, emerging as an increasingly important concern, *quality of care.*

In the early 1990s these same three issues prompted the Clinton administration to wage a high-stakes battle to radically change the health care system—a battle that was ultimately lost. Still unresolved, policies are continually being developed to address these issues. For example, quality of health care has captured the attention of policy makers from state capitols to the nation's capitol. Health care quality, the mantra that has historically set this country's health care system apart from so many others, has been called into question by purchasers, consumers, and providers of care, as well as policy makers. Attempts to maintain and improve quality of care and protect consumers from poor care are evident in a myriad of initiatives. Initiatives range from legislative backlash to managed care in states across the country to the creation of an advisory commission on consumer protection and quality in the health care industry by President Clinton in 1996 in order to recommend policies that would maintain and strengthen health care quality.

## A PREFERRED FUTURE

Absent simple solutions to this complex and interwoven triad of cost, quality, and access issues, two predictions about nursing can readily be made. First, as health care continues to be buffeted by turbulent change, windows of opportunity and serious challenges to the nursing profession will emerge. These same changes that affect health care broadly, and nursing specifically, will often result from or serve as a catalyst for new public policy initiatives.

The second prediction follows, in that nursing's future is inextricably linked to public health policy. Consequently, the extent to which nurses individually and collectively engage in the public policy-making process will determine the form and substance of nursing's future, that is, who practices nursing and how and where that practice occurs. For nurses to fully engage in the policy debate, they must understand the problems driving policy initiatives and position the profession as part of the solution to these problems.

### Nursing's Involvement in Health Policy

With a multitude of demands on the nursing profession, skeptics may question how nurses can afford to markedly increase their public policy efforts. However, a preferred future reveals nursing leaders who recognize the challenges facing both the nursing profession and the profession's ability to fully contribute to the health care of consumers. In this future, nurse leaders will commit themselves and their organizations to serve as architects of change through public health policy rather than functioning as passive recipients of policy crafted by others. By building and expanding efforts to influence public health policy, nurses ensure that the practice of nursing does not become a marginalized invisible part of the health care system. This commitment involves a recognition that exerting significant influence in the public policy arena is a complex undertaking, ". . . involving the interactive participation of many members of the health policy community in several interconnected and interdependent phases of activities" (Longest, 1994).

At an individual level every nurse in this preferred future will recognize that he or she has an opportunity and an obligation to influence the health care of society by being informed and involved in public health policy. To that end nurses will be as well versed in the components of the policy-making process as they are in the nursing process and, commensurate with their education and expertise, will be engaged in influencing policy outcomes. Furthermore, public health policy will serve as a point of convergence for nurses, whether they are engaged in practice, research, education, or administration.

Resulting from nursing's expanded activism in the policy arena, a common understanding will emerge from both the public and policy makers regarding nursing's contribution to decreasing costs, increasing access, and improving the quality of health care. Furthermore, nursing expertise, research, and opinions will be sought to educate the public through mass media and to inform policy makers, purchasers, and other providers of health care. Nursing associations will create an overarching entity that links nursing organizations, establishes priority policy aims, develops a comprehensive plan, and incorporates an array of strategies that will serve as catalysts for and responses to health policy crafted at multiple levels. If influencing public policy in a comprehensive and significant way is our goal, then what are the structures and processes that take us there?

Although there is a wide range of strategies that can enhance the linkages between nursing and public health policy, three specific areas are discussed in this chapter. These areas of emphasis include linking nursing organizations, enhancing educational content in nursing programs, and using nursing research to inform public health policy. Nursing should focus its efforts on these areas to position the profession to inform policy makers and shape health policy.

## The Role of Nursing Organizations

The mechanism for taking collective action is generally a professional organization activity (Cohen and others, 1996). With more than 80 professional organizations, nurses align themselves with associations that focus on interests ranging from nursing history to the care of patients with head and neck pathology. With headquarters across the country and membership ranging from a few thousand to more than 250,000, the scope of interest and influence of nursing organizations varies considerably.

Longest (1996) notes that there are direct and powerful links between public policy crafted at both state and federal levels and the strategic decisions that shape and direct health care organizations. At least indirectly, public health policy influences the interests and agenda of every nursing organization. Although each organization exists to meet the special interests of its membership, there is significant variation in the extent to which organizations engage in public policy–related activities as a means for addressing member interests. For example, most committed to broadly influencing health policy, ". . . the American Nurses Association (ANA) has been the major voice for nursing at the federal level. At the state level, state nurses associations typically take the lead in determining preferred policy and lobbying on most issues . . ." (Cohen and others, 1996).

Historically, the ANA has allocated a significant amount of its resources to affect a broad spectrum of public health policies, ranging from occupational safety to enlisting federal funding for the Nursing Education Act. This comprehensive policy agenda stems from one of the stated purposes of the ANA, which is to "ensure that health care public policy is consonant with the goals of nurses, nursing, and public health" (American Nurses Association, 1997). Most other organizations that value and engage in public policy initiatives narrowly target their policy agenda and often reflect different policy priorities. For example, the relationship between nursing research and public health policy is a concern to the American Academy of Nursing (AAN), which has considered ways to facilitate the work of nurse scientists at the national policy level.

Whereas the American Association of Colleges of Nursing (AACN), representing baccalaureate and higher degree programs, lobbies for funding for the National Institute of Nursing Research and the Nursing Education Act, internally the association strongly prescribes health policy as a curriculum focus for its member schools. To position future nurses to maximize their contribution to health care, AACN believes that health policy and legislative advocacy should be an educational priority for all nursing curricula. Offering guidance to its member schools, AACN (1997) states that,

> While nursing education must prepare expert practitioners, schools also have the responsibility to produce nursing professionals who can participate as full partners in health care delivery and in shaping health policy . . . It is critical that nurses be prepared with the skills to negotiate the political system and to remove artificial barriers that limit the profession's ability to practice in the best interest of consumers.

With a view toward the future, AACN (1997) believes that "nurses' responsibilities increasingly will include educating the public and policy makers of nursing's role within the overall scheme of health care, of the range of nursing's skills and scopes of practice, and of the relationships between nursing care and positive outcomes for patients."

Public health policy is also identified as a priority for nurse executives by the American Organization of Nurse Executives (AONE). AONE (1996) indicates that new competencies necessary for contemporary nurse executive practice include participating in public policy related to health care.

## Transcending Organizational Goals

Although each nursing organization rightly pursues its own unique interests, the overall strength of the profession lies in the ability to identify and work toward common policy goals that transcend nursing organizations. Collaboration is essential. The power of the profession is contingent on a critical mass of nursing organizations that are willing to commit to selected public policy priorities through political action and by influencing policy development. Policy development is a process used by society to make decisions about problems, choose goals and the appropriate strategies to reach them, manage conflicting views, and allocate resources (Institute of Medicine, 1996).

The ability of nursing organizations to influence policy development rests with nursing's expert power and ability to reward. That is, through collective action, the nursing profession can help to position and draw on the power of many nurses with diverse expertise in health care who can provide valued information necessary to solve policy problems. This expert power, accessed through an overarching nursing entity, may influence policy development in numerous ways. For example, nurse experts, drawn from a range of nursing organizations, could assist in drafting and critiquing legislative proposals or providing public comment on proposed federal regulations. Furthermore, by combining the efforts of multiple organizations, the ability to give or withhold significant rewards increases. These rewards can take many forms, from providing political support through involvement in reelection campaigns to supporting proposed legislation by committing financial resources to media advertising campaigns.

To position nursing so that the profession contributes to and benefits from public policy, organizational leaders must anticipate both the emergence and impact of relevant public health policy on nursing organizations specifically and the profession more broadly. Longest (1994) notes that accurately analyzing the public policy environment requires that organizations (1) assess the effects of public policy on the organization in terms of opportunities and threats and position the organization to adjust to these effects, and (2) identify public policy objectives that are consistent with the organization's values and mission and help shape those public policies. Specific analytic steps (Longest, 1996) include the following:

- Identifying and monitoring public policy of strategic importance
- Projecting future directions of strategic public policy issues
- Assessing the implications of these strategic issues
- Diffusing information produced about public policy throughout the organization

The challenges associated with developing and implementing public policy include "conflicting and competing values and goals, struggles with defining and resolving problems, and obstacles to the implementation of programs" (Institute of Medicine, 1996). As part of the family of nursing, both the members and leaders of every nursing organization must directly confront these challenges both within and across nursing organizations. Although individual interests of nursing organizations may vary, ultimately nursing's influence is only as strong as the unifying commitment of nursing organizations to bridge differences, set common public policy goals, and develop a plan and related strategies to achieve those goals. In addition, the ongoing education of organizational members to public policy processes and emerging policies should be an organizational priority. Whether by devoting newsletter space to a public policy column or ensuring that at least one plenary session of every sponsored conference relates to health policy, there are a host of strategies that all nursing organizations should employ to educate their members about the direct relevance of health policy to their practice and the health of their patients.

## Coalitions With Nonnursing Organizations

Although nursing and health care will directly benefit from the development of a shared commitment across organized nursing, nursing's influence also markedly increases by participation in coalitions that encompass nonnursing organizations, which has much more power to influence policy than any one organization does (Brownson and others, 1997). Interest groups commonly join coalitions to increase visibility, credibility, and power in the political process. Also, coalition members benefit by pooling resources, sharing information, and representing a broader constituency (Schauffler and Wikerson, 1997).

Coalitions are often fluid and temporary. They are designed to address specific policy issues and, once resolved, coalitions generally disband. Typically, policy makers have heightened sensitivity to views that are broadly held by large numbers of people.

Critical to working effectively in the public policy arena is the development of relationships between organizations that withstand differences of opinion and changing alliances. For example, on policy issues such as provider scope of practice or reimbursement, the American Medical Association and any number of nursing organizations may advocate very different policy solutions. However, on a range of public health issues, as well as a host of other issues, both nursing and medicine should encourage cultivation of collaborative relationships to highlight health concerns or advocate policy solutions from injury prevention to teenage obesity.

Nursing involvement in broad health and social issues does not preclude pursuing policy that directly relates to nursing practice (Cohen and others, 1996). In addition, whether working across nursing organizations or in coalitions with other groups, the likelihood of policy success is enhanced when public opinion supports the perspectives of interest groups (Weissert and Weissert, 1996). Through the collective effort of nursing organizations, the profession's policy interests need to be defined, policies that advance these interests need to be developed, and specific efforts, including work through coalitions, must be made to build and maintain the support of the public and policy makers. Throughout these efforts, an underlying objective should include promoting a greater understanding by the public and policy makers regarding the contributions nurses are making to health care.

## Nursing Education

### Teaching Health Policy

Expanding the depth and breadth of the nursing profession's orientation toward public health policy should largely emanate from nursing education, the standard bearers responsible for ensuring that the next generation of nurses is well equipped to influence health care. Imparting fundamental information about political and policy-making processes and structuring meaningful interactions with policy makers are essential. To position nurses for the future, Cohen and others (1996) state that "today's visionaries must actively cultivate and educate the next generation about the workings of the legislative, judicial, and executive branches of government."

Students need experience in planning and implementing strategies useful for educating and influencing government officials. Whether nurse educators are expert in critical care or community health nursing, incorporating public policy content and activity related to their areas of expertise provides students with concrete examples of how to link practice and policy and why creating these linkages is critically important to both their profession and the patients for whom they care. Policy content should be a part of every class discussion, and nurse educators should include their own examples of policy-related activities.

Although faculty embrace the value of disseminating ideas and research findings to the nursing community through professional nursing journals, little is said about the need for and value of communicating information to the public and to policy makers. The potential and far-reaching impact of a well-written letter to the local newspaper editor that provides a nursing perspective on a proposed health policy, for example, should be highly valued and encouraged. Radio and television call-in programs and today's easy access to public forums via the Internet are other avenues to promote nursing's perspective.

### Communicating With Consumers

Communicating health-related information to consumers and policy makers is as valuable and important to influencing health care as communicating one's research findings or opinions to an audience of peers. Health care consumers have never had access to the depth and breadth of health-related information that is available to them today—from sources as accessible as their daily newspaper, which reports new discoveries weekly, to information available on their home computers. These information vehicles, coupled with emerging public and private sector initiatives designed to inform consumers about issues ranging from which health plan to select or which hospital has the best outcomes to which health care provider has the highest patient satisfaction ratings, provide nurses with the opportunity to create, influence, and communicate useful information.

Students need to witness their faculty, working individually and through professional organizations, communicating with and educating policy makers and other key stakeholders about health care issues and ways that nursing can be part of the policy solutions developed to solve health care problems. Ensuring that students include policy implications in papers or presentations helps to lay a foundation for understanding. In fact, speaking about graduate education, Cohen and others (1996) suggest that "every graduate of a doctoral program in nursing should be able to articulate the policy relevance of his or her research."

In addition to encouraging the publication of dissertation findings in nursing journals, communicating the information in the popular press should also be considered. To the extent that nursing's contribution to health care is known within the profession but invisible to the media and policy makers, the goal of nurses to serve as informed resources on health policy matters and to actively participate in setting health policy agendas will remain elusive. Furthermore, faculty should strongly encourage nursing students to actively participate in student organizations. From city government to state capitals, nurses are underrepresented. Student organizations can provide a training ground for building the confidence, skills, and knowledge necessary to campaign for elective offices or to seek political appointments.

## Research

Given the phenomenal rate of change in the health care system, ranging from the reconfiguration of provider mix to the utilization of genetic information, the impact of scores of new innovations on cost, quality, and access to care is simply unknown. Change is producing an insatiable need for sound research that can be used to make decisions. As Greenfield and others (1996) note, "Without incorporating research findings into policy, there is no sound method to ensure that the quality, type, availability, and cost of health care are appropriate."

Numerous factors influence public policy; among them are political ideology, special interest groups, public opinion, the media, and research. The strength of any one of these factors to influence policy varies considerably. Research findings, the gold standard from which expensive and far-reaching policy should emanate, are often either unavailable or available but not influential in policy discussions. For example, during the 1993-1994 debate over the Clinton health care reform plan, "the level of debate was set more by the infamous television ads starring Harry and Louise than by careful research on the costs and benefits of various systems of health care finance and delivery" (Wilensky, 1997).

There is a range of strategies that nurses, both researchers and nonresearchers alike, can use to increase the likelihood that policy will be developed based on sound research. Strategy decisions begin with an understanding of the relationship between public policy and research. Doctoral students (who are tomorrow's researchers) should be encouraged to minor in public policy or public affairs, and doctoral programs should include this content.

In spite of the tremendous potential for nursing research to influence public policy, few research articles are published with policy implications and even fewer nurses incorporate strategies needed to increase the likelihood that policy makers will capitalize on their research findings. To improve the use of research findings in forming policy, a number of considerations are in order:

1. *Nurses must understand the policy-making structure and process, including activities of the executive and legislative branches of government.* Both use research to make decisions. Research findings are often provided to legislators and their staff, especially by special interest groups, as Litman and Robins (1997) note, within the executive branch: "The entire thrust of a piece of legislation may be muted, if not reversed, in the writing of the regulations or administration of [the legislation]." Consequently, nurse researchers should not overlook the very significant role that state and federal agencies play in designing public health policy and informing the the executive branch.
2. *Nurses need to present research findings in a way that can be used by policy makers.* Just as researchers may not be initially familiar with the lexicon of public policy, policy makers are often unfamiliar with the research lexicon. Consequently, when nurse researchers communicate with policy makers through correspondence or in meetings, a discussion of policy-relevant research bears little resemblance to a traditional research presentation. Policy makers are not in a position to critique the quality of a research study; their focus is on application of the study findings. Therefore the information essential to informing policy makers should be the primary subject of conversation or the highlighted content in correspondence. Although background

information (e.g., research design, or statistical analysis) can always be appended, nurse researchers should refrain from using research or nursing jargon and distill the problem, context, findings, and conclusions of a study in a letter that does not exceed two pages. Policy makers will not read more.

Furthermore, researchers often communicate findings in tentative rather than absolute terms; however, policy makers frequently enact legislation or regulations based on limited information. The pressure to address complex health problems does not allow time to do more. Policy makers often enlist support from the public and relevant stakeholders by attempting to base their arguments on conclusions and recommendations that are research based (Davis, 1986). In speeches, correspondence, interviews, and other forms of communication, policy makers citing research findings generally do not provide an accompanying discussion of the mechanics or limitations of the research study.

Given that policy makers are interested in application of findings, it is up to the researcher to ensure that information provided to policy makers is based on sound science. Within this context, "policy researchers must balance scientific rigor with the need for public health action" (Brownson and others, 1997). In testament to the imperfect nature of policy making, if the policy problem is serious enough, policies will be enacted that may be based on little or no scientific information. The challenge for the researcher is to know when enough evidence has accumulated to draw conclusions and to recognize that research is just one factor used to inform public policy makers.

3. *Research must be policy relevant.* Although a nurse may produce research findings that highlight a relevant health problem not currently debated in the policy arena, such research could serve as the stimulus for debate, and the researcher is more likely to be successful if the findings relate to an identified or emerging policy concern. For example, in addition to tracking policy developments and proposals in nursing publications and columns designed to monitor political activity, nurse researchers can stay abreast of likely policy topics by familiarizing themselves with health problems discussed in the mass media. Not infrequently, policy makers pursue legislative proposals based on information presented in the press. For example, an article that describes how managed care organizations deny access to certain medical procedures can quickly become the stimulus for the introduction of a bill. Given that media reports can serve as the stimulus for health policy proposals, universities and health care institutions should encourage nurse researchers to publish their findings in the press, as well as peer-reviewed journals.

   Another strategy to link research with policy is to identify the priorities of state legislatures or the agenda of the Congress when priority issues are highlighted at the beginning of each legislative session. It is important to note that the leadership of political parties will likely identify different priorities (e.g., access to insurance for children versus expansion of medical savings accounts for Medicare beneficiaries).

   Nurse researchers also need to remember that, like research, policy is incremental. For example, although a new initiative may be launched to increase the availability of health care providers in underserved areas, rarely does one legislative initiative provide the complete answer to a public health problem. Therefore, although research findings should be presented in a timely fashion, public health problems are generally solved incrementally, and policy work on any particular issue is rarely final.
4. *Policy makers are typically under tremendous time constraints.* Consequently, most policy makers and their staff are not generally in the habit of perusing nursing research journals (or most other health-related journals, for that matter). Likewise, policy makers do not usually contact individual nurse researchers

or nursing organizations to identify current research findings that might help them fashion sound public health policy. Instead, it is incumbent on nurses to disseminate findings from nursing research and to package them to increase the likelihood that they will be reviewed.

In addition to conducting policy-relevant research, another role that may be assumed by nurse researchers is to conduct policy analysis. Policy analysis is concerned with "summarizing the best available information bearing on choices among policy alternatives . . . In the absence of hard information . . . informed judgment must be relied upon" (Davis, 1986). For example, rather than initiating an empirical study, nurses can influence health policy by relating findings and their policy implications from published research that is not likely to be reviewed in its original form by policy makers. Through the process of disseminating research findings, opinions, and expertise that inform policy makers and improve health care, the nursing profession enhances its own visibility and expands its worth to the public and to policy makers.

## CONCLUSION

The value assigned to nurses, as individual providers and collectively as professional organizations, will be based on a standard that simply states: what is valued in health care is that which enhances access and achieves the highest quality at the lowest cost. To optimize the profession's contribution to health care and, more fundamentally, perhaps to even survive, nursing must fare well measured against this standard. Equally important, when nursing provides sound evidence and successfully communicates that it is a high-quality, cost-effective health care provider, there is an increased likelihood that the public, purchasers of health care, and policy makers will acknowledge and act on that information. Without a commitment to engage in public health policy, health care providers invite their own obsolescence and fail to fully use their knowledge to positively affect the health care of entire populations. Nurses, acting in public health policy arenas today, can determine a positive and preferred future for consumers of health care, as well as the nursing profession.

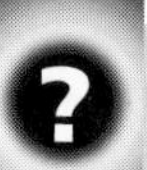

## *Discussion Exercises*

1. The value of organizations joining together for the public good is described in the chapter. Why might such collective action *not* succeed?
2. What changes in nursing education would you suggest to encourage policy participation? Be specific about content and experiential learning activities, and include all levels of education.
3. What opportunities have you had to influence public policy? Describe public policy efforts you could make now and in the future.

## References


Affara FA, Styles MM: *Nursing regulation: from principles to power, a guidebook on mastering nursing regulation,* Battlecreek, Mich, 1992, International Council of Nurses with the support of the WK Kellogg Foundation.

American Association of Colleges of Nursing: *Executive summary, a vision of baccalaureate and graduate nursing education: the next decade,* Washington, DC, 1997 The Association.

American Nurses Association: Legislative, political, and grassroots programs: fact sheet, Washington, DC, 1997, The Association.

American Organization of Nurse Executives: The evolving nurse executive practice, issue brief, Washington, DC, 1996, The Organization.

Brownson R and others: Policy research for disease prevention: challenges and practical recommendations, *Am J Pub Health* 87(5):735, 1997.

Cohen S and others: Stages of nursing's political development: where we've been and where we ought to go, *Nurs Outlook* 44(6):259, 1996.

Davis K: *Research in health policy formulation in applications of social science to clinical medicine and health policy,* New Brunswick, NJ, 1986, Rutgers University Press (edited by Aiken L, Mechanic D).

Greenfield L and others: *Evaluating the quality of health care: what research offers decision makers,* Battlecreek, Mich, 1996, Milbank Memorial Fund.

Institute of Medicine: *Healthy communities: new partnerships for the future of public health,* Washington, DC, 1996, National Academy Press.

Litman T, Robins L: *Health politics and policy,* ed 3, Albany, NY, 1997, Delmar.

Longest B: *Health policymaking in the United States,* Ann Arbor, Mich, 1994, AUPHA/Health Administration Press.

Longest B: *Seeking strategic advantage through health policy analysis,* Chicago, 1996, Health Administration Press.

Schauffler H, Wilkerson J: National health care reform and the 103rd Congress: the activities and influence of public health advocates, *Am J Pub Health* 87(7):1107, 1997.

Weissert C, Weissert W: *Governing health,* Baltimore, 1996, Johns Hopkins University Press.

Wilensky G: Promoting quality: a public policy view, *Health Aff* 16(3):77, 1997.

Wilensky H: Social science and the public agenda: reflections on the relation of knowledge to policy in the United States and abroad, *J Health Polit Policy Law* 22(5):1241, 1997.

# 5 Nursing in the Public Domain: The National Perspective

**Marla E. Salmon**

*America is great because she is good; when America ceases to be good, she will cease to be great.*

**Alexis de Tocqueville**

When de Tocqueville made this observation more than 160 years ago, he captured the essence of what has been a fundamental part of the character of the United States: a generosity of spirit, a caring for its peoples, and a system of public office and action that was built on the values articulated in the Declaration of Independence and in the U.S. Constitution.

Although de Tocqueville's comments do not specifically relate to nursing, their meaning does provide an important lens through which the past, present, and future of caring can be viewed. It is this socially mandated capacity for caring, particularly as it relates to health care, that gives meaning to nursing in the public domain. The purpose of this chapter is to explore the future of America's capacity to care and the roles that nursing might play in the public sector in support of that societal function.

## DEVELOPMENT OF NURSING IN THE PUBLIC DOMAIN

### Nursing as a Public Good

The concept of nursing as a public good formally emerged in the United States around the turn of the century with the recognition of the need for public programs aimed at promoting and protecting the public's health. When one considers the health problems facing the country during that period, it is not surprising that nursing was an important intervention. The massive influx of immigrants, coupled with the spread of contagious diseases and premature death, created an environment in which community and public action were needed to promote and protect the well-being of the public. Beginning in the early part of the twentieth century (Mullen, 1989), the U.S. Government formally offered nursing services as a public health measure through the U.S. Public Health Service in settings such as merchant marine hospitals, leprosariums, and Ellis Island.

Lillian Wald, the mother of American public health nursing, formalized caring at community levels and national levels in other ways. She began her work with the founding of the Henry Street Settlement House in 1893 and proceeded through the next four decades progressively advancing the impact of nursing as a public good. She convinced boards of education and city officials to hire nurses as part of their public health efforts and helped to found the National Organization of Public Health Nurses. She also encouraged government officials of the United States and other countries to incorporate nursing into their public health programs (Coss, 1989).

Lillian Wald was not alone in these efforts, although she was certainly among the most visible. Her success was, in part, a reflection of the maturation of the United States as a nation. As the country increased its awareness as an entity and as social programs at a national level progressed, nursing presence in the public domain increased.

## Nursing in the Public Sector

The development of a formal nursing presence in state and national government mirrored what was happening in the broader social context. As nurses were being individually called on to provide services for the public and supported by public dollars and programs, the need for leadership and the resources to ensure nursing's ongoing ability to provide service resulted in the creation of offices and nursing leadership positions within the government.

Offices of public health nursing were established as a fundamental part of state health departments in the early part of this century. These offices initially provided centralized direction for the work of public health nurses across states. As state health departments moved away from direct control of public health services, the roles of the nursing offices and their directors moved more toward influencing policy at state levels and providing advice and consultation to local health authorities and their nurses. As a group the state and territorial directors of nursing played an important role in influencing national policy relating to nursing.

The regulation of nursing practice also emerged as a presence for nurses in the public domain. State boards of nursing formed across this country in the early part of this century to serve important functions for the public good by helping to standardize education and practice and ensure a minimum level of safe practice.

## The Federal Domain

The formal presence of nursing within the federal government took root during the twentieth century as well. The most visible of these was the creation of the Cadet Nurse Corps in 1943 (Willever, 1993), which was the foundation upon which national nursing workforce development was built. Through the Cadet Nurse Corps, the federal government became directly involved in ensuring that there was an adequate supply of nurses to meet the needs of the United States during a time of war. This program had a major impact on the expansion of educational opportunities for nurses, the overall improvement of nursing services, and the development of nursing education. It was a highly visible example of how nurses and the federal government could improve the health of the public.

The Cadet Nurse Corps was an example of one of the three types of roles or functions that evolved for nurses in the federal government over the course of this century. Perhaps the most easily understood is the role of nurses in the provision of health services by the federal government as part of the executive branch. This role includes health programs for members of the armed services and programs for special populations, such as veterans, Native Americans, and federal prisoners. Nurses also can be found in federally funded community, migrant, and other health programs. For each of the branches of the armed services and for the Commissioned Corps of the U.S. Public Health Service, there is a chief nurse officer who serves as the focal point for nursing within their respective organizations.

The second function of nurses in the federal government is to provide nursing expertise to other types of federal programs and activities. Nurses can be found in virtually all branches of government. The most common location is within the executive branch, where nursing expertise contributes to health-related research, education, financing, regulation, and policy setting. Nurses can be found in a variety of roles in the Health Care Financing Administration, the Agency for Health Care Policy and Research, the Food and Drug Administration, and the Health Resources and Services Administration. Nurses also can be found in the legislative branch in the Senate and the House of Representatives, where they serve as both elected officials and staff members. In addition, nurses play important roles in the formulation of legislation relating to public health programs.

The third type of federal function relates directly to the development and improvement of the national nursing workforce and the services delivered to the public. There are two major focal points for these activities. The first, the Division of Nursing, was created in 1946 as an outgrowth of both the Cadet Nurse Corps and previously less visible federal programs aimed at improving nursing services. The Division of Nursing has the primary responsibility for national nursing workforce development. In this work, the Division provides leadership in national nursing workforce planning and analysis, development of projects and programs aimed at expanding and improving nursing education and services, enhancement of ethnic and racial diversity in nursing, financing of educational programs and student support, and improvement of the infrastructure needed to ensure an ongoing supply of well-qualified nurses to meet the health care needs of the public.

For the first four decades of its work, the Division of Nursing also funded nursing research, providing the foundation for what became the National Center for Nursing Research and was later renamed the National Institute of Nursing Research (NINR) at the National Institutes of Health (NIH). This Institute is the second major federal focal point for nursing. Because of the fundamental relationship between the development of nursing science and the improvement of nursing practice, NINR plays a central role in federal public health efforts. In its national leadership role, NINR stimulates the improvement and expansion of nursing research, fosters the development of nurse researchers, and provides a focal point for investigation of key health issues for which nursing interventions have significance (see Chapter 26.)

## THE PROBABLE FUTURE

The probable future for nurses in the federal government is best understood as a reflection of the emerging roles of the federal government and the social forces shaping them. The federal government is experiencing what will likely be an extended period of massive change. In his 1996 State of the Union Address, President Clinton proclaimed that: "The Era of big government is over!" (Gore, 1996) The evidence to support this statement includes the significant reduction in spending and the size of the federal workforce, closure of military bases and field offices, and adoption of strategies aimed at eliminating, overhauling, and reengineering the work previously performed by the federal government. Clearly, the federal government as it was known before Clinton's presidency has been significantly altered.

### Reduction in Clinical Services

The forces driving these changes include public distrust of "big government," the drive to balance the federal budget and reduce the deficit, and the increased emphasis on the marketplace or corporate America as likely solutions to problems in the health and social arenas. The net result is that the federal government is increasingly less likely to provide direct health services. Rather, the government will likely downsize, discontinue, or contract for provision of these services. This means that nurses employed in clinical roles may find fewer opportunities. Those in managerial and policy roles may be looked upon to develop the strategies, contracts, and partnerships that will enable these transitions to occur.

The emerging trends affecting nurses with clinical services responsibilities also will have an impact on nurses whose roles relate to other types of programs. For example, nurses who are involved in policy, financing, and regulatory roles will be challenged to help achieve a balance or appropriate regulation and policy that is in the interest of the public and fosters a climate in which the health marketplace thrives. As the federal government moves to a more "hands off" stance with respect to its programs, such as Medicare and Medicaid, nurses also will be challenged to find ways to actually assess and measure the impact of these developments on the health of people.

## Legislative Branch

For nurses in the legislative branch, it will be increasingly more important that health and nursing expertise be available in Congress, either with nurses as elected officials or as staff members. The emergence of a market-driven health care system has significant implications for the roles that Congress plays in ensuring the well-being of the nation and its people. It appears that there is increasing concern on the part of the public about the impact of changes in the health care system, especially the effects of managed care with regard to the adequacy of care. Congress is being asked to legislate in a way previously unheard of in health care. Legislating such things as length of hospital stay after a normal vaginal delivery, for example, and access to certain procedures and benefits is an indication of a growing need for a broader policy and regulatory framework in which the good of corporations and the good of the people are balanced.

## Nursing Workforce

The probable continuing current involvement of the government in structuring and managing the nursing workforce is questionable given the push to balance the federal budget, the increasingly strong reliance on the marketplace to solve health problems, the decrease in discretionary spending, and the devolution of programs and responsibilities to states. For the near-term future, it is possible that there will be decreased federal involvement in nursing education, practice improvement, or overall ongoing analysis and assessment of the nursing workforce. However, future shortages of nurses, problems with health care quality and access, concern by the corporate sector, and political activism by nurses might provide a reaffirmation and basis for increased involvement in the nursing workforce development.

## Nursing Research

The probable future of federal involvement in nursing research is somewhat brighter. Given the importance of science and technology to the health care industry, it appears that there will be continuing support for the overall mission of the National Institutes of Health. However, NINR may be challenged to assume roles that may go beyond those traditionally found at NIH. For example, public concern about the quality and organization of health care delivery may result in more pressure to do health care outcomes research rather than basic research aimed at diseases, disorders, body systems, organs, or treatments. In addition, if the Division of Nursing becomes less involved in nursing workforce analysis, NINR may be asked to assume some of its former responsibilities.

## Opportunities in the Probable Future

The probable future for nurses in the federal sector is one in which there are likely to be far fewer opportunities relating to nursing specifically but possibly more that relate to utilizing nursing expertise to carry out the increasingly smaller, more efficient federal functions. Nursing opportunities also will be shaped by the willingness and ability of nurses to move away from a federal career mentality. Unless nurses currently in the federal government are willing to change their roles, their workplaces, and even their relationships with the federal government (e.g., contract work), it will be very difficult for many of them to make the transitions required to take advantage of emerging opportunities.

In the longer-term future, some of the change we are seeing today may reverse itself. It is possible that society may call on the federal government to resume some of the roles and functions it currently plays in response to widespread social concerns that states may not be able to manage, such as access to health care and social equity. It is highly unlikely, however, that the federal government will return to the ways in which it operated before 1992. Thus the future will require a great deal of flexibility and creativity in nurses who are functioning in that federal public domain.

## THE PREFERRED FUTURE

The federal trends of downsizing, devolution, reinvention and reengineering offer many opportunities for nurses who are able to see change as the condition in which opportunity thrives. This is to say that virtually everything in the federal government at present and near term is going through dramatic change. For those who focus only on what nurses have previously done, future opportunities may be less apparent. For those who view these changes as the forces that create new opportunities for nurses, however, the future holds great promise.

### Using Nursing Expertise

The preferred future for nurses in the federal government is one in which nursing expertise will be of great value. The types of nursing expertise needed will include competence in politics and public policy; regulation; functioning in interdisciplinary workgroups; and managing change, resources, people, technology, and one's career. Nurses who will do well in the future public domain are those whose commitment to the public good and whose understanding of nursing's role in its service provide an anchor for their flexibility, creativity, and optimism. For example, although the federal government has been a direct provider of nursing services for decades, it is moving away from that role. Nurses' understanding of clinical services and how to meet the needs of groups and populations will be very important to determining how the federal government makes its current transition and ultimately ensures and manages those services that it ends up providing. Whether services are provided directly, contracted for, or financed, nurses will play important roles in the planning and implementation of the strategies that move the government forward in this regard. This holds true for all areas in which the government has provided clinical services, including the military, Indian Health Service, and other areas. Nurses with an understanding of emerging federal roles in health care will have tremendous opportunities for formulating and carrying these roles out.

It is important to emphasize that technology and its application will be a major part of all future federal work. It will be extremely important for nurses to be adept in using technology in the improvement of effectiveness and efficiency of federal work. In addition, as nurses assume more and more responsibility for developing programs and strategies and for assessing effectiveness, expertise in technology and in the development of information systems will be extremely important.

The roles of nurses in executive branch programs relating to health outside of direct service provision will be similar to those emerging in the direct service areas. There will be tremendous opportunity for nurses whose knowledge and skills allow them to function comfortably in rapidly changing work environments in which uncertainty and creativity go hand-in-hand. The federal government's role in health policy, financing, regulation, and research will continue; however, the changing health care system and social climate will require the expertise of people who are well grounded in a variety of sectors. It will be important for nurses interested in the public domain to be experienced in other sectors, such as working in a health care system or research and development firm. The experience across sectors and the ability to move in and out of government roles will be very important in the future.

## Workforce Research and Development

Roles for nurses interested in nursing workforce research and development also will continue, but it is likely that these roles will become increasingly focused on developing overarching human resource policies and strategies of which nursing is a component. This means that there will be a need for nurses with strong policy and analytic skills and with the ability to work well across health disciplines, as well as an understanding of the federal role in workforce development as one in which nurses are a resource that is important to the public's health. "Evidence based" will increasingly be the phrase used to describe how policies and programs will be formulated in nursing workforce development. This means that nurses in the future will need to be knowledgeable about the relationship between the organization and the delivery of nursing services and health outcomes, as well as capable of encouraging outcomes research.

## Executive and Legislative Opportunities

Nurses in the future should look to actually running the departments and agencies of the executive branch. Several examples come to mind. Carolyne Davis served as the administrator of the Health Care Financing Administration, and Shirley Chater was Commissioner of the Social Service Administration. Other natural fits for nursing expertise include director of the Bureau of Health Professions in the Health Resources and Services Administration and various positions in Federal Drug Administration, Department of Justice, Department of Education, and Department of Agriculture with its extension service focus on health.

Whether serving as political appointees or career bureaucrats, nurses will have much to offer in the management of these public institutions. This type of work, however, requires the leadership development necessary to understand how public administration is done well. As political appointees, nurses need to understand how to lead bureaucracies and foster positive change in the public's interest. Becoming a political appointee requires expertise and significant work in party politics. Becoming a successful public administrator requires knowledge in the field, the ability to bring nursing expertise appropriately into the work of the agency, and an abiding commitment to the public's good.

Although there will be significant opportunities for nurses in the executive branch, the greatest emerging need for nurses may be in the legislative branch. Nursing has become fairly adept at helping to shape legislation through lobbying and other political action, but there are far too few nurses actually involved in the legislative process, either as elected officials or staff. Because Congress will continue to focus on health-related issues, it is important for nurses to be well represented in the Senate and House of Representatives. For this to happen, nurses will need to become involved in politics beyond the helping others to be elected. Nursing organizations and individual nurses need to work together to develop the pool of nurses seeking public office. These are long-term commitments that require unflagging strategy and work.

## CONCLUSION

The preferred future for nursing in the public domain is one in which nurses are visible across the government in all of its functions and that both individual nurses and the profession understand that nursing has a great deal to offer beyond its clinical application. The preferred future is one in which nurses and educational institutions understand that the education of nurses is lifelong and must go well beyond notions of a profession unto itself. The nurse of the preferred future is one whose commitment to the public good is unflagging and who understands that nursing is a precious resource to the public's health and that nursing is important to the future of this country. The nurse of the preferred future is a professional who is creative, flexible, and able to work beyond personal and professional self-interest in the service of the nation. The nurse of the future in the public domain is someone who will ensure that greatness in the United States will continue to rest on its ability to care for the well-being of its people.

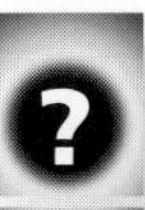

### *Discussion Exercises*

1. Discuss the roles and functions of nurses in the public sector today.
2. What is the difference between future roles for nurses described in the probable future and those described in the preferable future? Do you think the preferable future will come true? Why or why not?
3. How will political, social, environmental, economic, and technologic forces interact to affect the public's interest in supporting health care services in the future?

### References

Coss C: *Lillain D. Wald: progressive activist,* New York, 1989, Feminist Press.

Gore A: *The best kept secrets in government,* Washington, DC, 1996, U.S. Government Printing Office.

Mullen F: *Plagues and politics,* New York, 1989, Basic Books.

Willever H: *The Cadet Nurse Corps in historical perspective: 50th Anniversary Celebration Booklet,* Washington, DC, 1993, Office of the Chief Nurse, U.S. Public Health Service.

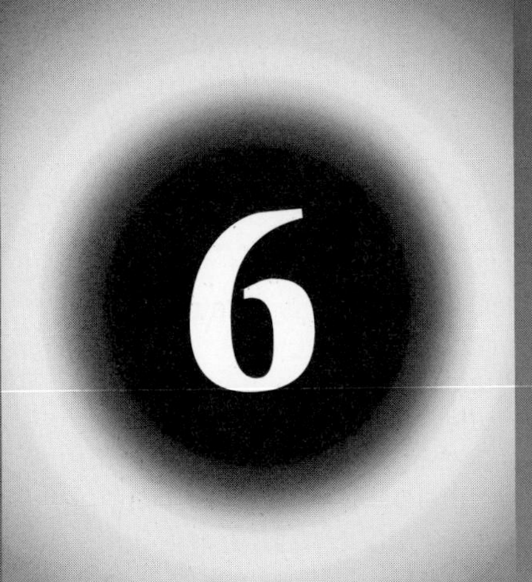

# 6 Nursing's Public Image: Making the Invisible Profession Visible

**Suzanne Gordon**

*You miss 100% of the shots you don't take.*

**Wayne Gretzky**
Hockey player

A probable scenario.

The year is 2006. Fifty-two-million Americans have no health insurance, up from 48 million in 1997. Millions more are underinsured. Most Americans with private, employer paid insurance benefits are insured by huge for-profit, managed care companies. In each metropolitan area two or three health maintenance organizations (HMOs) and giant for-profit hospital chains control the market. The use of health care services and deployment of health care personnel are tightly controlled by executives of large, nationally run health care corporations.

Hospitalization is strongly discouraged. In the 1990s patients were increasingly having mastectomies, hernia repairs, and other surgeries on an outpatient basis. Now, most procedures, from hip replacement to prostecthomies, are performed in the outpatient setting. Only desperately ill patients are admitted in the hospital, and they are discharged as soon as their most serious symptoms are treated.

The hospitals to which they are admitted have become giant intensive care units, staffed largely by machines rather than people. Robots and high-tech machines have replaced the aides who, in the mid 1990s, replaced registered nurses. Robots deliver patients' food and clean their rooms. Patients are tethered to high-tech equipment that monitors their vital signs and any changes in their status. A few advanced practice nurses manage patient care—charting their hospital stay, supervising the machines and the few aides on site, and executing discharge planning—but do no hands-on caregiving.

Nursing in the hospital seems to have faded from the organizational chart. Starting in the early 1990s, vice presidents of nursing became vice presidents of patient care services. Nursing managers on individual wards and nursing executives at the highest echelons of the hospital administration were replaced by MBAs, social workers, or even physicians. After all, as one CEO of a hospital said, "It's clear a nurse has to be vice president of nursing. But why does a nurse have to be in charge of all patient care services?"

> There was a great deal of talk about integration of care in the last decade of the twentieth century. Instead of integrating care, care of the sick has become increasingly fragmented. When they leave the hospital, some acutely ill patients are sent to one of the "subacute facilities"—the new acute care hospital of the twenty-first century. There they are tended by either machines or aides who are supervised by a smattering of registered nurses. Choice of subacute facility is made by the patient's HMO, and the facility may not be located near the patient's family or community.
>
> Most patients still needing care go home. The cost-cutting trends of the 1990s have merely accelerated, and year by year, insurers have cut back on home care benefits. Thus patients in the home are largely cared for by unpaid, female family caregivers who bear the social and financial costs of this care themselves. Some advanced practice nurses, who are employed by for-profit home health agencies that have supplanted the nurse controlled nonprofit visiting nurse agencies, supervise the few bedside nurses and aides sent into the home for a short time. Care in the home has become such a rapid-fire affair that nurses have little time to precept and mentor a new generation of caregivers. Schools of nursing find that they have difficulty educating those students who want to become nurse practitioners in the community because working nurses have so little time to spend on the education of either students or colleagues.

Sound far-fetched?

If current corporatization of health care continues, this may be the kind of health care system we will have in the year 2006. If price competition becomes a health care system's guiding principle and for-profit health care the dominant force, erosion of care will not only take place in the hospital but also everywhere that care should be given—the community clinic, nursing home, home care agency, and even in hospice and palliative care. We will see an increase in the uninsured and an even more severe decline in the number of nurses working in hospitals. As a prominent Princeton health care economist recently told a private sector conference held at Duke University, "I view the war on health care costs and the quality issue as (thus far) basically some skirmishes on the fringes. . . . They took out a few machine-gun nests, but . . . the pill boxes are still there, fully manned. We're in one of them—an academic health center . . . . I predict a second major war is going to come." (Iglehart, 1997) Or as Malik M. Hasan, chief executive officer of Foundation Health Systems, said, "A war is coming which will make what has happened until now look practically like a picnic." (Iglehart, 1997)

# HEALTH CARE WARS

## Health Care for Profit

War is the metaphor of choice for those who govern health care today, so let's be perfectly clear: the war we are in is for the very soul of health care. Increasingly, health care is being controlled by executives and boards of large for-profit corporations. Although one might argue that profit has always existed in health care (nonprofit hospitals, after all, served as a conduit for profit to physicians and drug and medical equipment companies), the scope of corporatization and privatization is overwhelming.

More than 70% of HMOs are for-profit and many nonprofit HMOs are converting to for-profit organizations. For-profit HMOs' share of the market has increased from 46.1% in 1991 to 61.1% in 1995 (Nelson, 1997). Over the past 7 years, group- and staff-model HMOs have declined from 18% of plans to 9.5%. Of the 150 million Americans covered by some form of managed care, very few are in staff- or group-model HMOs. Most so-called HMOs are, in fact, independent practice associations (IPAs) or preferred provider organizations (PPOs), in which physicians are gathered simply for the purpose of reimbursement. These physicians are not part of cohesive organizations that can educate them about effective care delivery. In HMOs today, what should be education about caregiving is replaced by the policing and denial of care. There is no culture of care created but rather a culture of competition in which specialist physicians compete against generalists, generalists against nurse practitioners, nurse practitioners against bedside nurses, and everyone competes for resources with patients.

Nonprofit hospitals are merging and consolidating into giant networks that are competing on the basis of cost rather than quality and compassion. Many nonprofit hospitals are converting to for-profit status. Moreover, large for-profit hospital chains are gobbling up nonprofit and public hospitals.

This causes a serious problem for patients and caregivers. Although the marketplace model may be fine for large retail chains, it is simply inappropriate for health care. Why? A health care system should be designed to keep people healthy and prevent illness and care for people when they are sick, old, infirm, and dying. These are labor-intensive, expensive activities that are in conflict with the mandate of the for-profit corporation. What is that mandate? The legal obligation of the CEOs and boards of directors of for-profit companies is neither to customers nor patients but to shareholders. The content of that legal mandate is not to provide quality care but to maximize the return on their shareholders' investments. This is why the morality of the marketplace is "buyer beware," not "do no harm." It is also why corporations that say they are promoting something called "managed care" and "health maintenance" are really in the business of promoting and maintaining profit.

The nature of this conflict is becoming increasingly apparent in the United States. More and more of those who become ill in this country recognize that the kind of care management that was originally practiced in the early nonprofit health maintenance organization is in jeopardy. It has always been crucial for nurses to communicate their important work to the public. In an environment in which concern for profit supersedes the concern for care, educating the public about the critical importance of caregiving becomes a moral obligation that should be part of every nurse's and nursing organization's or union's moral mission.

## The Inevitability of Mortality

To advocate for patients, nurses must help patients and the general population to face our cultural amnesia about the irrevocable facts of the human condition, that is, vulnerability and mortality. In our culture, we have invested physicians with the belief that there is some final solution to all of our physical afflictions and that infirmity, aging, and even death can be vanquished. We teach physicians to hide behind a shield of technology and invincibility and to focus on diseases rather than the people who have them. Hospital administrators and insurance executives exacerbate our national exercise in denial by claiming that the mission of the health care system is to manage care from afar rather than to get up close and actually deliver care to those who need it.

## Nursing's Vital Role

In the present health care environment, nurses must explain what they do and why they do it. They must explain that nurses are educated, not born, and that they are neither saints nor angels who move into patients' lives on invisible wings and practice their mysterious arts through intuition or instinct. What the public must understand is that nursing is intellectual, emotional, and social work. It is not simply an individual intervention but an organizational and social intervention. There is a lot of talk in nursing today, for example, about how to produce competent nurses who can serve the needs of a complex society. There is little talk, however, about how to produce competent institutions that will allow these competent nurses to practice quality care. Even the most competent nurse can be defeated by an incompetent organization.

Nurses must explain to the public that their care is not a matter of "TLC" but rather a matter of life and death. Nurses are the ones who monitor patients' conditions and prevent catastrophes, who educate patients about how to live with their illnesses, and who help family members cope. Those who don't understand nursing often argue that nurses do "those nice little things" that matter to patients. These "little things" that matter are hardly trivial. It is the nurse who makes sure that a red spot on a patient's hip does not become a bedsore, who ensures that a patient receives adequate pain medication after surgery, who makes sure a patient walks or drinks enough so he or she doesn't develop a pulmonary embolus, and who makes sure that a patient coughs so that he or she does not develop pneumonia.

Nurses are also the ones who help patients scale the molehills of life that illness has turned into mountains. Virginia Henderson defined nursing as helping patients perform the routine activities of daily living that they would do themselves if they had the strength, will, or knowledge. Most people hearing this definition don't get it. Many people question why nurses should be paid $40,000, $50,000, or $60,000 a year to bathe and feed patients or to go into their homes and lay out their medications. This view reflects the fact that the healthy superimpose their vision of life on the sick and those who care for the sick. They don't understand that when a person is sick, the routine activities of daily living often become difficult, impossible, and sometimes lethal. Patients need educated, expert nurses who continue to study and to research and be at their side.

Patients require a nurse because illness sometimes jeopardizes their ability to perform everyday activities. Nurses can help patients negotiate the intimate spaces nurses enter while maintaining the patients' dignity. It may be mortifying for adult patients or even children, to recognize that they need someone to bathe them, help them to the toilet, clean them after using the toilet, or take them for a walk. Patients express their fear of dependence or of being a burden by rejecting help or apologizing for their need of it. To help patients tolerate care requires skill, tact, and emotional intelligence.

Patricia Benner and Judith Wrubel (1989) maintain that nurses are the compassionate strangers who share patients' and families' secrets at their most vulnerable moments, and tolerate their pain and suffering when they are overwhelmed and out of control. Nurses recognize that illness may represent an assault, not only on patients but also on their families and friends, and that these loved ones may be too frightened and anxious to provide the kind of compassionate care patients so desperately need. Nurses understand that there are times when compassion may be possible only from a stranger.

Nurses mobilize their skills of involvement and engagement to provide care for more than just disease. Nurses know that illness not only attacks the body but also the soul. Because of their history and daily work, nurses live through this day-by-day, minute-by-minute attack on the soul and realize patients have not only sick or infirm bodies but also lives and families that are disrupted and need to heal. They know that the healing goes way beyond the healing of the body. When patients are sick, they don't just ask what pills they should take or operations they should have. They ask, Why me? Why now? How can I deal with this? How can we, as a family, cope? Is there hope? Is there meaning? Is there God?

In their book, *The Primacy of Caring: Stress and Coping in Health and Illness*, (1989) Benner and Wrubel distinguish between illness and disease. "Disease is the aberration at the cellular, tissue or organ level." On the other hand, "Illness is the human experience of loss or dysfunction." Benner and Wrubel quote from Oliver Sacks, who says, "Animals get diseases, but only man falls radically into sickness."

In the self-enclosed world of the high-tech hospital where ordinary men, women, and children are confronted with people who wear alien costumes, adhere to peculiar customs, and even speak a different dialect, nurses can help patients deal with fear and anxiety—not only of their diseases but also of the people who are supposed to cure them.

## PROMOTING NURSES AND NURSING

### Why Nursing Is Invisible

One fact of health care is that nurses are often reluctant to educate the public about their work. Sadly, many nurses have been taught to be silent rather than exercise a genuine voice of care. Both traditional female and nursing socialization have told women/nurses that virtue should be its own reward and that it is unseemly or unprofessional to trumpet their individual and collective accomplishments.

Worse still, many nurses have been programmed to believe that communication is an act of betrayal. In nursing school, nurses are taught not to talk about the work they do with patients because this might betray patient confidentiality. Some nurses are taught that when a patient or family member compliments them on their work, they should not respond with, "Thank you" and an explanation of that work but with, "That's just my job." Other common responses to a grateful patient or family member are, "Oh, it was nothing" and "I'm just a nurse."

When nurses are employed by health care organizations, their schooling in deference is often exacerbated. Some are asked to view themselves as employees who have no right to talk about their work without permission from hospital administration. Many are told that loyalty to the organization takes precedence over loyalty to either patients or their profession. Some nurses also are fearful of distinguishing their work from that of physician colleagues because they think that telling the truth about their role in health care will "make doctors angry." In addition, some nurses are afraid of talking about their work because other nurses will view them as "tooting their own horn," or trying to "stand out from the crowd."

For many registered nurses, this programming in deference creates a kind of communication phobia. Many nurses today are understandably reluctant to talk about the erosion of care in their institutions for fear of reprisal. Some are also afraid to discuss their positive contributions because they may be perceived as vain or unprofessional. The result? When doctors talk about their heroic efforts to save patients, they are hailed for their nobility. When nurses want to talk about their accomplishments helping these same patients to cope or to die with dignity, they are sometimes warned against being boastful. That pernicious double standard must end. Only nurses can end it. Nurses must view communication as an act of commitment, connection, and invitation.

## Telling Nursing's Story

To talk about the work one does with a patient is not an act of betrayal but rather one of commitment. Only by explaining nursing's mission and contributions can one protect caregiving. Only by talking about the essence of patient care can one save the patients one is trying to protect. If nurses are afraid to betray patient confidentiality, they have only to change the details that would identify their patients. In the book, *Life Support: Three Nurses on the Front Lines* (1997), for example, Suzanne Gordon turned men into women and altered patients' ages and significant details of their lives to protect their privacy.

If one has a commitment to discussing one's work, it is always possible to tell the story while protecting one's patients. For example, a nurse in a small rural community, where people really do know each other's business, can always say, "When caring for a patient who has had a stroke, or has cancer, a nurse will do . . ." and explain the work. If hospitals and other health care organizations do not permit relationships with journalists or other members of the public, nurses can speak without an institutional affiliation or can speak as a member of an organization such as Sigma Theta Tau International or the Oncology Nurses Society. Nurses also can ask patients for their permission to talk about their care. Nurses should explain that they will not use patient names or significant identifying details. Many grateful patients will be delighted and say yes. They may even want their names to be used.

It is also important for nurses to understand that distinguishing their work from physician's work is not an act of aggression. When nurses explain that doctors are usually with hospitalized patients for only a few minutes every day but nurses are usually with patients 24 hours a day, this is not a judgment or criticism. It is merely a statement of fact. When nurses describe the difference between the medical model's view of death and the nurses' view, this is a constructive comment about a critical social issue not a vicious assault. Nursing is a different discipline from medicine. Nurses are not simply doctors with less education; they have been schooled in a different art and science. Nurses can help the public understand the difference between the two most important disciplines in health care by making critical qualitative distinctions. In drawing these distinctions, nurses can create a constructive public discussion about the nature of health care and how it is organized.

Communicating nurses' work is also an act of connection and invitation. It is a way that nurses can connect themselves to colleagues and to the profession. It is an invitation to other nurses, physicians, patients, and the public to engage in an informed debate about a subject of critical importance.

Inside of each nurse is a voice of care that lies somewhere between the fear of self-aggrandizement and the false humility of self-effacement. Nurses should look inside themselves and find that authentic voice of care, liberate it, and exercise it daily. Whenever someone says, "Isn't it depressing being an oncology nurse, a psychiatric nurse, or a nurse practitioner who works with the poor or the elderly?" A nurse should not respond with anger or despair but reply instead "On the contrary, let me tell you what I did yesterday." When a nurse is thanked for doing an extraordinary job, the response should not be, "Oh, it was nothing," but rather, "Thank you. I was very honored to have been able to help save your father's life . . . teach your wife how to take her medications . . . help you and your family cope." Nurses should explain their work. The stories will move and enlighten people and shouldn't be kept a secret.

Nurses must mobilize the voice of care and utilize the power of persuasion. When talking about nursing work, it is critical that nurses paint a vivid picture rather than speak in jargon or generalities. When nurses are asked to describe what they do, too many will use professional jargon. "I am a patient educator or advocate," a nurse may say, "I assess, monitor, and evaluate patients."

Although these words may be comprehensible to nursing colleagues who, after all, have a sense of what nursing practice is and how it is done, they are meaningless verbiage to an outsider. Thus it is critical to paint a picture. Jeannie Chaisson, one of the nurses in the book, *Life Support* (Gordon, 1997), describes her work with an elderly stroke patient:

> Feeding a stroke patient is an extremely complicated process. If not properly done, it is risky for the patient. You must constantly assess the patient's ability to swallow. Swallowing is a complex series of voluntary and automatic processes. It utilizes six nerves and 25 facial and oral muscles that propel food to its proper destination—the stomach. This ostensibly simple act has four distinct phases. With a stroke victim, something can go wrong during any, or every, one of these four phases. Brain damage can be so extensive that a patient has no muscular control of the mouth and no automatic gag reflex. In this case, anything eaten has a clear shot right into the lungs, where it can create a pneumonia.
>
> Because some patients who seem to be in control of their swallowing may, in fact, be a "silent aspirator," nurses must always evaluate each stroke patient's ability to chew and swallow. If the patient has aphasia and is thus unable to understand language, the nurse can't just tell such a patient, 'Now close your mouth. Chew. Now, swallow for me.' They are unable to understand or comply with the simplest instructions. So this assessment process can be very difficult.
>
> I must first see if the patient's gag reflex functions by slowly feeding him specially thickened food that won't go down the wrong way too easily. If the patient seems to be choking and changes color, he may well be aspirating. Some patients don't choke because they have lost that reflex. To determine whether this kind of patient is aspirating, I carefully watch for changes in color and any increased difficulty breathing or increased respiratory rate. Patients who have no cough reflex are particularly in danger and you have to really know what you're doing and have the time to observe closely if you're going to keep them safe.

Consider how nurse practitioner Ellen Kitchen describes the process of taking care of patients in their own homes. To Ellen, managing her "cases" involves carefully studying each patient's living situation, understanding who the patients are, and what care is appropriate for them. She delivers much of this care and coordinates all the help her patients are receiving so that everyone works as a team on both medical and social problems.

> Elderly, house-bound patients are often confused or inarticulate about their problems. But, when you go into their homes, there it is in front of you. You can see exactly how they are responding to treatment and care. You can see if it is safe and then do things to make the environment safer. You'd be amazed what you learn by just walking into a bathroom, bedroom, or kitchen.

When Ellen goes into a patient's kitchen to wash the dishes or quickly scrambles an egg, she says she is doing a lot more than simple housework. She is discovering if the house is clean, if it conceals health hazards, if the patient has enough clean linen and food, and if the food is the kind the patient should be eating. This kind of health care and personal safety detective work could easily be conducted like—and perceived as—a total assault on an individual's privacy and autonomy. No matter how needy, frail, or confused many of Ellen's elderly patients may be, they don't necessarily welcome with open arms the succession of well-intentioned helpers—nurses, social workers, home health aides, and homemakers—who come their way. For many elderly people, it is bad enough that they must spend so much of their final years in hospitals, pharmacies, and doctors' offices. To have the health care and social service systems invade their homes as well adds insult to injury. Ellen is acutely aware of this tension. "What I've found, for the most part, is that so-called 'difficult patients' are either terrified that you're going to place them in a nursing home or that you're going to come in and try to make tremendous changes in their lives. A lot of times, these patients are just trying to hang on to their independence."

Ellen explains that she views each patient as a special challenge. Her approach is to go slowly. "You enter the house as a guest not as a general imposing martial law. At first you make little suggestions that will change things for the better and produce immediate, perceptible benefits. Perhaps you order a commode for the bedroom, a toilet seat extender, the installation of rails that helps the patient safely enter or exit the bath, or someone to help the patient with laundry. Gradually, most patients come to appreciate the help and feel less threatened by it."

There are, of course, exceptions. A patient may say, "I'm sorry; I don't want this any more." If patients are adamant in their refusal of home care services, the burden will inevitably fall on family members, if they have any. If patients are isolated and alone, they will fend for themselves until their next medical emergency. "The longer you're a nurse," Ellen says, "the better understanding you have of human nature. So you do your best to get them to see that you're only trying to help. Sometimes, it just doesn't work" (Gordon, 1997).

Nancy Rumplik describes how she protects patients against medication errors (Gordon, 1997). Both legally and ethically nurses are responsible for the medications and treatments they administer. Nurses are patients' last line of defense in a system that is supposed to protect patients against potentially harmful, or lethal, human errors. The actual administration of chemotherapeutic drugs is the last phase of the multistep process that Nancy engages in with every patient to whom she gives medication.

Before Nancy even approaches a patient with her medication, she has checked it against the physician's written order. "According to an old-fashioned saying in nursing, we check the Five Rights—right patient, right drug, right dose, right method, and right time," Nancy explains.

When it comes to chemotherapy, Nancy looks at the physician's order and then does her own calculations to make sure it is correct. "First, of course, you make sure it's the right drug. All nurses are educated in a general knowledge of pharmacology. But, when you specialize, as I have in oncology, then you add specialized knowledge of the specific drugs used in the field. For example, you have to know that you wouldn't give a breast cancer patient CHOP (a chemotherapy regimen for patients with lymphoma) or

CMF (a chemotherapy regimen for breast cancer) to patients with lymphoma. Then you have to check the dose. To do this I calculate the patient's BSA—body surface area."

Nancy uses a body surface area calculator and the patient's height and weight to get the correct BSA. Using a computer program, she enters the patient's height and weight, and the program computes the body surface area in meters squared ($m^2$). One patient, for example, is 5′7″ and weighs 140 lb. This makes her 1.72 $m^2$. To calculate the correct dose of cyclophosphamide, which is 600 $mg/m^2$, Nancy multiplies $600 \times 1.7$.

This method of calculation is used because weight itself is not an accurate measure in determining the dosage of chemotherapy drugs. What is critical is the actual volume over which the drug will be distributed. If, for example, a patient is very thin and very tall, his or her body weight alone would lead to an underdose of medication. Conversely, if a patient is short and fat, using body weight alone to calculate the dose might lead to a fatal overdose.

"You have to check everything yourself," Nancy says. "Although it's rare, sometimes the weight recorded is incorrect. Sometimes patients lose weight and you have to recalculate their BSA. If I think there is a question about body surface area, I will weigh the patient again and recalculate. And believe me, sometimes the dose needs to be recalculated."

Then Nancy makes sure it is the right time to give the drug. "If patients are supposed to receive their drugs every 3 weeks, you have to check to make sure they have come in to the clinic at 3 weeks not 2 weeks. Again, there are mistakes. I've sent people home because they've come in at the wrong time to take their drugs."

If she is sure she is giving the right drug, to the right patient, at the right time, with the right method, she must also make sure the patient's blood counts are in the right range. Nancy thus checks the patient's white counts to make sure it's safe to administer the chemotherapy at that particular moment. "Chemotherapeutic agents make patients' white counts drop. To avoid neutropenia—a state in which patients' white counts are dangerously low and they don't have enough neutrophils (i.e., mature white cells) to fight infection—you have to make sure their counts are okay."

Once all this is checked, Nancy gives the medication order to the pharmacy (located right in the clinic), the pharmacist mixes the drugs, then Nancy comes back to get them. She checks the vials—patient's name, drug name, and dosage are all marked clearly on the label—and then, with the top copy of the physician's order, she goes to the patient to give the drugs. At this point she also pays attention to any questions or reservations the patient may have. "You always listen to a patient. If someone says, 'I've never taken a blue pill before,' then I never give them that blue pill without checking." Her motto is the patient is always right (Gordon, 1997).

To describe care in vivid, comprehensible language, as the nurses did in *Life Support,* helps people understand how important nurses' work is. One can augment these descriptions with statistics that further illuminate nursing's importance. For example, one of the many things a nurse does is protect against bedsores. Five hundred thousand Americans suffer from decubitus ulcers each year. Sixty thousand die from bedsores, and it can cost between $5000 and $40,000 to heal just one bedsore. Deep venous thrombosis affects 600,000 patients a year, of whom 100,000 die from pulmonary emboli.

Nurses are instrumental in preventing the hospital acquired infections from which 2,000,000 people suffer and from which 77,000 die each year; they also prevent medication errors and other treatment acquired injuries, which can kill some 180,000 patients each year (Lazarou and others, 1998). Statistics about the cost of the pneumonias that are produced because a nurse has not had adequate time to help a patient walk or cough, about the importance of nurses' role in pain management, in preventing deep venous thrombosis and pulmonary emboli, and in preventing falls and the inappropriate use of restraints should all be marshaled to help the public understand what nurses do.

Finally, to the power of persuasion, nurses must add the persuasion of power. There are 2.1 million nurses in the United States. Nurses are members of the largest female profession in the country and its second largest profession. Nurses outnumber physicians four to one. To be strong, they must do more than practice their profession, they must engage in the practice of citizenship. Imagine the impact if each and every nurse in the United States devoted 10 minutes a month to making two or three telephone calls to a political representative. If every other month nurses devoted an hour to attending one political meeting; wrote one letter to the editor of a newspaper; spoke to 10 friends, neighbors, relatives, or to the media about their vision of health care; or pledged to work individually as well as through their professional associations, unions, and other organizations then we could finally create a genuine health care system in this country.

## CONCLUSION

Without assertive efforts on the part of nurses in every community and at every level of nursing, we will never achieve genuine health care. We will never be able to truly protect and serve patients if nurses do not assertively share their insights, vision, and moral passion. In her book, *Notes on Nursing* (1859), Florence Nightingale argues, "If we were perfect, no doubt an absolute hierarchy would be the best kind of government for all institutions. But, in our imperfect state of conscience and enlightenment, publicity, and the collision resulting from publicity, are the best guardians of the interests of the sick."

This has never been more true than it is today.

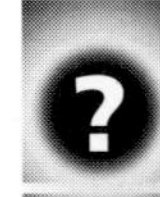

## *Discussion Exercises*

1. How likely is the probable scenario described in this chapter? What conditions or events would make it more likely to occur? What would make it less likely?
2. Describe your experience with nursing's invisibility.
3. Create a plan for your participation in making nursing more visible. Include your goals, action plan, timeline, and evaluation of outcomes.

## References

Benner P, Wrubel J: *The primacy of caring: stress and coping in health and illness,* Reading, Mass, 1989, Addison-Wesley.

Gordon S: *Life support: three nurses on the front lines,* Boston, 1997, Little, Brown.

Iglehart J: Listening in on the Duke University Private Sector Conference, *NE J Med* 336(25): 1827, 1997.

Lazarou J and others: Incidence of adverse drug reactions in hospitalized patients: a meta-analysis of prospective studies, *JAMA* 279(15):1200, 1998.

Nelson H: *Nonprofit and for-profit HMOs: converging practices but different goals?* New York, 1997, Milbank Memorial Fund.

Nightingale F: *Notes on nursing,* New York 1859, Dover.

# II

# The Future of Practice and Education

# 7 Practice of the Future

**Karen L. Miller**
**Susan C. Fry**

*There is not a more difficult problem in the world than the education for a particular profession.*

**Peter Mere Latham**
Nineteenth Century

Florence Nightingale wrote in *Notes on Nursing* (1859) that nursing has as its most critical work the caring required to promote the health of the individual. More than any other profession, nursing has the distinction of being responsible for the caring that patients receive in our health care system. Physicians, therapists, and other specialized caregivers care for patients as part of their unique contributions to the cure and treatment of illness; however, caring is described as the "essence of nursing" and the most central and unifying focus for the nursing profession (Leininger, 1984).

Since Nightingale's time, nurses have developed the caring skills to complement the technologic and assessment competencies at the heart of modern nursing practice. Anticipated changes in the environment of health care, demands for a workforce that can support the needs of a diverse population, and the impact of information technologies on clinical work create unprecedented challenges for nursing practice and education into the twenty-first century. Given nursing's fundamental tradition, both the probable and preferred visions for the future direction of nursing practice and education must be considered in light of the most severe consequence: Will nurses' capacity to be caring survive into the future?

## PROBABLE FUTURE

The future of any profession reflects both its past and present values and the environment that influences its work. The predominant sociocultural values of the present health care environment emanate from the economic realities of our nation's free market. Competition for economic survival among health care organizations, payers and health insurers, and care providers has become the driving force of health care delivery. Profitability, efficiency, quality, service, reductionism, competition, and standardization with decreased individual variation describe desirable industrial assets. Yet these same assets applied to health care often create philosophic disharmony when compared with the traditional altruistic, public caretaking missions espoused by health professionals, hospitals, and other health care organizations.

## Economics

Nurse scientists have explored the economics of caring (MacPherson, 1989; Nyberg, 1990). Nurses value their ability to give good care to their patients and to be caring to individuals and families. Studies show that threats to nurses' abilities to be caring can adversely affect patient outcomes (Valentine, 1991). Replete with alarming statistics and trends, experts have predicted the future of health care to be precarious and dependent on inflationary economic projections (Fubini, 1997). At the same time, nurses are enjoying unprecedented opportunities for clinical practice in a variety of settings and renewed trust by the public for advanced practice expertise (Cronenwett, 1995). This situation is likely to lead to a paradox for nursing in an environment for practice that is rapidly evolving and focused on financial resources.

Consequently, a political mandate currently exists to reduce the cost of health care to individuals through tax cuts and to employers through lower-cost health care benefit options. Consumer-friendly, service-oriented companies that provide the best-quality product for the lowest cost have the advantage in today's corporate marketplace. Competition among systems of care, payers, and care providers is central to the probable future regardless of the nonprofit, altruistic past traditions of our health care professions. As the single largest health care profession (more than 2.5 million registered nurses nationwide), nurses will see increasingly more changes to their practice environment as a result of future economic pressures on the health care industry.

## Advances

Simultaneously, advances in biomedical sciences and information technology have created approaches to medical care that extend lifespan, decrease chronic disease, and save the lives of the critically ill. New medicines allow successful treatment of previously devastating mental illnesses, infectious diseases, cancers, and endocrine and reproductive disorders. Rapidly improving technology in radiology and laser techniques supports surgical intervention, including older adults and younger infants, more than ever before.

State-of-the-art information systems allow tracking of individuals and families as they utilize the health care system. Physicians, nurses, and clinical support service personnel can communicate patient information electronically whether the individual is in the hospital, the emergency department of another institution, an ambulatory care center, or a physician's office. In the next few years elaborate health care data tracking systems will be available that will help care providers track the health status of family members in the home through personal television or computer hookups and even alert employers to prevent injuries. The concept of health promotion will take on new meaning as nurses and other care providers contribute the human element in a highly technologic system of health communications.

## Quality

The paradox in the future practice for nurses and all health professionals will be to keep up with the latest technologic and clinical wonders of contemporary nursing and medicine while creating new approaches to care that decrease cost. In today's market, employers and payers of health care expenses are most interested in the lowest-cost care; however, increasing pressure from consumers is causing a slow shift to consideration of quality and effectiveness of health care.

Tomorrow's nurses will be people who are energetic, quick learners, adaptable, and willing to sacrifice some degree of "form for substance." Traditional approaches to nursing care must change to incorporate the possibilities of advanced information, fast responses to needs of the public, and community-based systems of health promotion. Ultimately, the public will select care providers in whose expertise there is trust and confidence and whose practices are efficient and effective in meeting both basic and advanced health and illness needs.

## Future Workforce

In the past, nurses often saw themselves as outside the discussion of the economics of health care. Patient advocacy and caring for patients at the bedside were activities hidden in the room charges of most hospital bills. In the last decade, however, nurses were directly affected as hospitals and other health care institutions struggled to survive economic challenges. A trend toward economics in clinical care, begun in the mid 1980s, will continue to cause changes in the way care is delivered. Nursing was at the center of many of the changes made by hospital administrators and executives of managed care companies to streamline the work of health care providers. More than 50 million fewer inpatient hospital days in the last decade resulted in restructured hospital services (Aiken, 1995). The number of registered nurses as a proportion of total hospital personnel is decreasing with a concomitant increase in unlicensed assistive personnel among nursing departments.

There is also evidence that patients in hospitals will be only those with life-threatening illnesses. Computer monitoring of nonhospitalized acute care patients will allow early discharge from inpatient institutions. Consequently, more nurses will find employment outside of the traditional hospital setting. In 1992, 66% of all employed Registered nurses (RNs) worked in hospitals. By 1996 that number declined to 60% as nurses moved from traditional care settings to a variety of outpatient and community-based practices. In the probable future there will continue to be a shift of nurses to non–hospital care sites, but there will be many jobs available in more traditional roles as well.

Today the numbers of people being cared for by home health agency staff have increased dramatically. Home-based health care, such as hospice care, acute and chronic nursing care, and physical and respiratory therapy, has tripled in the last decade. In the future, sophisticated robots, capable of monitoring vital signs and blood electrolyte and oxygen levels, will replace many home care personnel. More professional nurses will find themselves in the role of clinical evaluator, using expert assessment skills to help families and primary caregivers make decisions about types of treatment or referrals to other levels of care. Already nurses are being recruited for phone triage services by managed care companies and vertically integrated health care systems in some regions of the United States. This kind of nursing practice requires confident knowledge of complex clinical and psychosocial and cultural variables.

## Educating for New Roles

According to Aiken (1995), the United States has an adequate supply of nurses, although the mix of nurses by educational background is not sufficient to meet future health care challenges. Not enough nurses are being educated at the baccalaureate and graduate levels, while too many associate degree nurses with no clear avenue for degree completion continue to graduate from 2-year programs. Today more than half of all new nurse graduates are practicing nursing before they have completed their college degrees. The future need for individuals with high levels of responsibility and the capacity to absorb rapidly changing medical science and technology means that the nursing workforce must be better educated. Aiken makes the case that as a result of the absence of nationwide shortages and reduced employer demand, "the relative surplus of nurses at present provides the profession with an opportunity it has not had in the past to make sweeping changes in nursing education." It seems logical that innovative approaches to the education of nurses across programs that can integrate student learning toward advanced degrees are not only possible but also necessary for nursing's future contribution to health care.

Unfortunately, educators are no closer to active cooperation to revise the nursing educational system than in the past. Accreditation arguments currently threaten to widen the gap between university and community college faculties. Present and future requirements for enhanced community and public health content in the curriculum make competition for student clinical experiences more severe. Inability of most faculty and administrators to create interdisciplinary educational programs among the health professions limits students' visions of collaborative practice that could benefit the health of the public. Predictions of less need for the numbers of nurses being graduated today and increased need for more graduate and advanced practice nurses jeopardizes the job security of nonuniversity faculty. Unless there is an era of innovation and collaboration among groups of nurse educators, the probable future is one of opportunity lost for a nationwide, cooperative system of nursing education.

Nevertheless, many progressive changes are underway in the curricula of individual nursing programs. One of the most significant is the movement to a community-based curriculum for undergraduate students. Many schools have incorporated concepts of community nursing practice at earlier stages of nursing education, including epidemiology, public health, family systems theory, primary care, and home health care. Initial reports from these programs indicate that students respond very well to a nontraditional curriculum (Connors, 1998). Early clinical practice experiences in the community give students an opportunity to learn how to interact with individuals where they live and work, before the hospital or illness episode. Earlier emphasis is being placed on communications and assessment skills for nursing students rather than on plans of care that coincide with a particular patient diagnosis or pathophysiology. This approach is expected to help nursing graduates be more comfortable in a variety of clinical settings and more open to the many possibilities for nursing practice in a diverse future health care environment.

## PREFERABLE FUTURE

The preferable future builds on predictions of the probable future but adds innovative suggestions based on emerging possibilities. New challenges and opportunities are evolving but many questions regarding implementation exist.

### Preferred Workforce

As baby boomers mature, the values of that generation will become dominant and the desire to recreate some of the 1960s peace and harmony will emerge. In developing countries, however, a growing force of teenagers and youth are emerging (Swartz, 1991). Most of these teenagers live in Asia and Latin America and will contribute to a combined force of over 2 billion teenagers in the world by the year 2001. This group will have a different impact on the world from the baby boomers because, as Swartz points out, they will be interconnected by a communication technology that was not available to the 1960s generation. Given the nature of teenagers worldwide to be exuberant, confused, explorative, and rebellious, in addition to the sheer numbers of them, they will create an impact that will be felt worldwide.

The coupling teenagers of developing countries with the mature and elderly of the developed countries by the communication systems available today could lead to some interesting and dynamic changes, especially as they relate to healthy communities. A concern often heard by today's health care providers is: Who will take care of us in our old age? This question relates to both personnel and monetary resources. If the youth of developing countries will be the manpower to care for the elderly of the developed countries, will they need to leave their countries or will the technology and communication systems of the future allow them to remain in their own countries? Will they want to remain in their own countries? If they are needed in the workforce in developed countries, will public policies and immigration laws support it? Clearly, many policy issues must be debated and resolved to implement this creative idea for the future.

## Educating the Preferred Workforce

The melting of the cultures under this scenario leads to some interesting education and service challenges. If the developing countries begin to export labor to developed countries, these new providers of the future also become consumers. The educational needs for language and cultural sensitivity training become even more critical than they are today. Are our educational systems ready to train and retrain providers? What about the needs of the consumers to accept culturally diverse providers?

Moore (1997), in his article "Medical Mecca," describes a project in Miami in which nine hospitals formed a coalition to promote international health care. Entitled "One Community, One Goal," the project hopes to draw paying patients from other countries and match them up with providers in Miami who can meet their medical needs while also understanding their cultural needs and, frequently, speaking to them in their native language. Nurses with foreign language skills and multicultural knowledge serve as case managers to facilitate housing and appointments and provide health information as needed. Are boards of nursing ready to deal with foreign nursing graduates whose specialized body of knowledge may be needed by the consumer but is not part of the repertoire of skills practiced by today's nurse? What about the licensing boards of other health care providers?

While we are possibly importing youth to care for the elderly, there also will be a large number of elderly who will be active and altruistic and interested in volunteerism. The depth and breadth of their expertise will reflect their work experience and could complement nicely the paid workforce. Productive and active volunteers contribute to the health of the community, as well as to their own health and well-being. Will the working nurse know how to use and appreciate this new supplemental labor force? Working with volunteers requires a different set of skills to motivate and manage. As nurses learned to move from an all RN staff to one using unlicensed assistive personnel, the use of more volunteer assistance could be equally as challenging and stressful. This area also needs attention in both undergraduate and graduate education programs.

Another trend in nursing education is the opportunity for students to participate in "internships" or "transition" programs, often in collaboration with an acute care institution. In these programs students spend time as seniors or new graduates in special, precepted clinical nursing roles that allow them time to become familiar with a clinical area before they are expected to undertake full employment responsibilities. Some of these programs involve salary to participants and some do not. New graduates like these clinical opportunities because they are able to learn a clinical specialty, such as critical care, operating room, or maternal-child care, which would traditionally require years of general medical-surgical care experience before nurses can move to these areas of practice. Nurse administrators like "intern" programs because they can hire these nurses in clinical areas where staff vacancies are more difficult to replace. In addition, costs for new nurses decrease and the organization has a cadre of nurses with better clinical competencies than they normally would with new graduates.

## Knowledge-Based Power

In *Powershift: Knowledge, Wealth, and Violence at the Edge of the 21st Century* (1990), Toffler, describes the shift and redefinition of power from the industrialized superpowers to a knowledge-based economy. He illustrates this by describing some of the decline in physician popularity in his exploration of the "punctured power of the god-in-a-white-coat." He explains that when physicians held onto their knowledge very tightly, even "providing the profession with a semi-secret code" by writing prescriptions in Latin, they could command a dominant role in society. The advent of information systems that allow general access to a vast body of medical knowledge, for example, *Physicians Desk Reference (PDR)* and the *Journal of the American Medical Association,* has served to demystify the profession. This provision of ready information allows patients to question medical advice and make informed decisions, thus "thoroughly smashing" the monopoly of the medical profession and "dethroning" the physician.

The same information/knowledge sources that have affected the physician community are also affecting nursing. One of nursing's privileged roles was reading prescriptions and interpreting them. Nurses fostered advocacy roles to interpret medical jargon for patients and families. Given all the sources of medical information available to the public today and the confusing and sometimes editorialized presentation, there is an emerging role for the nurses of tomorrow to be information brokers for patients and families as they access the Internet and mass media medical information. The shift to knowledge-based power is a movement that nursing and nurses cannot afford to overlook.

In "Old Wine in New Bottles: Nursing in the 21st Century," Bulger (1996) sees health care "as three things: preventing, curing and caring . . . We might argue that of the three, caring is the greatest." He further states, "In my view, of all the major health professions, nursing is the one most broadly engaged in all three areas of health care." With the changing health care environment, providers are scrambling to find their niche in the new marketplace. While the scramble is going on, market forces are demanding a more user-friendly, efficient system with lower costs and better outcomes.

Collaboration is a must, but few health professionals have been educated or mentored in a collaborative practice environment. Bulger further challenges academic health centers to "exemplify the collaboration and teamwork the service sector is demanding even as we seek to criticize and improve the status quo in the practices of health care." Nursing should take a leadership role in the collaborative education of health care professionals if in fact we have the broadest-based practice for preventing, curing, and caring. Nurses must remain true to these basic tenets of nursing in the face of a system with such a strong focus on reducing costs and documenting outcomes. Can the impact of caring on outcomes be demonstrated in time to preserve this basic essence of nursing? Miller (1995) in her article, "Keeping the Care in Nursing Care: Our Biggest Challenge," encourages the profession to hold true to "the very essence of nursing and what our patients and families need most."

Technology and new knowledge will change the job descriptions of all health professionals over the next decade; however, the public's need for caring, compassionate, competent health professionals will remain. The caring professional of the future will have very different skills from those embodied in the current concept of caring. With electronic advances and the focus on keeping populations well and in their homes, the care professional of the future will need to be able to convey an attitude of caring and compassion via the telephone and computer. Although this may sound cold and impersonal to today's nurses, there is already a developing skill in this with some mail order businesses and some web site developers (see Chapter 11). It is clearly a different skill set from the direct touch taught and practiced by many today but is no less "personal" when practiced well over the phone or computer. There will, of course, still be direct hands-on care for those times when there is direct contact between patient/client and nurse.

## CONCLUSION

Keeping populations well in an information age will mean less direct contact and more and more use of technology from the home. These practice and educational issues require careful thought, planning, and implementation to ensure the adequate preparation of future nursing graduates. Regardless of the setting for care or education, the care embodied in nursing's history can remain. It is up to all involved in health care to ensure that it does.

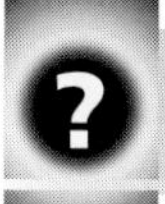

## *Discussion Exercises*

1. What strategies can you suggest to create new approaches to nursing care that combine the latest advances with compassionate care?
2. How would you restructure nursing education to prepare nursing students for the future?
3. How can nursing practice and education be more reciprocal and collaborative? Be specific.

## References

Aiken LH: Transformation of the nursing workforce, *Nurs Outlook* 43(5):201, 1995.

Bulger RJ: Old wine in new bottles: nursing in the 21st century, *J Pro Nurs 12*(6):338, 1996.

Connors HR: Telecommunications and rural healthcare: the Kansas example, *Adv Nurs Pract* 6(5):40, 1998.

Cronenwett L: Molding the future of advanced practice nursing, *Nurs Outlook, 43*(3):112, 1995.

Fubini S: Whither go health care costs? *Healthcare Trends Rep 11*(5):1, 1997.

Leininger M: *The essence of nursing and health,* Thorofare, NJ, 1984, Slack.

MacPherson K: A new perspective on nursing and caring in a corporate context, *Adv Nurs Sci 11*(4):32, 1989.

Miller KL: Keeping the care in nursing care: our biggest challenge, *J Nurs Adm 25*(11):29, 1995.

Moore JD: Medical mecca, *Mod Healthcare* 27(20):30, 1997.

Nightingale F: *Notes on nursing,* New York, 1859, Dover.

Nyberg J: The effects of care economics on nursing practice, *J Nurs Adm 20*(5):13, 1990.

Swartz P: *The art of the long view,* New York, 1991, Doubleday.

Toffler A: *Powershift: knowledge, wealth, and violence at the edge of the 21st century,* New York, 1990, Bantam Books.

Valentine K: Comprehensive assessment of caring and its relationship to outcome measures, *J Qual Assur* 5(2):59, 1991.

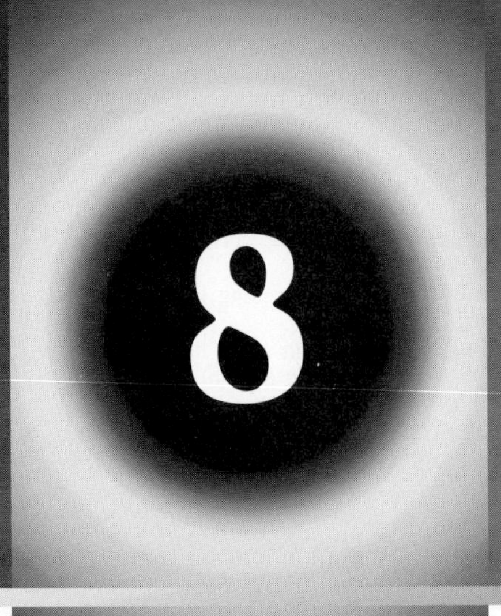

# 8 Advanced Practice Roles

**Carole A. Anderson**

*Socrates, you will remember, asked all the important questions, but he never answered any of them.*

**Dickinson W. Richards**
1953

Since 1993 the world of health care has experienced significant turmoil as a result of massive changes driven primarily by the payers (insurers, employers) for health care demanding that costs be reduced. This reform of the health care system was initially stimulated by President Clinton's Health Security Act—an initiative driven by the White House and developed by experts with consultation from special interest groups. The plan was never enacted not so much as a result of the plan itself but primarily because of the lack of wide-spread consultation with the public and its representatives (Yankelovich, 1995). Nonetheless, the public's awareness was piqued, and health care became a topic widely discussed. Reform measures began to occur at the state level in response to the same factors that had stimulated the federal initiative—rising and uncontrolled costs, diminished access, and outcomes that were not commensurate with the costs. These measures have continued, as have modifications in the federal Medicare and Medicaid programs as payers, an aggressive force, began to demand lower costs, stimulating the development of new initiatives to reduce costs, of which managed care, hospital restructuring and reengineering, and prospective payment became the linchpins.

## PRIMARY CARE

Implicit in the concept of managed care is the need for primary care providers who are able to assume the role of gatekeeper to expensive services, provide relatively low-cost care for common illnesses, and offer prevention and health promotion services. Yet the country found itself with a shortage of primary care physicians and an oversupply of specialists in almost every medical specialty. Nursing and others saw this situation as providing enormous opportunity for the greater utilization of nurse practitioners, which has occurred.

Concomitantly with the drive to reduce costs, many of which were inextricably tied to inpatient care, technology has allowed for more medical care to be delivered outside of hospitals, thereby reducing both the number of inpatient days per patient admission and the number of inpatient beds that were needed. To economize, hospitals began to merge and consolidate and make internal changes in their staffing mix, with the net effect of reducing the total number of beds and the number of RN employees. So, as the need for nurse primary care providers was increasing, the demand for staff RNs was decreasing. Also, internally, hospital reengineering reduced the numbers of staff and line administrative and consultative positions, including those of nurse managers and clinical specialists.

The demand for nurse practitioner programs increased, which was driven by clinical specialists desiring to retool and other nurses who saw the need for further education as hospital-based staff nurse positions decreased. Existing programs were quickly filled to capacity (AACN, 1997) and the ability to expand was compromised by a shortage of faculty and clinical teaching sites. In spite of this situation, however, there was an increase in the number of new and planned nurse practitioner programs (AACN, 1997) and a decrease in enrollment in programs that prepared clinical specialists, administrators, and community health nurses (AACN, 1997) (see Appendix B).

A successful model for predicting the demand for various types of health care professionals has yet to be developed. The reasons for this are many and complex but do not include having never tried. Numerous attempts have been made to develop a model to accurately predict the demand for various types and kinds of nurses (as well as other professions), but either they have insufficient predictive power or the results have been ignored.

Certainly nursing has never tried to regulate the supply of nurses. Not only is there currently an overall surplus of new graduates entering a field that has been and is downsizing, but there is also an existing undereducated labor pool. The models developed by the industry predict an existing and continuing need for more primary care providers and a continuing shortage of nurses prepared at this advanced level. This prediction, however, is predicated on a continuing demand for primary care providers, but it does not factor in the increasing numbers of medical school graduates entering primary care. So, what exactly is the future for advanced practice roles and what is their optimal preparation?

## ADVANCED PRACTICE NURSING

Advanced practice nursing is the overarching term introduced in the early 1990s to differentiate it from basic, that is, entry level, clinical nursing practice. Advanced practice nurses include nurse practitioners, clinical nurse specialists, nurse midwives, and nurse anesthetists. In the American Nurses Association's *Social Policy Statement* (1995), advanced practice is described as "involving both specialization and expansion and is characterized by the integration of a broad range of theoretical, research-based, and practical knowledge that occurs as a part of graduate education in nursing."

Nurse anesthetists and nurse midwives were the first nursing specialties to be developed. Nurse anesthetists actually date back to the mid to late 1800s, with the first postgraduate course being offered in 1909. Nurse midwifery training began in 1932 in connection with the Maternity Center of New York City (Bigbee, 1996). However, in both instances, early postgraduate training did not lead to an advanced degree in nursing.

Nurses have been prepared as clinical nurse specialist (CNS) in masters programs since the 1940s, with psychiatric nursing being the oldest and most well developed. The development of the psychiatric CNS, stimulated in large measure by the 1960 Community Mental Health Center Act, gave rise to other clinical specialties. A large number of nurses prepared in masters programs took positions in education or administration because the CNS role was slow to develop in many settings.

In the mid 1960s the role of nurse practitioner was introduced. Initially, nurse practitioners, like nurse anesthetists and nurse midwives, were prepared in both masters and non–degree-granting, certificate programs. In addition to diversity in the types of educational programs engaged in postgraduate training, over the years, many different titles or specialty foci in graduate programs also emerged, with the net effect of creating confusion. This confusion in turn created difficulties for policy makers and regulatory bodies.

## Supply and Demand

Health care reform initiatives depend heavily on primary care providers, but a shortage of primary care physicians existed. However, managed care health care organizations, such as Kaiser Permenente, have for many years provided services with models of care delivery that included a mix of physician and other primary care providers, including nurse practitioners and nurse midwives. New managed care organizations looked to these models for guidance in developing their cost-effective staffing models. Given the changes in hospitals and the obvious need for increased numbers of nurse practitioners, graduate programs in nursing are experiencing an increased demand for nurse practitioner education. Consequently, enrollment in these options has increased and other program options preparing clinical specialists or administrators are experiencing enrollment declines. New programs have opened and existing programs have converted their curriculum to prepare nurse practitioners. These trends, however, have generated concerns among regulatory bodies, nurse practitioner faculty groups, and professional associations regarding the need to develop appropriate standards for graduate education for all advanced practice roles and to reign in the diversity of titles.

## Education for Advanced Practice

In 1990 the American Association of Colleges of Nursing (AACN) undertook a project to develop a comprehensive data set describing graduate education in nursing, which had never been available (Bednash and others, 1990). This report offered comprehensive data on all aspects of the graduate enterprise in nursing, including characteristics of students, programs, and institutions. Interestingly, the report found that the vast majority of students were enrolled in a specialty area having a clinical focus. However, almost a quarter of these students reported having no direct care experiences as part of their program. This finding began to raise questions regarding what is and what should be a standard curriculum for advanced practice.

The National Organization of Nurse Practitioner Faculty (NONPF) has as a part of its mission the promulgation of standards to guide the development and implementation of nurse practitioner programs. Their standards are designed as a curriculum guide for nurse practitioner preparation (NONPF, 1995).

The diversity of programs for advanced practice is reflected in the regulatory environment and requirements for legal recognition by the various state boards of nursing. Virtually all states now regulate advanced practice through such mechanisms as title recognition, an identified scope of practice, curriculum requirements, requirements for relationships with physicians, and required experience. The regulatory environment and the position of these regulatory bodies is fundamentally one taken as a response to the lack of standardization in both the educational program and the certification process.

The various regulations and requirements are an attempt to provide evidence that programs preparing advanced practice nurses contain the same elements deemed essential requirements for advanced practice. In this way they attempt to establish comparability of competencies and ensure, for example, that individual *A* prepared at program *X* is similar to individual *B* from program *Y.* For many, the diversity of programs in terms of title, length, and content made this comparability difficult to discern. When certification is used as a proxy for uniformity, and it is in some states, those states desire evidence that the certification process is sound. This led to an opening up of the certification examinations for external review.

Barbara Safriet (1992), a lawyer interested in health care, published a report on the role of advanced practice nursing in health care. In this report Safriet argues that the problems of the current system of care are "too little care, too late, for too few people at too high a cost" and that a fundamental restructuring of the system and more effective utilization of all health care personnel is needed. She argues persuasively to reduce restrictions on advanced practice nurses who have been proven providers of cost-effective, high-quality primary care. She notes the "crazy quilt" of regulation that currently exists and the diversity of titles used to describe advanced practice nurses. While calling for reducing the variances in state-by-state regulation and federal barriers, she also strongly recommends that the profession take steps to clarify titles and standardize educational requirements for these roles.

To bring further clarification and standardization to the educational programs, in 1995 the American Association of Colleges of Nursing established a task force to develop the "essential elements of master's education for advance practice roles in nursing" (AACN, 1996). Using a consensus-building process with input from all relevant groups, the basic elements of a masters curriculum were identified. These standards were designed to apply to programs that prepare nurses for advanced practice in a direct care role. This curriculum model consists of three essential elements: a graduate nursing core, an advanced practice clinical core, and specialty courses. These standards, although designed to be used as guidelines rather than dogmatic requirements, are unprecedented in their specificity in the history of masters education in nursing. As written, they should make a valuable contribution to the standardization of graduate education for advanced practice.

## Advanced Practice Roles

The role of an advanced practice nurse (whether as a nurse practitioner, midwife, clinical specialist, or nurse anesthetist) includes functions unique to that specialty and those that are generic to advanced practice. In a rapidly changing system of health care delivery, educational programs must maintain a broad perspective, resisting the temptation to design programs for narrow specialties and specific roles. Furthermore, academic programs need to ensure that the knowledge base in graduate nursing programs mirrors that expected of all masters-level programs and also contains strong clinical preparation. This combination is needed to prepare a clinician for a variety of emerging roles. Regulatory bodies should strive to avoid developing a "laundry list" of functions/tasks for this level of practice. Doing so reduces this level of practice to a technical level and restricts the scope of practice—a most undesirable and unprecedented outcome for any health professional.

In an evolving and ever-changing health care system, new roles for advanced practice nursing have emerged and will continue to emerge. Advanced practice nurses function as primary care providers, acute care nurse practitioners, clinical specialists, case managers, and clinical care coordinators. Importantly, these roles now transcend institutional boundaries. For example, nurse practitioners functioning as case managers might be responsible across the care continuum beginning with an inpatient stay and continuing through rehabilitation and eventual return home. As hospitals develop their own home health agencies, they increasingly are employing nurse practitioners to provide clinical care in people's homes, often avoiding a hospitalization. Forward-thinking long-term care agencies also utilize nurse practitioners to provide clinical management for their residents' chronic illnesses. Primary care also is being provided in nontraditional settings such as schools and the workplace.

The traditional hospital-based clinical specialist role, focused on education and consultation, is being transformed into case management and care coordinator roles. These roles require in-depth knowledge of specific patient populations, as well as expertise in moving people through complex systems.

A relatively new role for nurse practitioners is in acute care. Initially, in the late 1970s this role was introduced in neonatal intensive care units in response to an undersupply of neonatologists. As graduate medical education began to shift out of hospital settings, the acute care nurse practitioner role expanded to other critical care areas. The role is still developing and expanding but, in general, is designed to provide care across the continuum of acute care services to acutely and critically ill patients (Lott and others, 1996). *Standards of clinical practice* and *scope of practice for the acute care nurse practitioner* have been developed by the American Association of Critical Care Nurses and the American Nurses Association (1995). It will be interesting to watch the continued development and expansion of this role in light of changes in graduate medical education and in choice of medical specialties by medical school graduates.

## Competencies of Advanced Practice Nurses

The scope of practice of advanced practice nurses has been well delineated by specialty organizations, educational organizations, faculty groups, and certifying bodies. In general terms, advanced practice nurses should possess the competencies to provide primary care, manage common acute and chronic illnesses, educate patients, design health promotion and disease prevention programs, clinically manage patient care across the continuum of an illness episode, utilize and interpret information to make decisions, engage patients and families in collaborative decision making, utilize research, understand the systems of health care, utilize frameworks for ethical decision making, and, increasingly, prescribe selected medications.

In addition, it is expected that advanced practice nurses function with a high level of professionalism that includes a commitment to continue to learn and an allegiance to the profession. It is also highly desirable for advanced practice nurses to be competent to educate future generations for advanced practice.

## Regulation and Certification

Regulation of advanced practice nursing has had an interesting history. For the most part, practice has been regulated by various specialty groups such as the American Association of Nurse Anesthetists and the American College of Nurse Midwives through a certification by examination process. The American Nurses Credentialing Center also provides certification for a wide variety of specialties. As noted earlier, the educational requirements for many of the specialties were varied and the certification examinations were developed and administered by each group. However, masters preparation is now required in each of these instances.

State boards of nursing have traditionally regulated only *entry* level practitioners. However, as advanced practice groups used the legislative process to gain title recognition, authority to practice within their scope, and prescriptive authority, state boards of nursing were typically given the authority and responsibility to enforce the legislation. In so doing, state boards of nursing have greater power to regulate beyond the entry level than is typically the case in other health professions that rely on a standardized certification process by a separate professional (c.f., regulatory) organization. For example, all physicians are licensed by the state to practice medicine, but a professional organization such as the American College of Surgeons certifies surgeons in their chosen specialty. The state board of medicine neither delineates the scope of practice for surgeons nor certifies them to practice the specialty.

It appears as if nursing has reached consensus on the masters degree being required educational preparation for advanced practice. Although the road getting to this point has been bumpy and convoluted, the profession has finally arrived at the desired standardizing preparation.

# CONCLUSION

There is little doubt that the health care system will require greater numbers of nurses prepared for advanced practice. In 1996 only 10% of 2.5 million nurses had with masters degrees (Moses, 1996), which is a tremendous disproportion to the numbers of nurses prepared in basic programs. The systems of care being developed need and will continue to need more nurses with masters degrees. Even if the numbers of physicians going into specialty fields decrease significantly (which is already occurring), nurses will still be needed to deliver primary care because they enhance the care provided and are cost effective.

Within hospitals and integrated health systems, new and emerging roles can be filled only by nurses with graduate education. These new systems are as complex as the needs of their patients. Providing care across the continuum is simply a level of practice beyond that obtained in a basic educational program.

Graduate programs will continue to be challenged to develop and implement quality programs that produce well-prepared masters graduates for practice. New models of programming and faculty roles will need to be developed within the context of the quality standards of graduate education.

Practicing nurses and faculty will need to invest themselves in furthering or continuing their education to remain competitive in a demanding and changing job market. Nurses have enjoyed substantial job security in a growth industry that, for the most part, was left to its own devices. Because of the massive changes in the industry, nurses must confront the need for more or different education to stay viable and qualified for new roles. Faculty, too, need to redefine what competencies they need to be credible and effective teachers. Academic institutions need to develop new models of faculty preparation and appointment to provide the mix of faculty and associated competencies that will produce a quality graduate.

The future bodes well for the nursing profession. Well-educated, clinically competent nurses at all levels have been one of the strengths of our health care system, which is the envy of the world. We must ensure that status remains while correcting some of the well-documented problems and continuing to produce quality advanced practice nurses for expanding and exciting roles in that system.

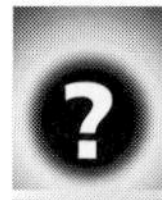

## *Discussion Exercises*

1. What are the arguments for and those against the use of advanced practice nurses in primary care?
2. What roles and settings, other than primary care, can you envision in the future for advanced practice nurses?
3. What do you think is missing in the education and regulation of advanced practice nursing?

## References


American Association of Colleges of Nursing: *The essentials of masters education for advanced practice nursing,* Washington, DC, 1996, The Association.

American Association of Colleges of Nursing: 1997-1998 enrollment and graduation in baccalaureate and graduate programs in nursing, Washington, DC, 1997, The Association.

American Nurses Association: *Nursings' social policy statement,* Washington, DC, 1995, The Association.

American Nurses Association/American Association of Critical Care Nurses. *Standards of clinical practice and scope of practice for the acute care nurse practitioner,* Washington, DC, 1995, American Nurses.

Bednash and others: *A data base for graduate education in nursing: summary report,* Washington, DC, 1990, American Association of Colleges of Nursing.

Bigbee JL: History and evaluation of advanced nursing practice. In Hamric AB and others, editors: *Advanced nursing practice,* vol 1, Philadelphia, 1996, WB Saunders.

Lott JW and others: Acute care nurse practitioner. In Hamric AB and others, editors: *Advanced nursing practice: an integrative approach,* vol 16, Philadelphia, 1996, WB Saunders.

Moses EB: *The registered nurse population,* Washington, DC, 1996, Department of Health and Human Services, HRSA Division of Nursing.

National Organization of Nurse Practitioner Faculty: *Advanced nursing practice: curriculum guidelines and program standards for nurse practitioner education,* Washington, DC, 1995, The Organization.

Safriet B: Health care dollars and regulatory sense: the rule of advanced practice nursing, *Yale J Regul 9*(2):417, 1992.

Yankelovich D: The debate that wasn't: the public and the Clinton plan, *Health Aff, 14*(1):7, 1995.

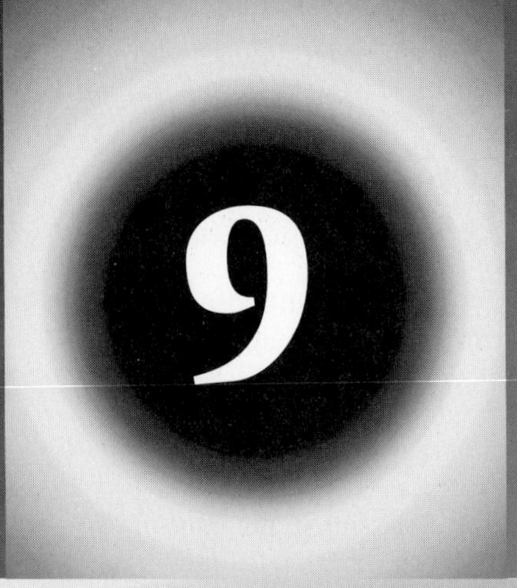

# 9 Clinical Learning Settings for the Future

**Andrea R. Lindell**

*The future ain't what it used to be.*

**Yogi Berra**

Much can be learned from history that can serve as a basis for predicting the future. How different are we from yesterday, and how different will we be tomorrow? Perhaps today we are better prepared than people of years ago. We have a global view. We can compare and contrast. We like to believe that history does repeat itself, even if in a modified form. It is a natural curiosity to look at the historic patterns of education to predict how nursing programs will or should design clinical settings in the future. Will there be a significant difference in the learning methodologies for the nursing student in the twenty-first century, or will a historic pattern be seen by educators living in the twenty-second century?

## THE PAST

A brief look at early medical education practices will provide a framework for what educators practice today and into the future. Davison, in his book *Everyday Life Through the Ages* (1992), explains that Egyptians primarily prepared individuals for the medical field by mentorship with an established physician, but there did seem to be an early forerunner of medical schools attached to Egyptian temples. Records show that there was at least one school for midwives. Most health care practitioners were prepared as "general practitioners" to work in the community. Midwives and physicians were "taught when making a diagnosis to first observe the patient closely, then ask questions, inspect, feel, smell, and probe" (Davison, 1992). Davison reports that the Greeks treated sickness by asking priests to interpret the patient's dreams. The priest then prescribed treatments such as diets, gymnastics, and baths. Learning occurred from observing patients during baths and periods of rest. Mental imagery was a popular method of self-learning. The Romans used female and male models and actors for observation and identification of normal body functioning. Chinese women used dolls to indicate the sites of their ailments to the health care worker. Storytelling formed the basis of most early learning. Teaching/learning strategies from the past ranged from simple observation to experiential learning. The learner participated in experiences such as meditation, imagery, biofeedback, aromatherapy, crystal healing techniques, virtual reality, and simulation with the use of models or actors.

Are we progressive in the design of new teaching/learning strategies and clinical settings today or do we prefer to continue to use past strategies and clinical settings that change little from year to year but make us feel comfortable? We should step back from "the way we have always done it" and be creative while still providing quality nursing education.

## THE PRESENT

Nursing and nursing education continue to be faced with numerous changes. Of particular importance today is the impact of health care reform. This reform has forced nursing educators to debate, hypothesize, and even theorize what the nurse's role should be for the next year while grappling with the uncertainty of what the role will be years from now. Faculty have stood firm about the necessity of a curriculum that stands for quality. However, debates continue about what constitutes a quality nursing education program and what requirements are critical for well-educated and trained graduates to meet the ever-changing health care needs of the population.

Historically, nursing curricula experienced many evolutionary phases from traditional multiple entry/exit points to the current quasiintegrated, open/with walls, community-based focus. Additionally, graduate-level programs have moved from specialist to generalist then back to generalist with a specialty-focused major. Curricular nursing roles have expanded from inpatient to outpatient, to home health care, community-based care, primary, secondary, and tertiary care.

There is no doubt that health care change has led us to a state of uncertainty and confusion. One can speculate what the future holds for nursing education. What does the future mean for nursing education in clinical settings in the next century? What types of learning can be developed if there is a paucity of patients? Where can we obtain clinical sites when the traditional ones have virtually disappeared? How should students be prepared? Can we capitalize on downsized, right-sized, consolidated, and developed health care alliances?

## THE FUTURE

### Survival Strategies

At present, educational institutions are in a constant state of flux because they must be prepared to meet the trends taking place in the business world. It is too easy to develop survival strategies to meet the problems of the moment rather than consider long-range implications and planning. Decisions must be made quickly but thoughtfully.

Consolidation of hospitals, alliances between and among health care institutions and the closings of hospitals have had a tremendous effect on the health care environment. Inpatient care days have shortened and in many cases been eliminated. New modalities of intervention/treatment techniques have created uncertainty and havoc in the availability of traditional, off-campus, or clinical learning experiences for students.

#### Settings and Roles

Nursing faculty can no longer expect to find nurses in traditional roles and locations for the required learning experiences. With the shifting forces that affect the health care environment and the unavailability of typical or traditional learning experiences, faculty must work to alleviate traditionalism and move to creativity and innovation to achieve the desired learning competencies of present and future nursing students.

### Changes in Higher Education

As we become a more global, knowledge-based economy, higher education also will have to keep pace with the corporate world. Professors will be more like tutors, distance learning will expand, and robotic helpers will assist with clinical applications. According to Jennifer Jarratt, a futurist for a Washington-based consulting firm, "In corporations such as IBM many employees work from their homes. Learning will no longer be linked to a specific time or place as colleges and universities develop distance learning" (Moore, 1997).

Higher education will become more responsive to students who come to college with a sound knowledge of technology and the ability to use it. Unique partnerships will be developed between universities and segments of the community. The relationship between teaching and learning in the community will expand as universities and colleges work side-by-side with individuals to overcome the impersonal nature of technologic education.

### Distance Education

Distance learning will become the norm. Students could be on campus for only part of a semester or perhaps not at all. Distance learning may be profitable for universities, but it will be difficult for some traditional faculty to adapt. Faculty will continue to teach students, but their role and major teaching strategy will be as a tutor and a coach. In this new role faculty will be seen as facilitators of student learning. Students will have primary responsibility in a self-directed learning relationship and process.

### Individualized Instruction

Nursing programs must design clinical learning programs that meet the needs of each student. We have made some progress; however, more must be done to individualize learning. Students must be placed in proper learning settings and be given timely feedback from faculty. Multiple assessment of students' performance throughout the learning experiences will be critical. New technologies and new creative clinical learning experiences will accelerate the evolutionary process by allowing faculty to assess student progress using a variety of methods. Student performance will be collected over time in an electronic portfolio for long-term assessment of the learning and competencies acquired. Grades will be meaningless. More time will be spent in purposeful learning by students in accessing information and also interacting with faculty by using electronic or other forms of telecommunication.

### Learning Sites

Learning will take place wherever and whenever it is convenient for students and meets the learning objectives: at home or at sites (kiosks) away from faculty and a typical classroom. Emphasis on student responsibility and self-directed learning in the new health care environment will emphasize the importance of a key psychosocial attribute: learner autonomy. Faculty will help students master autonomy and increase learner independence. Autonomy is central to the development of becoming a critical thinker with the ability to prioritize and then delegate professional responsibility and tasks. New teaching-learning strategies will be coupled with new technologies to assist students to acquire greater responsibility for their own learning and gain greater self-confidence and independence (University of Cincinnati, 1997).

## The Relation-Centered Care Model

Nursing educational programs must forge a stronger link between their curricular activities and learning experiences with the community at large and employers of their graduates. Both the probable future and the preferred future are moving us toward the relation-centered care model. This care model proposes that practitioners' relationships with their patients' community and with other practitioners are central to health care. This model is the vehicle for putting into action a paradigm of health that integrates caring, healing, and community (Tresolini, 1994).

The Pew-Fetzer Task Force report identifies dimensions of the relation-centered care model (Tresolini, 1994). There are three interrelated relationships: patient-practitioner, community-practitioner, and practitioner-practitioner. These dimensions form the foci within which clinical learning sites can be developed and/or established.

- The *patient-practitioner relationship* is based on the practitioner's relationship with the patient. Work relationships include assessing the biopsychosocial aspects of the patient, organizing the information, and promoting health and treatment of illness in the individual and family.
- In the *community-practitioner relationship,* the community is central for health and human development related to the patient within the context of the community. The focus of the practitioner's relationship with the community is assessing the direct impact on client care. This requires the practitioner to have a working knowledge of the community and its social, political, cultural, and economic determinants. It also requires the practitioner to recognize and act in accordance with the values, norms, and social and health concerns of the community. The practitioner should develop a sense of community responsibility, work within the community, and try to change harmful aspects of the community to promote overall health.
- *The practitioner-practitioner relationship* emphasizes the interrelationship of practitioners who are committed to working together to meet individuals' needs to promote health and prevent illness. Practitioner-to-practitioner relationships are both within and across disciplines and include established practitioners, as well as those practitioners engaged in learning. These relationships require teamwork. Individuals share values, learn from each other, and assist in the self-development of team members. To be successful in this approach, personal viewpoints of specialism, hierarchy, and rights of principle must be cast aside (Tresolini, 1994). It is the movement toward community-based relationships in the provision of health care that gives hope and direction for new educational and clinical learning experiences.

## Experiential Learning

The future preferred methodologies of educational and clinical learning will most likely occur in the experiential learning arena, linking the classroom with the community. These methodologies will contribute to greater educational productivity for the faculty and the student. Cantor (1995) has identified the major factors to increase interest in experiential learning:

(1) Develop a strong relationship between classroom learning and the realities of our global community.
(2) Understand learning theory, cognitive development, social development, and emotional development.
(3) Broaden the teaching styles used by faculty to more effectively relate to the multiple learning styles of the older, nontraditional student.
(4) Acknowledge that knowledge base and career skill needs are changing so rapidly in our society that it is increasingly important to educate students on how to be self-learners.
(5) Increase importance to the overall reputation of an academic program or institution to forge a stronger link between academic programs and the employers of their students and their community.

The future of nursing schools rests on their ability to adjust and adapt quickly to change. A futuristic educational program requires faculty and administrators who are risk takers and able to respond quickly to change. The changing health care environment has decreased the amount and type of perceived ideal clinical settings in which students attain objectives and competencies. Faculty must be innovative and creative in the design of new and different learning experiences. In addition, the sites currently in existence may be modified to increase the availability of clinical settings.

## Clinical and Educational Learning Strategies

To develop a clinical learning experience in a community-based model that has the three dimensions of relation-centered care, one must move from the traditional format and mindset that students are able to learn only in a hospital-based facility. The community format permits faculty to become flexible and innovative.

When faculty accepts that learning occurs in an independent and self-directed manner, they will have a wealth of opportunities to draw on for student learning experiences. An assessment survey of the surrounding community and its geographic area must be conducted. What services are available in all types of settings, for example, shopping malls, health care agencies, and businesses? Identify corporations and industrial plants and their needs. What are their products and what kind of workers characterize local industries? Describe community programs and agencies, school systems and their activities, the business leadership and its members and goals, political resources, and religious institutions. These are only a few of the numerous opportunities for potential learning sites in the community.

As the future is upon us, the nursing profession must make decisions about what is essential learning for each individual nursing student. In what clinical experiences must every student engage? How can students learn from each other? What can be learned only from a nursing type of learning experience versus what can be learned from a clinical experience that can be extrapolated to a nursing-focused plan of care? All of these factors plus many others must be identified and described within each and every nursing program to prepare nurses for practice in a rapidly changing health care environment. The biggest challenge facing us is the need for our own personal transformation—to understand and promote change within ourselves.

The availability of traditional educational clinical learning settings in the hospital-based clinical arena has virtually disappeared. With fewer patients on pediatric units, in labor and delivery rooms, and long-term psychiatric wards, we have lost traditional hospital-based clinical sites. The hospital, however, still is in many instances the "end product" designed for the achievement of clinical learning objectives. The probable evolution will result in nursing programs trying to "fit" health agencies' philosophy of patient care and types of available care into the new learning objectives and different program outcomes. It is the round hole and square peg syndrome. The preferred evolution is for nursing programs to realize and accept that the patient/individual, not the health care setting, is the focal point of the student's learning experience. The environmental setting, then, will not be the primary learning focus and will serve only as an important factor having direct and indirect influence on the needs of the individual patient.

## Clinical Learning Settings

Faculty must shed traditionalism. The present clinical environment requires a program of study that moves the course plan of classes and clinical times from Monday through Friday during the hours of 8:00 AM to 4:00 PM to a modular, self-directed approach. As long as program faculty believe that learning can occur only in a classroom with faculty as prime lecturer, that clinical rotations cannot exceed 1:6 to 1:8 ratios, or that students can learn nursing content only from nurses, opportunities for planned change will be missed. The Pew-Fetzer Task Force report identified that didactic instruction in itself is insufficient. "Effective relationship-centered care and effective education programs and processes must parallel one another so that students, faculty, and practitioners are immersed in a learning environment. The educational environment we construct will reinforce our teaching-learning agency or belie our every intent" (Tresolini, 1994).

Faculty must become facilitators of student learning. The community's wealth of learning opportunities awaits the inquisitive faculty to recognize, revise, or enhance.

## Industry

Industrial plants and corporations are sources of clinical learning opportunities waiting to be discovered or enhanced. The auto industry lends itself to individual/client experiences and client/family/community health care activities. In one nursing program, a group of students were assigned to a Michigan-based auto body plant. The selection of this nontraditional site afforded students the opportunity to assess the health status of many individual clients and to intervene when appropriate. When attainment of optimal health necessitated family support and/or counseling or identification of community services for support of the patient or when health conditions necessitated home care, families were included. Thus students engaged in the health education of the worker, assessed and obtained services for the family, identified hazards in the occupational work environment, and worked with community and industrial services to identify available benefits and services for the patient.

## Camps

To establish a camp nursing experience for student learning, faculty should identify camps available within the local geographic area. Susan Praeger (1997) wrote, "Selection of a camp depends on a number of professional, educational, and logistic factors including timing, expectations, available opportunities, on-site support, distance and accommodations." Camps can range from camps for children with disabilities (e.g., wheelchair bound), chronic illness (e.g., diabetes), or acute illness (e.g., cancer) or to recreational camps with health as an indirect focus.

## Shopping Malls or Individual Stores

Clothing or merchandise stores are excellent clinical learning sites. These sites offer great opportunities for students to engage in health education activities. Two examples follow.

1. Students can work with employees to develop protocols for education in areas such as lifting techniques, strategies to decrease back strain or injury, and communication strategies between employees and with shopping customers. Shoppers are an excellent health learning and teaching resource for faculty and students. Health assessment kiosks can be set up in malls. Nutritional status can be assessed and proper nutrition guides can be distributed to shoppers. Nursing students can offer children games to play that focus on health while the parent is free to shop. Students can display health-related projects and serve as educational resources to answer questions. The learning opportunities are limitless.
2. Undergraduate and graduate-level students enrolled in community or health policy–related courses can engage in community-service activities to enhance the emergence of the educational program/community partnerships model approach. Students then become accepted as providers of health care, contributors to the health needs of the community, and ultimately as important links with the community.

## Schools

Students can provide health education to students from kindergarten to grade 12 on topics such as head lice, healthy nutrition, proper eye care, need for routine health care assessments, and eye examinations (Dr. Eyeball). Working with teachers and school nurses, students can design health programs and also assist in school-based health clinics.

## Community Projects

Project reports can consist of (1) defined goals; (2) measurable outcome parameters; (3) review of the literature and data sources; (4) project and evaluation plan; (5) presentation of findings and data analysis; (6) implications and recommendations; and (7) appendixes/ interventions/additional data for community leaders, agencies, and political and consumer groups. Examples of some clinical learning projects follow.

Assist a community center with an empowerment project to develop and implement a health promotion program for its older seniors.

Collect and analyze data for a subcommittee of a large community group conducting a community health status assessment.

Develop and implement a wellness program for older adults with alcohol-related illness.

Conduct a community analysis of emergency room use for a managed care group.

Develop, implement, and evaluate a documentation system for parish nursing.

Identify populations at risk in major Medicaid HMOs, and develop intervention strategies for those populations.

Develop an evaluation plan for a case management model for a working population.

Conduct a health needs assessment; develop an arthritis self-care program and integrate it into a wellness center for older adults.

## Disaster Management

Faculty can develop objectives and competencies to be gained by students assisting with the assessment of available community and federal services and providing first aid to flood victims. In addition to indepth nursing assessment and intervention techniques, triage methodologies and group multidisciplinary team strategies can be taught by student participation in actual and simulated disasters.

## Health Planning Projects

Student experiences for project objectives can be to (1) engage in holistic community assessment, (2) define a specific health prevention project for the community, (3) develop a budget to substantiate the project need, and (4) negotiate the project's financial requirements and other needs with community leaders. *Healthy People 2000* can be used as a reference source (U.S. Department of Health and Human Services, 1990). One project, based on a health planning project, was to purchase a mobile medical van to provide health care to underserved, rural clients.

## Cultural Diversity

It is important to expose nursing students to individuals from diverse cultural backgrounds. When the nursing program has limited access to individuals from a variety of cultural backgrounds, opportunities can be explored for clinical sites such as Native American reservations, migrant camps, public and private schools from kindergarten to grade 12, or religious institutions. Attendance at conferences or seminars on topics of culture and the use of simulation offer additional opportunities to enhance cultural knowledge.

In many geographic areas, it may be impossible for each student to have direct interaction with an individual from a cultural background different from his or her own. In this circumstance, faculty should design class discussions and preclinical and postclinical conferences and seminars to foster shared student learning. Students can learn from each other; for example, student *A* cares for an African-American child, student *B* cares for a Hispanic male patient, and student *C* cares for a 60-year-old Native American female. Strategic discussion led by faculty to assist students in sharing their experiences will increase sensitivity to cultural issues, foster assessment of cultural factors, assist students to plan culturally relevant care, and enhance students' ability to understand the diverse needs of the patient.

## Comprehensive End-of-Program Experiences

An end-of-program experience provides an opportunity for students to engage in a clinical learning site of their choice before graduation. During the last semester or quarter, preceptors work with students (one to one) for an assigned period. This learning experience generally is called an *internship* or *role transition* experience.

Students are in the clinical learning setting at times when the assigned preceptor works. The time may vary from 20 to 40 hours per week, depending on the number of credits assigned to the course. The overall objective for this type of experience is to allow students to implement all learned skills, abilities, and competencies in a complex, comprehensive manner.

Clinical agencies support this learning approach. They tend to hire such students because of familiarity with the agency's philosophy and procedures. An additional benefit to the participating agency is reduced orientation time for new hires, thus decreasing agency cost.

### Long-Term Patients

The student is assigned an individual in a family at the beginning of the student's first nursing course. The individual's illness and the family's response are followed by the student for the entire nursing program. Skills and content related to objectives that are not available may be supplemented by video simulations, patient simulators, nonparticipatory observation, or role playing.

## Created Clinical Settings

Using a strip shopping mall for clinical experiences is a creative approach that can offer increased learning opportunities. A strip shopping mall is designed for shoppers to stroll along an avenue lined with shops and to choose which store meets their needs. Providing learning experiences in created clinical settings helps to ensure that we take control of our future. Some other examples of created clinical learning environments follow.

### Patient Simulations

Using a simulated situation requires an actor to play the role of a patient. The actor will portray a patient having a history of illness, expressing appropriate signs and symptoms and responding to questions about psychologic and social needs according to the information detailed in the case history. The "patient" can be presented to an entire class, to a small group, or to an individual student. The advantage of this approach is the ability to create your own case study. Simulated situations are flexible in all types of patient care situations, which can provide practical opportunities in assessment, diagnosis, intervention techniques, and even evaluation strategies. The disadvantage of a simulated patient approach is cost, which may be prohibitive.

### Recruitment of Friend or Family Member

Friends and family members can serve as patients to assist students in developing health assessment skills and communication techniques. An advantage of this approach is that the students are responsible for obtaining their own partners. A disadvantage may be decreased availability of faculty when they are needed by students.

### Grand Rounds

Student and faculty participation in medical grand rounds offers numerous opportunities for learning. Grand rounds also facilitate the professional socialization process for nursing and medical students with preconferences and postconferences led jointly by nursing and medical faculty.

DeWolf-Bosek and Savage (1997) suggest some ethical teaching moments for grand rounds: do not resuscitate orders, advance directives, informed consent, conscientious objection, and requirements for resolution of ethical conflicts. Faculty can utilize actual situations to demonstrate the decision-making process. Use of nonparticipant observation of nurse/physician interactions can serve as an excellent foundation to further develop critical-thinking competencies related to subissues such as planning end-of-life care and appropriate actions when a medication incident occurs. When mock experiences are used in a post conference, role playing among the staff nurse, physician, patient, hospital administrator, orderly, housekeeping, and others will enable students to identify factors and emotional responses to ethical decisions or conflicts.

## Co-Op

A co-op curriculum pattern integrates a cooperative approach for the student. Many universities offer students in a variety of majors a cooperative educational program at the undergraduate level. The traditional 4-year program becomes a 5-year one. During the third year, or junior level, the program plan integrates a full-time work experience. At the conclusion of the 5-year program, the student has the equivalent of a 1-year work experience.

Students are assigned to or selected by participant agencies. Students receive an hourly salary and work full time under the supervision of a designated preceptor. Evaluation is given by the agency preceptor or co-op leader. The plan usually includes summer co-op work or course enrollment for a total 12-month design.

Many health care agencies have expressed interest in the co-op approach rather than the semester, summer, or quarter internship approach. The advantage of the co-op experience is the immediate and direct application of theoretic content in a health care setting. The student has learning experiences in the health care environment on a full-time basis, functions as a member of the total health care team, engages in the health care work role, and receives a salary. Health care agencies can develop "bonding" techniques to enhance their ability to recruit new employees and decrease their cost for orientation, as well as develop agency socialization to the organization. The disadvantage is a long program of 5 years with some academic years of 12 months for student and co-op activities.

## Alternate Spring Break Experiences

The College of Nursing at the University of Cincinnati offers students the opportunity to gain credit from a 5-day community experience in a country outside of the United States during their traditional spring break week. Under faculty supervision, students engage in direct care of patients living in Celeston and Cochol, Mexico. Students receive community health course credit. This approach increases the type and availability of learning experiences in community health clinical settings. The advantage is that students have increased opportunities to meet their community-focused learning objectives and work directly with patients from another culture. The disadvantage is the cost to the nursing program or student for travel and lodging.

## College/School Nonprofit Corporations

As health care agencies adopt a corporate model with increased emphasis on revenue income versus expenditures, cost containment, and cost-effectiveness, it might be beneficial for nursing academic units to form their own nonprofit corporation. Three years ago the College of Nursing at the University of Cincinnati formed a corporation that was not guided by the policies and procedures of the University. This corporation, *Nurses in Advanced Practice, Inc.*, is a nonprofit organization. The development of a corporation has enabled the College faculty to develop clinics and contract health care services for direct reimbursement without any financial obligation from the College's annual operating or endowment budgets. The nonprofit corporation increases the faculty's opportunity to create alternative learning experiences from existing clinical settings or to create new clinical settings. The opportunities for student learning at the undergraduate or graduate level can be numerous and exciting as faculty allow themselves to be creative and innovative.

## Faculty-Managed Clinics

Forming and operating a school-based clinic can be fun and exciting in addition to enhancing existing clinical experiences or creating new learning opportunities for students. Establishing a nurse-managed clinic can serve a multitude of programmatic needs and achieve numerous learning clinical objectives for the curriculum. Many nursing program clinics have evolved based on availability of federal monies or current goals of foundations. When goals or federal interest changes and funding diminishes, these clinics either close or limp along dependent on the faculty's commitment, with the assumption of a heavier workload or the sporadic "financial goodwill" of others.

Linkages and co-partnerships with the community are essential for success. Interest and support, financial and other types, are germane to the outcome in community/institution partnerships. The design of a clinic should be based on community needs, not the current funding priorities or the "bell and whistle" approach. The success of any nurse-managed clinic depends on the support of the community in the immediate geographic region of the nursing program. The clinics operated by the College of Nursing and Health at the University of Cincinnati provide examples for the organization of clinics and the opportunities they provide for clinical learning experiences.

For example, the Health Resource Center is a nurse-managed medical and psychiatric clinic serving primarily the indigent and/or homeless mentally and physically ill. The clinic is under the auspices of Nurses in Advanced Practice, Inc. The clinic serves clients on a walk-in basis at no charge. Most of the clients are marginalized from mainstream society and have no access to funds for care either through entitlements or insurance.

There were more than 8000 documented visits in the first 2 years of the Center's operation, with approximately 650 visits monthly. Staffing consists of three full-time staff, several part-time physicians, nurses and other support personnel, selected graduate and undergraduate students from five disciplines (nursing, psychology, medicine, social work, and education), and volunteers. The clinic is open 5 days weekly from 9:00 AM to 2:00 PM and is funded by the local mental health board, selected grants, contracts with health provider agencies, and private donations. The clinic is fully certified by the Ohio Department of Mental Health to provide five services: diagnostic assessments, counseling and psychotherapy, medical somatic, community support program services, and prevention services.

The specific services provided at the Center include psychiatric assessments, counseling and psychotherapy, medication management, case management or community support program services, individual or group therapy, family therapy, substance abuse treatment and referral, and testing and counseling for human immunodeficiency virus. Services are also provided for the mentally ill client offenders who are under the supervision of the Adult Parole Authority system. In addition, staff are able to provide medical services and referrals to a network of supportive agencies. When a client is no longer considered indigent, measures are taken to move the client to an appropriate agency.

This clinic affords learning experiences to nursing students from the undergraduate and graduate nursing programs, as well as students from other health professions, including social work, psychology, psychiatry, medicine, interns and residents, and nutrition and dietetics that together form the nucleus of student providers of health care. This multidisciplinary environment enables faculty to create interdisciplinary health care teams for learning, as well as establish patient-focused care.

Examples of student clinical learning activities in the Center follow.

- Students can have experiences that emphasize critical thinking and practical solutions for clients. For example, students experience the same uncertainty, stress, and fear that clients experience by riding on city buses to learn how clients must negotiate the transit system. This experience may help students develop a greater appreciation of how a mother with three children can get to a doctor's appointment if she does not have personal transportation.
- Students can observe and participate in the day-to-day management of a "one-stop service clinic."

- Students experience multiple options and flexibility in nursing interventions.
- Students experience some of the hopelessness that community-based mentally disabled or indigent persons experience on a daily basis.
- Students learn how to assess strengths and limitations of communication models by observation versus direct interaction.
- Students learn how to provide care within the community system.

At the Health Resource Center, students never just observe. They are part of the care given, and they function in an interdependent manner. Staff serve as resources to facilitate learning by fostering in-depth clinical analysis of client needs. Students are "pushed" to think critically while they are working with patients.

Students accompany clients to agencies by taking the elderly to the Social Security office, standing in line with them, and assisting them in getting identification. Students also plan and give health-related seminars in the treatment programs for women incarcerated for 3 to 4 months for drug and alcohol-related problems.

Some students attend court hearings with clients. This enables students to learn about the forensic system and experience the internal operations of the legal system. Relationships are established, fears are lessened, and misperceptions are erased through such experiences.

Other student activities such as "friendly begging," or the art of asking for donations or funds for the clinic or patients, may be new for the student. Knowledge about the mechanisms of philanthropy and why and how people give money or material goods is a valuable competency learned.

Graduate students are involved in more complex and comprehensive assessments and treatments regimens. Psychiatric-focused students are assigned a specific client caseload and update clinic staff regularly on client outcomes. They present case studies to the Department of Mental Health board, review and evaluate certification policies and procedures and licensure renewal policies, and sometimes serve on committees to select and rate volunteer medical students.

## More Opportunities

A clinical environmental setting can provide a variety of learning experiences that could articulate with many courses and clinical objectives inherent in the majority of nursing curricula. The degree of one's ability to be creative, innovative, or simply really "see" what is there will determine the extent that a nursing program will be successful in adapting to the changing health care environment.

### Multidisciplinary Care Teams

Many programs have multidisciplinary courses with students from nursing, medicine, pharmacy, and allied health disciplines. This multidisciplinary approach fosters increased knowledge of or about the roles of other health care disciplines. Additionally, it can be cost effective to consolidate like courses among academic units, thus decreasing duplication and cost. The multidisciplinary approach can be used, for example, in lectures, care conferences, and grand rounds.

This educational approach also prepares students to adjust quickly to multidisciplinary health care teams, the current movement in health care settings. Students will learn in an environment that is similar to the real world.

### Corner of Third and Main

On every street corner in every town and city there exists a collection of individuals who come together more or less on a regular basis for a specific purpose. The shops that line the corner change depending on the specific location of the corner. Shops range from laundromats, delis, convenience stores, fast food restaurants, department stores, pool halls, and liquor stores to rooming houses, churches, and retirement communities. The important factor is not the type of shop that will serve as the clinical learning experience but rather is the people who frequent the establishments. Shops may serve as ideal environments for the creation of many clinical learning opportunities.

### Support Groups

The formation of groups for support and mutual teaching/learning can provide a vast array of experiences for the graduate-level student. For example, groups of new mothers can help students develop skills in mother-child relationships, well-child growth and development, health teaching, health assessment, and establishing nurse/patient trust relationships.

### Hair and Nail Salons

These are potential educational environments that will challenge the creativity of faculty but have numerous possibilities for clinical learning activities. You can allow yourself freedom to design and develop new techniques.

### Teaching Modalities

In the absence of actual patients, some possibilities for learning include the following:

- Virtual reality
- Computer-based simulations, such as touch screen software programs
- Mentor/mentee relationship with nurse as a role model
- Simulated events such as accidents or natural disasters (e.g., floods, tornadoes, hurricanes)
- High-tech mannequins that respond to correct or incorrect nursing diagnoses and interventions and can signal increased pain and indicate inaccurate medication or inappropriate treatments

The learning strategies and clinical settings that have been described in the relationship-centered care model and its three dimensions, patient-practitioner, community-practitioner, and practitioner-practitioner, should not be construed as representing an exhaustive description of innovative and creative learning opportunities. They were described to tantalize the creativity that lurks within all of us.

Innovation does not preclude quality or the attainment of objectives by the learner. Whether the setting becomes available through modification of our teaching/learning methodologies or we establish our own setting, such as a nurse-managed clinic, the educational program must become an organization that pervades the community health care system. Programs must develop collaborative, interdisciplinary linkages. It is difficult to ascribe a specific learning activity for the patient-practitioner versus community-practitioner versus practitioner-practitioner relationship, for example. The inherent outcome for the learning activity will be determined by the specific relationships, and then the appropriate clinical setting can be selected.

## CONCLUSION

Nursing must engage in preferred change for the future. If we do not have the ability to secure clinical settings reflective of society, changes in nursing education will be greatly diminished. Why? Because other disciplines are beginning to vie for the same clinical settings. To simply float along doing what we have always done increases our chances that the availability of patients for learning experiences will be taken by others.

History teaches us that learning occurs in many ways. Patterns occur that are enhanced during each century. We must enhance and expand our creativity. We must take charge and control of our own destiny to design and implement creative and innovational educational clinical settings within the existing environment for our students and our future.

### *Discussion Exercises*

1. Discuss advantages and disadvantages of the clinical settings described in this chapter.
2. Describe any involvement you have had in the types of clinical settings described in the

chapter (e.g., as a student, practicing nurse, administrator, instructor).
3. Name three additional ideas for clinical sites for student learning, and indicate the pros and cons of each.

## References

Cantor J: Experiential learning in higher education: linking classroom and community, *ASHE-ERIC Higher Education Reports* 7:1, 1995.

Davison M: *Everyday life through the ages,* New York, 1992, Readers Digest Association.

DeWolf-Bosek S, Savage T: Teachable moments: integrating into clinical education, *Deans Notes* 18(5):1, 1997.

Moore GR: Futurist says global economy: new technology to force higher education to keep up, *University Currents* 6(27):37, University of Cincinnati, 1997.

Praeger SG: Establishing camps as clinical sites, *J Nurs Educ 36*(5):236, 1997.

Tresolini CP: *Report of the Pew-Fetzer task force of psychosocial health education, health professions and relationship-centered care,* San Francisco, 1994, Health Professions Commission.

U.S. Department of Health and Human Services: *Healthy people 2000: national health promotion and disease prevention objectives,* 1990, U.S. Government Printing Office.

University of Cincinnati: *Student development and the new technologies,* student affairs learning imperatives, Cincinnati, 1997, the University.

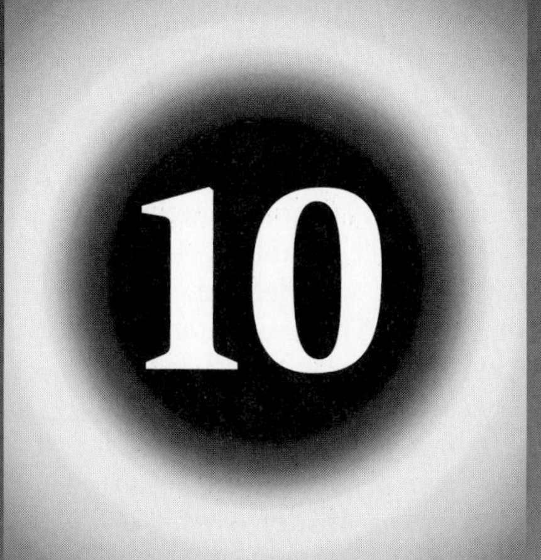

# The Impact of Scientific Discoveries and Technology on Practice

**Virginia L. Morse**

*Science without conscience is but the death of the soul.*

**Montaigne**
*Essays*

As we enter the twenty-first century, the nursing profession will partake in a difficult struggle to balance the pitfalls and possibilities of weaving increasingly sophisticated technology into daily practice. Advancements in computer technology are expanding the capabilities beyond the basic ability of storing and accessing information to become an increasingly important tool in the monitoring, diagnostic, and therapeutic roles for nurses providing health care. The increasing complex computational abilities of computers also have fueled the rapid growth of new discoveries in molecular biology, which are revolutionizing our knowledge of natural evolution. In the future we will move from passive observer of the genetic code to active manipulators and controllers of DNA and thus our genetic destiny. Controversies will emerge for the nurse delivering care within a highly technical global society along with new opportunities to restructure current approaches to nursing education, research, and practice.

This chapter explores the impact of future developments in computer technology and the scientific discoveries in molecular biology on the practice of professional nursing. In addition, the potential implications and ethical dilemmas associated with these advances are discussed. Finally, within a health care system composed of highly integrated computer sophistication and scientific ability to manipulate nature, strategies are offered for harnessing the benefits, avoiding catastrophic events, anticipating outcomes, and preserving the art of nursing as a humanistic, holistic, and caring profession.

# COMPUTER TECHNOLOGIC ADVANCES

Current trends in computer technology would lead you to believe that the increased availability and capability of computers will be a continuing significant influence on the health care industry. The Labor Department's Bureau of Labor Statistics (1996) published a report, "Tomorrow's Jobs," with projections of the labor force, industry, and occupational employment from 1994 to 2005. Computer technology and health services are projected to be the fastest growing occupations. The projections are based on the societal trend of a growing number of elderly and hospitals and insurance companies mandating shorter hospital stays. Computer engineers and system analysts will be needed to meet the expanding needs for scientific research and use of computer technology in business and industry, as well as in health care.

Nursing will find new roles and new job opportunities as advancements in computer technology are introduced into health care. Areas of increasing sophistication will include the availability of large databases that support measuring outcomes; expanded communication with international colleagues; the ability of computers to "learn" from information input; and increased options, many less invasive, to assess, monitor, and treat acute and chronic illness.

## Artificial Intelligence

Computers are well suited to rapidly analyze large amounts of data at an increasingly low cost. The question of whether computers will actually have the capability to out-think humans is an area of investigation termed *artificial intelligence.* "One common definition (of artificial intelligence) is the ability of a computer to imitate human problem solving, decision making, reasoning, and learning" (Schnider, 1996). Although still in the preliminary stages, in the near future, advancements in artificial intelligence will increasingly find applications in health care.

### Expert Systems

One branch of study in artificial intelligence is based on heuristics (Kaku, 1997) and sometimes referred to as *expert systems* (Schnider, 1996). The computer is fed a set of well-defined "rules of thumb" and outcomes. The computer can then analyze the information at the speed of light and derive a logical solution. Current health care applications for this kind of program are similar to algorithms for patient care. For example, a computerized telephone triage system with artificial intelligence capabilities would ask a set of questions based on the caller's complaint. In response to the caller, the program would generate additional questions and finally recommend a treatment plan, which may include directing the patient to seek medical attention. If limited by carefully defined boundaries, this type of program may be more accurate and up to date than its human counterpart. Critics frequently call this "cookbook medicine." The existing fatal flaw in this type of system is the ability to program the system with all possible "if . . . then" propositions (Schnider, 1996; Kaku, 1997).

### Neural Networks

Another branch of artificial intelligence is sometimes referred to as the "bottom-up approach" (Kaku, 1997). These computer models are based on biologic systems and resemble a simplistic nervous system. The computers are designed with a limited amount of hardware and software (neural networks) but have the ability to learn by interacting with the environment. They are equipped with input elements (sensory) and output elements (effector) that are interconnected with neural bridges. The neural networks produce output based on a sum of inputs after applying various weights or relative value to the information, very similar to how a young child learns not to touch a hot stove. Initially, the weight or value of the information is learned by training the network with a set of data with known results. The computer continually updates and modifies the output based on the amount of output error compared with the known outcome. Once they are "trained," the neural networks seem to be particularly adept at analyzing nonlinear data such as is found in many biologic systems (McGonigal and others, 1993).

Neural networks are currently in the development stage to predict patient outcomes based on clinical parameters. These systems may eventually serve the purpose of establishing benchmarking and perform quality monitoring functions (McGonigal and others, 1993). Demands for evidence-based practice will create a plethora of applications for both expert systems and neural networks.

### Assessment and Monitoring

Trends that will drive future development in assessment and monitoring technology include health care administrators' demands for cost effectiveness, consumer preference, and the need to bring health care to populations in new and diverse environments. Changes in the environment in which health care is delivered and consumers' preferences will demand developments that are less invasive, more compact, and increasingly portable. Technologies that are less invasive will be adopted by patients for the increased comfort, and health care providers will embrace them because of decreasing exposure to infectious diseases.

## TELEHEALTH

Computerization will expand capabilities and improve the efficiency of monitoring patients in traditional and new settings for health care ranging from home care to critical care and eventually to the far reaches of outer space. Telecommunications technology is a medium for the provision of health care services to sites that are distant from the provider. Telehealth applications are categorized into three areas: support for decision-making, remote assessment, and collaborative arrangements for the real-time management of patients at a distance (Scannell and others, 1995). Telehealth, which includes telemedicine and telenursing, uses technology ranging from the simple standard telephone service to complex communication systems combined with computers, fiber optics, satellites, and other sophisticated equipment or software. The more complex systems use high-speed, wide bandwidth transmission of digitized signals and provide for real-time management from distant locations.

In 1993 a survey conducted of telemedicine programs sampled only twelve active programs (McConnell, 1993). By 1997 Grigsby and Allen found 80 active programs. This rapid growth is in part due to the many applications and increasing sophistication of the technology.

Home health care is by far the most common division of health care that is overwhelmingly embracing this technology. Telehealth allows nurses (telenursing) to extend their reach by "visiting" more patients daily with video conferencing. Also the home health nurse has the ability to transmit information back to large databases quickly and efficiently when conducting on-site field visits.

This is a use of technology that literally takes the health care provider through cyberspace to be present with patients in their environment. It is rapidly evolving and new uses for computer software and hardware are developing daily. The original purpose of telehealth was to move information across distances, but it has increased access to remote or underserved populations needing health care (McConnell, 1996). In the future these applications may play an important role in our excursions into outer space.

## POINT-OF-CARE TECHNOLOGY

Point-of-care (POC) diagnostic technology is another emerging trend that spans distances and has the potential for improving the quality of care, enhancing cost efficiency, and providing information within minutes of a patient's rapidly changing condition. The laboratory results are accurate and available within 2 to 5 minutes at the patient's bedside with just a few drops of blood. Implementation of the technology began with the analysis of blood glucose levels, and continuing expansion has led to more complex laboratory diagnostics, including arterial blood gas analysis, electrolyte analysis, hematology profiles, and other testing (Lamb and others, 1995).

One example of bedside patient monitoring is the i-STAT System (McConnell, 1996). The technology uses a portable, hand-held, battery-powered analyzer, an infrared interface, a portable printer, and a central station. The system eliminates the exposure to blood-born pathogens by employing a single-use cartridge that does not come in direct contact with the analyzer. Currently this technology is primarily used in the critical care setting with patients who have rapidly changing conditions. Evolving health care markets will necessitate that this technology span distances, and future versions will interface with wireless technology for patient use in the home. Results will be transmitted to the health care provider's personal computer for evaluation and intervention (McConnell, 1996).

As with many new technologies, the benefits and drawbacks must be considered. It is important to take into account the resource utilization associated with POC technology. Although POC testing may be done at the bedside by nurses or other health care personnel, the central laboratory is responsible for the quality of testing. Compliance with quality assurance monitoring is regulated through the Clinical Laboratory Improvement Amendment (CLIA) and Joint Commission on Accreditation of Health Care Organizations (JCAHO). Time and resources spent on compliance with these regulations may be offset by the benefits of immediate results and time saved by not having to track down results from the central laboratory (Miller and Miller, 1997).

The issues that affect nursing practice include not only the economic cost of the technology but also how it effects the ability to provide care and ultimately improve patient outcomes. Conventional systems and POC technology must be compared to evaluate the time needed to carry out these additional responsibilities against time taken away from other responsibilities of direct patient care. Ultimately the time saved in the overall process of obtaining a laboratory result and the ability to intervene faster may result in better patient care management and overall cost that is comparable, or even less, than today's.

## NONINVASIVE TECHNOLOGIES

The trend toward more noninvasive technologies for monitoring and diagnostic testing will continue and compete with the invasive counterpart. Benefits of noninvasive technology include decreased risk of iatrogenic injuries, minimizing exposure to blood and body fluids, and the ability to apply the technology to a broader patient population in diverse settings. Examples of future innovations using noninvasive technology are a noninvasive glucometer, cerebral oximeter, computerized impedance cardiography, and online ischemia analysis (McConnell, 1996).

Current standards of care are being questioned and compared with their noninvasive counterparts. An example is the recent controversy over the use of pulmonary artery (PA) catheters. Less invasive monitoring is favored for some patients, whereas complex, critically ill or injured patients may require the more sensitive invasive monitoring of the PA catheter. Specific needs of patients will be balanced by the benefits of noninvasive technology. Choice of methods will be determined by considering the information patients provide, risks to patients, associated costs, and, ultimately, improved patient outcomes (Paladichuk, 1998).

### Therapeutics

Emerging trends in technology for therapeutic use will have many of the same attributes as monitoring and assessment technology. Overall there will be a tendency to be less invasive, and the technologies that are invasive will be small and portable. A few illustrations of technology that exemplify these principles include the automatic cardioverter internal defibrillator (ACID) and the left ventricular assist system (LVAS).

*Automatic cardioverter internal defibrillators* deliver electrical therapy for patients with ventricular dysrhythmias. The therapy may range from simple pacing for an abnormal heart beat to a 750-volt shock for total defibrillation of the heart. The pulse generator is implanted in either the patient's pectoral or abdominal region and is connected to the heart by a set of leads. The generator monitors the patient's cardiac rhythm and delivers the appropriate electrical therapy according to preprogrammed parameters (McConnell, 1996). Newer ACIDs are planted transvenously in the catheterization laboratory. The use of ACIDs has decreased the sudden cardiac death mortality rate approximately 2% annually in this population for the past 15 years. This long-term, chronically ill population has a new lease on life but must learn to accept technology as a means of maintenance (Burke, 1996).

The *left venticalar assist system* was originally designed to be used as mechanical circulatory support for patients awaiting cardiac transplantation. The majority of patients remained hospitalized awaiting a donor implant while connected to a large bulky electrical console system. An increasing need to bridge the gap for patients awaiting donor implants supported the drive for technologic advances in the LVAS, which led to the adaption for out-of-hospital use. Clinical trials are now being done to evaluate the wearable LVAS. The pump or energy system is implanted in the abdomen, and the power source, weighing approximately 8 lbs, is worn externally. In the future a permanent LVAS may be successfully developed that will benefit more patients and potentially provide an alternative to organ transplant (Moroney and Powers, 1997). These new advances will help to bridge gaps to transplantation or maybe to other new therapies yet to be imagined.

## SCIENTIFIC DISCOVERIES IN GENETICS

Genetic discoveries are changing health care from the current efforts to diagnose and treat disease to predict and manage illness. Health care as we know it promises to be nonexistent in the future.

Deoxyribonuclease (DNA) was first proven to be the molecule that encoded genetic material in 1944, but it was in the 1950s that Watson and Crick's historic description of DNA as a double-helix molecule held together by weak bonds between base pairs of nucleotides gave birth to the revolution in DNA technology we are now witnessing. The gene, a segment of the DNA molecule, is the fundamental physical and functional unit of heredity. Each gene produces a specific protein that has a unique function. Proteins—polypeptide chains categorized as hormones, enzymes, and antibodies—are required for the structure, function, and regulation of all body cells, tissues, and organs. Recently a variety of techniques have been developed to map the specific base sequence for each gene located on the human chromosome, manipulate the gene, and replicate DNA (Lewin, 1997). The array of procedures that are now commonplace have revolutionized molecular biology and will affect the future of modern science for many decades to come.

### Gene Mapping

The Human Genome Mapping Project (HGMP) is one ambitious scientific endeavor that will significantly influence health care in the next century. The $3 billion federally funded research project, located at the National Institutes of Health, is to develop a map of the human genetic code in its ultimate molecular detail by the year 2005 (Beardsley, 1998).

Gene mapping is the process of determining the relative position of a gene on a DNA molecule. There are over 100,000 genes on the 23 pairs of chromosomes in our cells. DNA sequencing was not performed on a large scale until 1996, and about 2% of the human genome has been sequenced so far. The pace has been accelerated and the overall cost has been reduced, with much of the sequencing being computerized and roboticized. Advances in the procedures used for DNA sequencing have the HGMP team optimistically projecting that overall sequencing will be 99% completed by the year 2002, significantly ahead of schedule (Kaku, 1997; Beardsley, 1998).

The ultimate aim of this project is to provide understanding and potential cures for the numerous genetic disorders known, as well as information about inherited normal human traits. Some of the genetic disorders that have already been isolated include cystic fibrosis, Tay-Sachs disease, sickle-cell anemia, Huntington's disease, Lesch-Nyhan syndrome, and Duchenne's muscular dystrophy (Kaku, 1997). Cures, unfortunately, are still not available. Genetic counseling of prospective parents is recommended, but aborting an affected fetus is presently the only intervention offered (Beardsley, 1998).

## Recombinant DNA Technology

Recombinant DNA technology is a mixture of techniques that is used to form a DNA molecule by joining together DNA segments from different sources in an environment usually outside the cell or organism. The recombinant DNA molecule, under appropriate conditions, can then be placed in a cell and replicated there. Recombinant DNAs are frequently used in cloning genes and in genetic modification of an organism (Alberts and others, 1994).

## Cloning

Cloning is one of the recombinant DNA technologies whereby a single DNA molecule is copied and then can generate numerous identical molecules. An active area of research, cloning has long been commonplace in plants, but the cloning of a mammal has eluded scientists until recently. In February 1997 Ian Wilmut at the Roslin Institute in Edinburgh, Scotland, reported to have successfully cloned an adult sheep by extracting cells from the mammary gland of an adult sheep. The clone was named Dolly, and the revelation shocked an unprepared world (Kaku, 1997). By June of 1997 a presidential ethics commission recommended a ban on human cloning (Alder and Fussel, 1998), and in mid 1998 successful cloning of mice was reported. The question is: How long before a human is cloned?

Although federal and private funding for research on human cloning has been banned, some predict it is only a matter of time before an underground laboratory creates a human clone (Kaku, 1997; Adler and Fussel, 1998). Cloning produces a carbon copy of an individual, much like an identical twin, but does not require two germ cells from the opposite sex to unite. A single cell source or parent is sufficient.

The ethical debate surrounding cloning will be heated over the years to come. Consideration of the advantages and drawbacks must be discussed. For example, the development of cloned organs is one potential option for the shortage of organ donors awaiting transplantation to save their lives. Although the concept of cloning a human raises many ethical dilemmas, it pales in comparison with dilemmas raised by advancements in genetic engineering.

## Genetic Engineering

Before the 1970s, attempts to isolate a single gene, a small region of the DNA molecule, seemed unsurmountable. The identification and purification of DNA restriction nucleases provided the tools to isolate and manipulate individual genes. These enzymes cut the DNA molecule at specific sites. It soon became relatively easy to identify a specific restriction nuclease that would create a DNA fragment containing a specific gene (Alberts and others, 1994). Once an individual gene that codes for a specific protein is isolated, the gene can then be injected into the cell of another plant or animal. Since 1978 insulin has been produced by injecting the human gene for insulin into *E. coli* bacteria.

These modified *E. coli* can then produce an unlimited quantity of insulin. Other proteins that were once available only in limited quantities—human growth hormone, factor VIII, erythropoietin, and somatotropin—are now produced cheaply and are readily available (Kaku, 1997).

Genetic modification of an organism is now possible, and the potential for creating entirely new species of plants or animals exists. As we identify the complete genome map of thousands of life forms, simultaneously with the Human Genome Mapping Project, the pace of creating transgenic animals will increase (Kaku, 1997). Gene therapy for humans is still in the experimental stages, but there are ongoing clinical trials for malignant brain tumors using gene therapy. Researchers are examining a variety of methods for introducing the specific gene into the host, including the use of retro viral-mediated gene insertion technology; directly injecting the tumor site with p53, a tumor suppressor gene; and intramuscular injection of a DNA package containing the normal gene (Gibbs, 1996). The development and refinement of these techniques will usher in new possibilities for gene therapy.

# NURSING IMPLICATIONS

## Practice

How will the increasing uses of computer technology and new scientific advances affect nursing practice in the future? Will the essence of nursing be preserved in a health care system that is becoming increasingly automated? Will new ethical and moral dilemmas be created with the upcoming technologic and scientific advances?

Technology is an important part of our everyday life and is an essential application in today's nursing practice. As with many frequently encountered entities, we become oblivious to technologic advances that only a few years earlier would have appeared out of the normal realm of possibility. Current trends suggest that the increased availability and capability of computers will be a continuing significant influence on nursing practice. The increasing use of computers has become important to the minute-to-minute function of most health care systems. Taken for granted, computers now perform many tasks quickly, efficiently, and accurately.

Expert clinical judgment and practice in nursing will become increasingly important as technology evolves and spreads to almost all aspects of health care. Micheal Dertouzos, Director of the Laboratory for Computer Science at the Massachusetts Institute of Technology projects that the future of computer science will never be able to transmit what he terms "forces of the cave: fear, touch, trust" (Leutwyler, 1997). Virginia Henderson (1985), a visionary leader in nursing, was prophetic in her statement describing the essential role nursing must play in a high-technologic health care system. "Nursing has never been more important than in this age when the comforting, caring presence and touch of the nurse enable the institutionalized patient to tolerate invasive, often frightening and sometimes painful technology."

Technologic advances have permeated health care since the advent of the intensive care units in the 1950s (Fairman, 1992). Improvements in technology and changes in the health care system have moved technologic care to settings outside of the hospital. Consequently, patients, families, and nurses have been forced to adapt to both the benefits and the undesirable sequelae of living with technology dependency. Patients and family members may experience fear and anxiety in the intensive care unit, but increasingly so if they are relying on technologic adjuncts or life support in the home setting (Halm and Alpen, 1993; Burke, 1996).

Benner and others (1996) have examined caring, clinical judgment, and ethics in the neonatal and adult critical care environment. Using selected critical incidents, the authors explain the importance of experience in developing clinical judgment. As nurses tell their stories, a clear differentiation between the advanced beginner in comparison with expert practice is revealed. Critical care nurses develop through stages from advanced beginner to competency to proficiency. The difference between proficient and expert nurses, according to Benner, is their use of "rules" (or prescribed protocols). A proficient nurse knows the rules and can implement them accordingly. An expert nurse, on the other hand, implements rules according to specific needs of patients and family members (Box 10–1).

## Education

Advanced technology can inhibit or facilitate nursing care. Nurses must have the knowledge base and psychomotor skills to use technologic tools. In the future, educators will design learning experiences using computer simulations and virtual reality (Neighbors and Eldred, 1993). (See Chapter 12.)

New discoveries in genetics are occurring daily and are discussed in academic circles,

### Box 10-1

***Being in Charge***

**Dana Marshall, RN**

I was first a Dental Hygienist for 3½ years, and then I went to nursing school. I received my RN and started working in a nursing home because my chosen field is gerontology. Because I chose to work the evening shift in order to continue my education, I was assigned to be charge nurse. Since I had to work evenings, I felt I had no choice. Besides, I rationalized to myself, I know the patients. They had been my dental hygiene patients. I was older and more mature than most newly graduated nurses, and the two LVNs that would be working with me had been RNs in the Philippines. Armed with my false sense of security, I made it through the first 1½ weeks without incident. The "honeymoon period," I like to call it.

We take our lunch breaks at different times to leave someone to cover the ward of 50 patients. On a good day, we have four to five staff; on a bad day, only three. This was a bad day. I was in the bathroom just finishing up when the nursing assistant called through the door: "I think Mr. D. just died." I hurried up and went into Mr. D.'s room. He was lying very peacefully in his bed. I hurried over to his chart to see if he was a DNR (do not resuscitate). While I was doing this I came to the realization that the LVN was at lunch, and I was the only licensed person on the floor, with only one nursing assistant to help me. I hate to admit it, but I was relieved when I saw the DNR order in his chart. We very respectfully cleaned him and prepared him in bed for his family to "view the body." We also called the Medical Officer on duty to pronounce the patient dead. All these thoughts were whirling round my head, my first dead patient, my first crisis, my first nursing job, maybe even my first nervous breakdown! Before the physician arrived, I got my stethoscope from my last school year (we do not wear them routinely), the one with the pink hoses that used to hold a clinging Alf for Peds two semesters ago. When I handed the stethoscope to the doctor, the diaphragm fell off. So much for professionalism. But that's okay, I found out that the physician in charge was a psychiatrist! I had to spell all of the big technical words for him when he wrote up the chart.

Against this backdrop of panic and false bravado, I also had a real problem, one that couldn't be solved by a DNR order in the chart, and rationalizations about leading a long, full life. In our ward, we also have a five-bed hospice unit. The philosophy of hospice is death with dignity, and comfort measures only. When I came on that day, both the head nurse and our ward physician explained that Mrs. S., a lady of about 60, had visited her daughter for a week, on pass from the hospital. She had leukemia and was receiving morphine for the pain. This made her very constipated and she returned from her visit with impacted bowels. The nurses had to remove the stool, and it had caused her rectum to bleed. Because of her platelet problem, the bleeding was uncontrolled, and I was informed that she would probably bleed to death on my shift. This was said in the gentlest of tones, but when I went into her bathroom, it looked like Charles Manson had been there. Apparently, she had sat down on the toilet, and that's when the bleeding had started. All of a sudden, "bleeding to death" didn't sound quite so gentle as the doctor had described it. I went back to the head nurse and asked her to redefine "bleeding to death" in more realistic over the Internet, and on the nightly news. Knowledge about genetics must be integrated into both nursing practice and education. Nursing must incorporate genetics into the basic nursing curriculum, as well as continuing education for nurses in practice (Lashley, 1997). Nursing educators must understand both the basic scientific concepts and the societal issues that emerging genetic technologies will present.

## Research

Investigations of the psychologic and physiologic implications of technology dependency are ripe areas for future research initiatives. As technology expands beyond the door of the hospital, it will be important for nurse researchers to address how to support the patient and family coping with ongoing acceptance of technology for support of life or with actual life-sustaining machines. In addition, identifying interventions

### Box 10-1
### *Being in Charge—cont'd*

terms. Would it be buckets? Should I get one? Would it be fast or slow? Should her family be there? Or would it be more humane to call them after she had died? These theoretical questions began to take on real proportions when I saw the blood on the bathroom floor. We put a diaper on her to contain the blood, and I called her family. I felt relieved that some things were done, and I repeated to myself the philosophy of hospice, as if I were reciting the Apostle's Creed or the Hippocratic Oath. It was apparent that this bleeding episode had really frightened Mrs. S., a former nurse herself. I tried to reassure her that we were doing everything possible to stop the bleeding. This was only partially true, because the doctor had told me that they had decided against a blood transfusion because of the advanced progression of her disease. "Comfort measures only" had been his last words when he left the ward that dark and stormy night. When her daughter arrived, I thought that I would get a little support for the "comfort measures only" philosophy of life. But to my chagrin, she was even more frightened and even less willing to let go of the little life her mother had left. She and I were about the same age, and I, too, had lost my mother, so I knew how she felt. This was clearly not a situation that fit any stereotype, and I was hard put to be objective about any decisions that I made.

Right about this time, the OD had been called in to pronounce Mr. D. Seizing the opportunity to unload my problems on someone else, even if he didn't know how to spell big medical words, I asked him to take a look at Mrs. S. and see what he thought. He spent a lot of time with both Mrs. S. and her daughter, just talking. Now I was glad he was a psychiatrist. He came back with a very concerned look on his face, a good sign. He called Hematology, and they decided that in spite of the comfort measures only order, they would do a blood transfusion. I was very relieved, because in this case, I just didn't feel that the patient or her family were ready to let go yet. This would give them a little more time to sort things out. I thought if I were going to err, as a new nurse, I would rather err on the side of a conservative decision, especially when the family seemed in favor of that decision. It was decided by the ward physician that Mrs. S. would get blood transfusions to carry her through the holidays, and then we would go back to comfort measures only. She died quite peacefully 2 months later and required no further blood transfusions. Her daughter and I became quite close, and I was able to share my experience of losing my mother. This helped her not to feel so alone in her loss.

I have thought about this often because it shaped my perceptions about death and dying. I still believe in the philosophy of death with dignity and letting go, when it is appropriate. But sometimes people aren't ready to let go just yet. As long as the measures don't create undue suffering and prolong someone's agony, we as nurses can respect someone's wishes with a clear conscience. Each case is an individual one, and each person must decide what is best. Sometimes you just have to throw away the book.

---

From Benner, PA and others: *Expertise in nursing practice: caring clinical judgment and ethics,* New York, 1996, Springer.

to decrease the negative impacts of technology and evaluate the impact on quality of life will be essential (Halm and Alpen, 1993; Burke, 1996).

Genetics will become an integral part of the delivery of health care as we discover the many effects our genes have in setting the stage for our health status. New areas of research will open for nursing that will consider the holistic view. Genes will be the canvas, and the paints and artist will come from the environment.

## ETHICAL ISSUES

Understanding the genetic contribution to disease and the ability to intervene will pose new ethical dilemmas. Who owns the genetic material? Will everyone have access to testing? Will testing be required? Knowledge that a patient has a certain gene for a disease process can potentially be used to discriminate against the individual. Forced sterilization or abortions could be considered in the best interest of society. Who will decide, the parents or society? Where will the line be drawn for abortion for the purpose of genetic enhancement of the human race? These very difficult ethical questions must be debated now. Our knowledge and ability to perform these genetic maneuvers are growing at a much faster pace than our critical reasoning to consider these difficult questions.

In the next decade we will move from passive observers of genetic information to changing the course of natural evolution. Society is both frightened and fascinated with the ability to clone animals. Questions will change from "Can we do it?" to "Should we do it?" A moratorium on human cloning may help us to pause and consider the ramifications, scientifically and ethically, of this genetic technology (see Chapter 25).

## CONCLUSION

Now and into the future, nursing will be faced with designing a value system to accommodate the many changes in knowledge from scientific discoveries and evolving technology. As with all scientific discoveries, knowledge itself is neutral, but how people choose to use the knowledge can be potentially dangerous or beneficial to the individual and society. Nursing research, practice, and education must evolve to meet the challenge of guiding nursing into the next century.

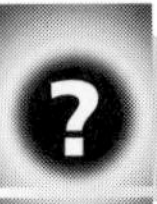

## *Discussion Exercises*

1. Discuss the advantages and disadvantages of (1) telehealth, (2) point-of-care technology, and (3) artificial intelligence in nursing care.
2. What nursing opportunities could you envision to take advantage of the technologic advances discussed in this chapter? What other advances can you imagine?
3. Genetic discoveries promise to eliminate many health problems in the future. Imagine such a health (care) system and describe it.

## References


Alberts B and others: *Molecular biology of the cell,* ed 3, New York, 1994, Garland.

Alder E, Fussell JA, Cloning: humans next? *Kansas City Star,* pp. A1, A19, January 11, 1998.

Beardsley T: Profile: where science and religion meet, *Sci Am* 278(2):28, 1998.

Benner PA and others: *Expertise in nursing practice: caring, clinical judgement, and ethics,* New York, 1996, Springer.

Bureau of Labor Statistics: *Occupational outlook handbook, ed 1996–1997* (bulletin 2470), Washington, DC, 1996, U.S. Government Printing Office.

Burke LJ: Securing life through technology acceptance: the first six months after transvenous internal cardioverter defibrillator implantation, *Heart Lung* 25(5):352, 1996.

Fairman J: Watchful vigilance: nursing care, technology, and the development of intensive care units, *Nurs Res* 41(1):56, 1992.

Gibbs WW: Explorations: gene therapy, *Sci Am* 276(10):2, 1996. 2-4.

Grigsby B, Allen A: 4th Annual telemedicine program review, part 2: United States, *Telemedicine Today* 5(4):30, 1997.

Halm MA, Alpen MA. The impact of technology on patients and families, *Nurs Clin North Am* 28(2):443, 1993.

Henderson V: The essence of nursing in high technology, *Nurs Adm Q* 9(4):1, 1985.

Kaku, M: *Visions, how science will revolutionalize the 21st century,* New York, 1997, Anchor Books.

Lamb LS and others: Current nursing practice of point-of-care laboratory diagnostic testing in critical care units, *Am J Crit Care* 4(6):429, 1995.

Lashley FR: Thinking about genetics in new ways, *Image J Nurs Sch 29*(3):202, 1997.

Leutwyler K: Profile: Michael L. Dertouzos—What will really be, *Sci Am* p 28, July, 1997.

Lewin B: *Genes VI,* Oxford 1997, Oxford University.

McConnell EA: The future of technology in critical care, *Crit Care Nurs* (suppl), p 3, June, 1996.

McConnell J: Medicine on the superhighway, *Lancet* 342(8883):1313, 1993.

McGonigal MD and others: A new approach to probability of survival scoring for trauma quality assurance, *J Trauma 34*(6):863, 1993.

Miller KA, Miller NA: Joining forces to improve point-of-care testing, *Nurs Manage 28*(8):34, 1997.

Moroney DA, Powers K: Outpatient use of the left ventricular assist devices: nursing, technical, and educational considerations, *Am J Crit Care 6*(5):355, 1997.

Neighbors M, Eldred M: Technology & nursing education, *Nurs Health Care* 14(2):96, 1993.

Paladichuk A: Life-saver or money waster? the PA catheter goes under the microscope, *Crit Care Nurs* 18(1):88, 1998.

Scannel KM and others: *Telemedicine: past, present future,* (GPO List ID: CBM95-4), Pittsburg, 1995, U.S. Government Printing Office.

Schnider SL: Artificial intelligence in emergency medicine, *Top Emerg Med 18*(1):15, 1996.

# 11 The Third Wave of Information Technology

**Betsy E. Weiner**
**Patricia A. Trangenstein**

*I think there is a world market for about five computers.*

**Thomas J. Watson**
Chairman of the Board, IBM
1943

Nurses have always been in the information business, using tools that have varied over time. Current technology tools allow practicing nurses to collect even more data and determine trends and relationships never before possible. It is therefore no surprise that technology and nursing practice have become so closely intertwined and interdependent as we approach the twenty-first century.

This chapter explores the growth of clinical practice needs compared with the advances made possible with technology. What were the initial technology needs for nursing practice? How did technology help to drive these needs to a level of information management? How can technology help us to revolutionize our nursing practice to encompass new client communities while providing comprehensive care based on identified nursing knowledge? Lastly, comes the ultimate question: Will nursing be able to orchestrate practice growth congruent with technology advances into the next century in order to survive?

## THIRD WAVE THINKING

Alvin Toffler has written a series of popular futuristic books that have become contemporary classics in social thinking (*Future Shock,* 1970; *The Third Wave,* 1980; and *Powershift,* 1990). *Creating a New Civilization* (Toffler and Toffler, 1995) integrates content from earlier works while synthesizing political events across time. The authors identify three great powerful influences (waves) of change. The *first wave* was the agricultural revolution and lasted for thousands of years. The *second wave* was the rise of the industrial civilization and took only 300 years. Today, the *third wave,* that of the information revolution, is upon us and likely to complete itself in a few decades (Toffler and Toffler, 1995). Central to their thinking is the assumption that technologic changes have been surging across the earth and have transformed everything in contact. As a result, a clash of the three waves during the next century will be inevitable, with dominance based on new ways of creating and exploiting knowledge. More information exchange will be required among health care providers and health care organizations, resulting in an increased need for computers and an expanded infrastructure to support higher-level transmissions. The globally competitive race will be won by countries (and professions) that most efficiently complete their transition into the third wave.

What does it mean to make the transition to third wave thinking? Transition requires a reexamination of our knowledge structure as we totally reorganize the production and distribution of knowledge. We will link concepts in ways never thought of before, build hierarchies of inference, derive new theories based on the unraveling patterns, and discover new logics. We will interrelate data in more ways in order to translate data into information; we will assemble the building blocks needed for our knowledge architecture. It is likely that technology will help us to achieve professional goals that have been impossible.

But what does this mean for nursing? The Tofflers view nursing in the middle of the "mind-work" spectrum as a job requiring the worker to perform physical labor but also handle information (Toffler and Toffler, 1995). Nurses deal with people but spend a considerable time generating, getting, or giving out information. They predict that the purely manual or task-oriented jobs at the lower end of the technology spectrum will begin to disappear, to be replaced by technology. A closer look into what this means for nursing helps to complete the picture.

## A Probable Scenario: Second Wave Thinking

One could argue that a probable scenario for the future would be that nursing as a profession chooses to continue to display second wave characteristics. It is easiest and most comfortable to assume that the world we know is the world that will continue to exist. At the same time this position ignores recent events, which illustrates that the world is being catapulted into the information age. Events such as the growth of electronic mail, the World Wide Web, and the recent establishment of Internet2 leave little doubt in the minds of the aware. To stay in second wave thinking would mean that nursing would stay largely unreformed, unre-engineered and unreinvented. To stay in second wave thinking means that nursing as a profession would cease to exist, not a very promising outlook for those of us who are vested in the profession.

## A Preferable Scenario: Third Wave Thinking

An alternative approach for consideration is the preferred scenario in which nursing embraces the principles of a third wave agenda. In doing so nursing will be reempowered and the concept of clients will be extended from the typical narrow institutional-bound view to that of a new civilization capable of more self-direction. Nurses today are witnessing the stress and tension resulting from the crosscurrents of the three waves, which puts nurses in the influential position to create our own destiny. That responsibility is ours, and if we do not continue our reconstruction, someone else will do it for us.

The importance of the Tofflers' works is the fact that they used historic events to provide a predictive framework (Gingrich, 1995). A similar situation can be constructed that will allow us to define nursing practice needs with accompanying technologic solutions. Comparing these events over time will allow us to take the prescriptive approach, which is necessary for third wave integration.

## THE HISTORY OF COMPUTERS IN NURSING

Even though Florence Nightingale made reference to needing a computer more than 100 years ago (Nightingale, 1859), it was not until the 1950s that the growth of the computer began to catch up with the needs of the hospitals (Saba and McCormick, 1986). These early uses were mostly business functions, such as admission information or billing. Little effort was required to move from handwritten or typed forms to a machine-readable format. Later efforts required much more work.

The influence of World War II spurred the growth of the computer industry, and during the late 1960s hospitals began using computers for patient care functions. The systems were mainframe based with terminal access from various units. The beginning hospital information systems began to emerge, but early developments again centered around automating the existing patient record.

### Merging Practice and Technology

Table 11-1 shows a model for merging nursing practice and technology. During this first period of growth, nursing care was focused on recording and automating specific tasks. Scheduling had long been a personnel problem for charge nurses, and because the logic of scheduling was easy to put into a decision algorithm, it was a natural first migration task. Patient classification systems also held early promise for success, although the methods for assigning acuity were varied and debatable. During this period nurses began to recognize the computer's potential for improving documentation of nursing practice. The computer could not only store a multitude of data, but it could order the data so that graphic presentations were informative. Trends in data patterns could be detected and further examined whether they were collected on individual patients or on groups of patients across time. The task-oriented needs of the nursing profession complemented the task automation strengths of technology. It was a simple beginning that would quickly explode into various levels of complexity.

The initial idea of automation was to enhance nursing efficiency and increase productivity. Increased accessibility to patient data; automated ordering methods; computerized entry of progress notes, care planning, vital signs, and medication administration; and online medication, dietary, or clinical references were but a few of the applications included in these systems (Yoder, 1992). Yoder further concludes that although the systems did not decrease the time nurses spent documenting care, research indicates that computerized systems improved the quality and accuracy of patient record documentation.

Computerization did not solve the problem of patient confidentiality; in fact, technology served to magnify the problem. Whereas only one patient chart had existed before, the computerized record was easily accessible by a number of different staff. Security issues immediately emerged as an important challenge. Although simple to solve with password protection schemas, this issue has been an ongoing challenge that continues to confront the information industry. With more sophisticated users, security firewalls have become necessary to keep unauthorized users from accessing confidential information. Although early systems were connected only to participating hospital units, most practice areas with technology today include Internet access for a variety of other reference tools. Greater network access further increases security concerns.

Driven by outside forces such as nursing standards, building the task automation functions became a consuming task. The Joint Commission on the Accreditation of Hospitals (JCAH, later JCAHO) asked that the nursing process be documented and by 1981 advocated that hospitals classify patient requirements to determine nursing resources and allocate nursing staff (Saba and McCormick, 1986). This request further stimulated hospitals to upgrade their medical and nursing record systems in order to take advantage of data processing capabilities.

**TABLE 11-1 Crosscurrents of Clinical Nursing Practice and Technology**

| Examples of Clinical Practice Focus | Emphasis | Examples of Information Technology Focus | Challenges |
|---|---|---|---|
| **Task Oriented**<br>Scheduling<br>Ordering<br>Patient classification<br>Computerized care plans<br>Patient data management systems<br>Physiologic signal processing<br>Medical imaging systems<br>Budgeting | **Collecting Data and Information**<br>Classification<br>Documentation<br>Monitoring<br>Trend projection | **Task Automation**<br>Hospital information systems (HIS)<br>Clinical information systems (CIS)<br>Nursing information systems (NIS)<br>Computerized patient records (CPR)<br>Point-of-care (POC) information systems | **Access**<br>Security |
| **Information Management**<br>Multisystem networks with online resources<br>Computer-assisted instruction for patients<br>Quality assurance<br>Health-oriented telecommunications | **Establishing Relationships**<br>Linkages<br>Outcomes<br>Coordination | **Database Creation: Elements and Connections**<br>Nursing Minimum Data Set (NMDS)<br>NANDA taxonomy<br>Home Health Care Classifications (HHCC)<br>Omaha System<br>Nursing Interventions Classification (NIC)<br>Uniform Minimum Health Data Sets (UMHDS)<br>Virginia Henderson International Nursing Library: *Online Journal of Knowledge Synthesis for Nursing* | **Integration and Synthesis**<br>Unified language<br>Minimum data sets<br>Longitudinal patient record<br>Registration of research<br>Knowledge synthesis |
| **Virtual Practice Arena**<br>Monitoring via modem<br>Medication administration from a distance<br>Patient and family computer support groups<br>Client-focused Web sites<br>Advanced simulations and decision support | **Autonomous Professional Nursing Practice from Generation of Nursing Knowledge**<br>Interaction of clinical nurse experts with clients in a variety of settings<br>Independent organization and delivery of nursing care | **Advanced Communication and Decision Making**<br>Web-based sites (see URL chart)<br>Decision/expert systems:<br>Creighton Online Multiple Modular Expert System (COMMES)<br>A Research-Knowledge System (ARKS) | **Revolutionary Revision of Nursing Practice Based on Nursing Knowledge**<br>Creation of new communities<br>Competency assessment via virtual reality<br>Online decision support<br>Advanced multimedia communications |

## Nursing Classification Systems

The American Nurses Association (ANA) advocates the nursing process model for nursing practice (ANA, 1980) and also recommends the development of a nursing classification system using this framework (Lang and others, 1995). The classification system is to be used in all areas of nursing practice and is to be integrated with other health care systems. The development of classification systems addressed assessments, diagnoses, interventions, outcomes and any combination of these steps in the nursing process. Organizing information in such a manner allows for relationships to be found and studied. For example, assessment classification systems study the relationship between nurses' assessments and decision making. Nursing diagnostic groups can associate cost with variation in outcomes. Intervention classifications allow nurses to determine the efficiency and cost effectiveness of nursing care, and outcomes help determine if the overall care was effective.

These classification needs marked the beginning steps in the quest for information management, the second column of the model in Table 11-1. Nursing's need to establish and explore these relationships through various linkages and outcomes coincided with technology's sophisticated growth in database creation and management. To take advantage of the databases, appropriate elements needed to be identified to help the nursing profession answer many of its practice-related questions.

The Nursing Minimum Data Set (NMDS) was designed to facilitate the abstraction of the minimum, common core of data to describe nursing practice (Werley and others, 1995). The data set was defined to be an essential set of items that have uniform definitions and categories concerned with nursing care. Many of the defined elements were collected as part of the Uniform Hospital Discharge Data Set (UHDDS).

Nursing nomenclature and taxonomies were critical to standardizing the databases, and many different databases were created and continue to be upgraded. Examples include the North American Nursing Diagnosis Association (NANDA) taxonomy (Warren and Hoskins, 1995), the Omaha System (Martin and Scheet, 1995), the Home Health Care Classification (Saba, 1995), and the Nursing Interventions Classification (Bulechek and others, 1995). The content of these databases directly relates to standards of practice against which quality of nursing care can be judged. The standards become measurable via identified criteria that can further be used to generate guidelines for patient care management. The influence of care thus goes outside the scope of one institution or patient.

## Virginia Henderson International Nursing Library

Although the work of developing national databases for nursing practice is ongoing, there recently emerged another event that illustrates how nursing leaders are embracing technology. Sigma Theta Tau International established nursing's first electronic library in 1989 and named it after the renowned nursing scholar Virginia Henderson (Hudgings, 1992). This unique library has electronic access to current nursing research and fugitive nursing literature. In addition, the Virginia Henderson International Nursing Library (VHINL) offers users the opportunity to network globally with nurses and other health care professionals, consistent with the organization's mission of knowledge development, dissemination, and utilization.

An electronic journal, *The Online Journal of Knowledge Synthesis for Nursing,* is another unique offering of the VHINL. As the first peer-reviewed online journal, this publication offers timely, synthesized knowledge to guide nursing practice and research. This new journal format attempts to capture and disseminate new nursing knowledge by linking new concepts, building hierarchies of inference, deriving new theories based on patterns, and discovering new logics. The journal is also available via the World Wide Web, and the hypertext link capabilities allow extensive navigation to other Web resources, full text searches, access to a variety of graphic figures and tables, and links to other electronic library resources.

Earlier search engines for the research registry component have recently been adapted for

World Wide Web access (www.stti.iupui.edu). As a result users may query the databases by researcher and demographics and study details, variables/concepts, and key words. The recording of the variable relationships is a critical step for the transition to knowledge-based practice, which stems from the work of Judith Graves, the former director of the VHINL. This registry allows the work of the VHINL to be expanded.

What we are beginning to see in nursing is the emergence of third wave thinking. For example, Graves and Corcoran (1989) had earlier set the foundation for this thinking with their classic article defining nursing informatics as the "management and processing of nursing data, information, and knowledge to support the practice of nursing and the delivery of nursing care."

Graves (1990) later described the relationship of nursing knowledge.

> Nursing knowledge and nursing data are the foundation for nursing practice. Both domain knowledge that is stored in the literature of nursing and related disciplines and knowledge of clinical data about single patients/clients and aggregates need to be accessible to nurses during the process of clinical decision making. Existing information and knowledge technology make it possible to bring both clinical data and the stored knowledge of the domain to the point of use.

Graves points out that although the hardware is currently available, the conceptual thinking lags far behind. She describes the contributions of her research toward knowledge engineering. This work has resulted in the development of a tool that prototypes the modeling of nursing knowledge, appropriately called "A Research-Knowledge System" (ARKS).

## USING TECHNOLOGY TO IMPROVE PATIENT CARE

Ball and others (1995) note that,

> Informatics will free nurses to assume the responsibility for systematic planning of holistic and humanistic nursing care for patients and their families, for continual review and examination of nursing practice, for applying basic research to innovative solutions to patient care problems, and for devising creative new models for the delivery of nursing care.

But wasn't that what nursing was trying to do with the early incorporation of technology in the task-oriented phase? Certainly, but what is missing is the conceptual creative thinking that expands the realm of nursing to include communities not possible to include before, practice arenas never before approachable, and independent nursing practice opportunities. These are all third wave thinking. The Tofflers (1995) remind us:

> Today we are living through one of those exclamation points in history when the entire structure of human knowledge is once again trembling with change as old barriers fall. We are not just accumulating more facts. Just as we are now restructuring companies and whole economies, we are totally reorganizing the production and distribution of knowledge and the symbols used to communicate it.

What does this mean? It means that we are "creating new networks of knowledge . . . linking concepts to one another in startling ways . . . building up amazing hierarchies of inference . . . spawning new theories, hypotheses and images based on novel assumptions, new languages, codes and logics" (Toffler and Toffler, 1995). Businesses, governments, and individuals are collecting and storing more data than any previous generation in history. But more importantly, we are interrelating data in more ways, giving them context and thus forming them into usable information; and we are assembling chunks of information into larger and larger models and architectures of knowledge.

Not all of this new knowledge is correct, factual, or even explicit. Much knowledge, as the term is used here, is unspoken, consisting of assumptions piled atop assumptions, of fragmentary models, of unnoticed analogies; it includes not simply logical and seemingly unemotional information or data but values, the products of passion and emotion, not to mention imagination and intuition (Toffler and Toffler, 1995).

Examine the third column of the model in Table 11-1. Although some of the applications listed in the information management level actually aid in transition to the virtual practice arena (and vice versa), evidence exists that nursing is moving toward this advanced level of thinking.

## Home Care

Practicing physicians and nurses have finally realized that clients do not need to be in a hospital to be treated. Hospitals are coming to grips with a shrinking census and the realization that their "clients" might actually be more comfortable and capable of health restoration in their home environment. This notion is fully supported in the Tofflers' (1995) notion of the third wave community, which reempowers the family and the home.

The Tofflers' definition of family is broader than in the past and includes families of many diverse types. Some are traditional nuclear families, some are extended and multigenerational, some are composed of remarrieds, some are big, some are small or childless, some families are couples who defer having children until later in life (Toffler and Toffler, 1995). This diversity is reflective of other areas such as culture, economy, and business. The Tofflers further advise providers that if we want to strengthen the family and make the home a central institution, we must accept diversity and return important tasks to the household.

Monitoring of many of the physiologic functions that were followed in acute care settings now occur via phone and modem. Medication administration from a distance is now possible with programmable devices capable of storing important data trends. The control of such devices is now in patient hands, but monitoring and manipulation by health professionals can occur from afar with today's technology. The future promises further expansion of patient care from a distance.

## Informed Consumers

Health care consumers want to be much more informed and not placed in the subordinate position of always asking for answers. Health care providers no longer have the time or comprehensive knowledge skills to be gatekeepers of patient information. Instead, client-focused community health sites on the World Wide Web provide virtual space for health care providers to learn more and clients to become more inquisitive and informed (again, in that third wave.). Examples of this can be found at the "Netwellness" site that was recently established at the University of Cincinnati (http://ovchin.uc.edu/) and at one of the Department of Defense's patient education sites (www.bce.army.mil).

The World Wide Web has expanded practice and patient arenas and made resources more available to all. The Web allows for access of resources that were typically accessed only by research universities, so that today all practitioners can receive the most current information. In addition, clients, including those challenged by disabilities, can expand their outreach to other patients and families who have already dealt with the same problems. Advanced search engines are being revised daily, and although present Web sites might contain only databases, the futuristic possibility exists for all of these to interrelate at a practitioner's command. Table 11-2 lists popular Web addresses.

## Expert Nurses

What about the nurse expert in this third wave arena? Thompson and others (1990) define expertise as a "phenomenon consisting of skill, knowledge, and the best possible performance in a limited field or endeavor." They point out that the essence of expertise is an ability to accurately perform the required mental or physical activity rapidly and with the fewest number of cues, a skill that develops over time as a result of relevant clinical and educational experience. Nothing about those statements leads one to believe that technologic expert systems could not be used to aid the clinician. The difficulty has been in creating an expert system that is equal to the level of decision making of our expert clinicians.

## TABLE 11-2 WWW Bookmark Sampler

| WWW Site | URL |
|---|---|
| Achoo-On-Line Healthcare Services | http://www.achoo.com/ |
| Agency for Health Care Policy and Research | http://www.ahcpr.gov/ |
| Aids Clinical Trials Information Service | http://www.actis.org/actihome.html |
| American Association of Colleges of Nursing | http://www.aacn.nche.edu/ |
| American Heart Association | http://www.amhrt.org/ |
| American Journal of Nursing | http://www.ajn.org |
| American Nurses Association | http://www.nursingworld.org/ |
| Centers for Disease Control (CDC) | http://www.cdc.gov/ |
| Chronic IllNet | http://www.calypte.com/ci_home.html |
| CU-SeeMe | http://www.goliath.wpine.com/cu-seeme.html |
| Genome Data Base | http://gdbwww.gdb.org/gdb/ideo/docs/ideogram.html |
| Hepatitis Information Network | http://www.hepnet.com/ |
| Martindale's Health Science Guide | http://www-sci-lib.uci.edu/HSG/HSGGuide.html |
| Morbidity-Mortality Weekly Report (MMWR) | http://www.cdc.gov/epo/mmwr/mmwr.html |
| Mother's Voices—United to End AIDS | http://www.mvoices.org/ |
| Multiple Sclerosis Foundation | http://www.icanet.net/msf/ |
| National League for Nursing | http://www.nln.org |
| NIH Clinical Center Nursing Department Standards of Practice | http://www.cc.nih.gov/nursing/standards.html |
| National Institute for Nursing Research | http://www.nih.gov/ninr/ |
| National Library of Medicine | http://www.nlm.nih.gov/ |
| New England Journal of Medicine | http://www.nejm.org/ |
| New York University Videos of Various Cardiac Surgical Procedures | http://www.cvsurg.med.nyu.edu/cvsurg/videolib/video.html |
| NetWellness—University of Cincinnati | http://www.ovchin.uc.edu/ |
| OncoLink—University of Pennsylvania Cancer Resource Center | http://www.cancer.med.upenn.edu/ |
| Research-It! | http://www.iTools.com/research-it/ |
| Sigma Theta Tau International | http://www.stti.iupui.edu/ |
| University of Maryland—Nursing and Health Related Web Links | http://nursing.ab.umd.edu/offices/opds/b&i/uomweb.htm |
| University of Oklahoma Health Sciences Center Cardiovascular Center | http://www.wailer.vahsc.uokhsc.edu/ |
| University of Washington—NW Regional Spinal Cord Injury System | http://weber.u.waghington.edu/rehab/sci/ |
| U.S. Department of Defense | http://www.bce.army.mil |
| Vanderbilt Pediatric Interactive Digital Library | http://www.mc.Vanderbilt.Edu/peds/pidl/ |
| Virtual Hospital | http://indy.radiology.uiowa.edu/ |
| Virtual Library | http://www.ohsu.edu/cliniweb/wwwvl/ |
| Virtual Nursing College | http://www.langara.bc.ca/vnc/ |
| The Visible Human Project | http://www.nih.gov/research/visible/visible_human.html |
| The Whole Brain Atlas | http://www.med.harvard.edu/AANLIB/home.html |

## Virtual Reality

A futuristic look would not be complete without recognizing the current and advanced capabilities of virtual reality. As practice arenas grow outside the bounds of typical institutions, the capability for peer review of clinical practice becomes even more complicated. A clinical simulation is one way to remedy this situation. Before this time, simulations used the subjective eye of the camera to bring one view into the nurse's field of vision. What has been missing has been the capability of controlling movement and tasks so that independent decisions can be made. Virtual reality simulations offer real-world models that can be manipulated by the participants. Certification and registration examinations can best be offered in this open, boundless arena of virtual reality.

As practice areas become less bound by physical space or time, new opportunities and possibilities will emerge that have never before been imagined. Growth, change, and learning will occur at phenomenal rates. Although this may seem both exciting and frightening, the use of information technology in this third wave to generate new nursing knowledge may well be the tool nursing has needed to advance the profession of nursing while maintaining core values and purposes.

# CONCLUSION

Neither nursing practice nor the integration of technology is a stagnant process. As nursing struggled to define its own practice, there emerged needs of such magnitude that they could be met only with the use of technology. At the same time, technology applications were building at a phenomenal rate, which made it difficult for nurses to stay current in their implementation strategies. Furthermore, authors such as Zwolski (1989) point out that technology at its incomplete and imperfect stages creates another set of problems. He mentions iatrogenic illnesses created by technologic advances, loss of patient autonomy, and prolonging life to be spent in ill health as three examples. It is no wonder that the practicing nurse, already stressed by the demands of today's workplace, can feel the tension created from this new merger of practice and technology, which was inevitable and is irrevocable.

This chapter described the changing clinical practice needs over the last few decades, highlighted major areas of emphasis, and showcased technology examples and challenges. The task-oriented and information management aspects of practice grew from second wave thinking. Many of the applications have the potential to continue their growth to the third wave thinking described by the virtual practice arena. Once the practice-based needs of nursing are determined and the possible roles of technology are identified, one can conclude that autonomous nursing practice might never have been possible without the merging of clinical practice and technology. As third wave thinkers we have to continue to create, to question, and to innovate.

This futuristic view of nursing practice merged with technology sounds exciting and challenging. Martha E. Rogers spoke in 1991 at the second annual Spero Lectureship on "Nursing Prepares for the 21$^{st}$ Century: The Science and Art of Irreducible People." Perhaps she summed up the situation best with her autographed message on that program cover. The message read, "Betsy, Drive on—The view is great—Martha E. Rogers." Perhaps more telling was her message to her former doctoral student Dr. Trangenstein, which read, "Trish, See you in space!" Please join us in our quest for "third wave" contributions to nursing practice.

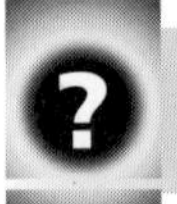

## *Discussion Exercises*

1. The chapter describes first, second and third wave thinking. What do you think will be the fourth wave?

2. What additional problems are inherent in using information technology in practice?
3. How can technology be used to teach nurses new skills?

## References

American Nurses Association: *Nursing: a social policy statement,* Kansas City, Mo, 1980, The Association.

Ball MJ and others: What is informatics and what does it mean for nursing? In Ball MJ and others, editors: *Nursing informatics: where caring and technology meet,* ed 2, New York, 1995, Springer-Verlag.

Bulechek GM and others: Nursing interventions classification (NIC): a language to describe nursing treatments. In *Nursing data systems: the emerging framework,* Washington, DC, 1995, American Nurses Publishing.

Gingrich N: A citizen's guide to the twenty-first century. Foreword in Toffler A, Toffler H: *Creating a new civilization: the politics of the third wave,* Atlanta, 1995, Turner.

Graves JR: A research-knowledge system (ARKS) for storing, managing, and modeling knowledge from the scientific literature, *Adv Nurs Sci* 13(2):34, 1990.

Graves JR, Corcoran S: The study of nursing informatics, *Image J Nurs Sch* 21(4):227, 1989.

Hudgings C: The Virginia Henderson International Nursing Library: improving access to nursing research databases. In Arnold JM, Pearson GA, editors: *Computer applications in nursing education and practice,* New York, 1992, National League for Nursing.

Lang NM and others: Toward a national database for nursing practice. In *Nursing data systems: the emerging framework,* Washington, DC, 1995, American Nurses Publishing.

Martin KS, Scheet NJ: The Omaha system: nursing diagnoses, interventions, and client outcomes. In *Nursing data systems: the emerging framework,* Washington, DC, 1995, American Nurses Publishing.

Nightingale, F: *Notes on nursing: what it is and what it is not,* New York, 1859, Dover.

Saba V: Home health care classifications (HHCCs): nursing diagnoses and nursing interventions. In *Nursing data system: the emerging framework,* Washington, DC, 1995, American Nurses Publishing.

Saba V, McCormick KA: *Essentials of computers for nurses,* Philadelphia, 1986, JB Lippincott.

Thompson CB and others: Expertise: the basis for expert system development, *Adv Nurs Sci 13*(2): 1, 1990.

Toffler A: *Future shock,* New York, 1970, Random House.

Toffler A: *The third wave,* New York, 1980, Bantam Books.

Toffler A: *Powershift: knowledge, wealth and violence at the edge of the 21st century,* New York, 1990, Bantam Books.

Toffler A, Toffler H: *Creating a new civilization: the politics of the third wave,* Atlanta, 1995, Turner.

Warren JJ, Hoskins LM: NANDA's nursing diagnosis taxonomy: a nursing database. In *Nursing data systems: the emerging framework,* Washington, DC, 1995, American Nurses Publishing.

Werley HH and others: The nursing minimum data set (NMDS): a framework for the organization of nursing language. In *Nursing data systems: the emerging framework,* Washington, DC, 1995, American Nurses Publishing.

Yoder ME: Computerized nursing information systems: benefits, pitfalls, and solutions. In Arnold JM, Pearson GA, editors: *Computer applications in nursing education and practice,* New York, 1992, National League for Nursing.

Zwolski K: Professional nursing in a technical system, *Image J Nurs Sch 21*(4):238, 1989.

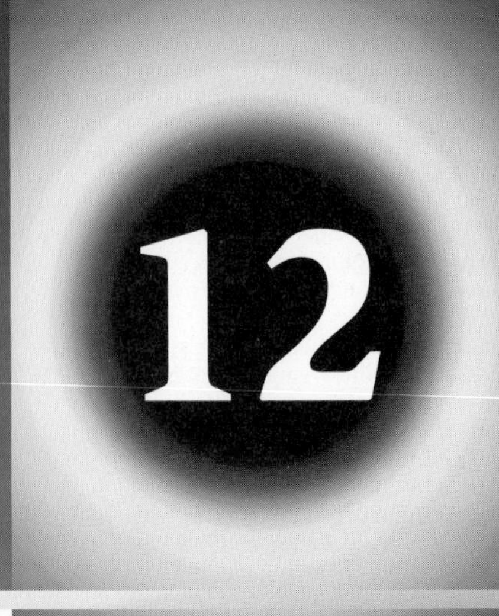

# 12 Using Technology to Teach

**Helen R. Connors**
**Linda L. Davies**

*The electric [electronic] age . . . establishes a global network that has much the character of our central nervous system.*

**Marshall McLuhan**
Understanding Media

The gradual evolution of distance or distributed learning in the United States, defined most simply as any case in which a teacher and learner are not in the same place at the same time, started with written correspondence courses in the 1920s, followed by television courses in the 1960s. Distance learning has evolved to include the use of advanced telecommunications technology such as e-mail, live two-way video/audio courses, and World Wide Web–based courses on the Internet. Unprecedented in its distance-unifying ability, this new technology actually provides more than the tools for downloading information and timely student and faculty communications. Its use also establishes a base for developing skills in knowledge acquisition from ever-expanding electronic information sources, eliminating distance in terms of time and space as an impediment to higher education.

During the last two decades personal computers have changed our work habits, but it is the evolving telecommunications and information technology and advanced computer applications such as the Internet that will change our educational system. Just like business has driven the changes in health care, business more than government is driving the changes in education (Davis and Botkin, 1994).

Dolence and Norris (1995) present a view of higher education as a growth market that is unable to keep pace with rising demand. They project that by the year 2000 the demand for postsecondary education will increase by 20 million full-time enrollments (FTE) in the United States and by greater than 100 million worldwide. This anticipated growth will not come from traditional on-campus students but from those already in the workforce: those whose knowledge and skills need continual updating or those who need to acquire new skills for career changes.

Traditional institutions must transform if they are going to step up to the challenges of lifelong learning. Institutions need to redesign learning experiences to reflect a shift from teaching content to assisting learners to develop skills to enhance lifelong learning. Recent advances in telecommunication technologies have radically altered the world of education, greatly increasing the choices and opportunities for learners. For the purpose of this chapter, distance learners are people who, because of time, geographic, or other constraints, choose not to attend a traditional classroom. Also, this technology has application to all types of pedagogy and should not be reserved for distance learners only.

**Box 12-1**
***Student Demographics***

| Former | Future |
|---|---|
| Student | Learner/consumer |
| 18 to 22 years of age | 18 to 80 years of age |
| Front-loaded learner | Lifelong learner |
| Set body of knowledge for career | Changing workplace/changing career |
| Single responsibility | Multiple responsibilities |

## THE FORCES OF CHANGE

Education is the single most important element in our nation's future; yet old models of education no longer address the realities of most students' lives in our rapidly changing technologic and multicultural society. There are many forces behind this call for educational transformation, and central to this movement is the learner.

### Time-Out Education

Student demographics are not what they used to be (Box 12-1). Students today do not take time out for education. Education is no longer front loaded, with all of education occurring in 4 years of college. Traditional institutions of higher education were originally designed for students ages 18 to 22 years and just out of high school. Many of these students left home and other responsibilities to take time to study and develop or expand knowledge and skills necessary for their future careers.

Today students in both undergraduate and graduate programs are increasingly older. They approach academics with a set purpose, a desire for efficiency in learning, a perception of what they need to learn, and most importantly a planned set of outcomes. Many are coming to academia for an education to advance an existing career or to meet the demands of a changing workplace. For workers to remain competitive in the workforce, they must continue to learn. There is no set body of knowledge to be mastered that will sustain graduates throughout their career.

### Just-in-Time Education

Today's employees are knowledge workers rather than skilled personnel who will return to educational programs several times throughout their careers. Many major companies spend millions on employee education. These employees have family, business, and lifestyle responsibilities that do not allow them to attend full-time traditional educational programs. This is not "time-out" education but rather "just-in-time" education.

Today's students perform these other responsibilities while they attend school. Their educational needs demand quality programs, flexible scheduling, and reasonable and affordable fees (quality, access, and cost). These students want to learn what they know they need and in a way that is best for them. They perceive themselves as consumers in the purchase of their educational products. This is frequently a difficult concept for faculty to understand. Faculty often believe they know what is best for the student, and they are reluctant to customize education for the learner.

With the explosion of information, students need high-level thinking skills, strong interper-

**Box 12-2**
***Industrial Age Versus Information Age***

| Industrial Age | Information Age |
|---|---|
| Teacher franchised | Learner franchised |
| Provider driven | Individual driven |
| Time-out education | Just-in-time learning |
| Traditional courses | Unbundled learning |
| Front ended | Point of access |
| Technology push | Learning vision pull |

sonal and communication skills, and knowledge of how to obtain and use information. They need to learn the tools necessary to be successful in a fast-changing global economy. They need to be able to use advanced technologies to put data and information together to help them work smarter. Educational institutions that meet the individual's need to learn quickly and conveniently can expect to reap tremendous rewards in the years to come. Education is likely to shift to high-tech learning as opposed to low-tech lecture methods to meet these consumer demands. Box 12-2 demonstrates the changes in the delivery of education from the industrial age to the information age.

## Challenges to Change

This change in direction is not without challenges. The shift to consumer-focused, high-tech education comes at a time when government leaders and citizens are demanding, and in some states imposing, reductions in tax dollars directed toward higher education. This makes it almost impossible for some institutions to establish the needed technologic infrastructure, to purchase and maintain appropriate hardware and software, and to develop faculty to teach with technologies. However, if educators do not respond by changing the delivery of education and curricula, businesses and entrepreneurs will successfully capture this growing market.

Currently schools are lagging behind business and industry in responding to the changing world. For the most part, changes in education have been piecemeal and therefore have not made a major impact on the system as a whole.

With the advent of affordable and widely available information and telecommunication technology, a paradigm shift is expected. The shift is movement from a teacher-centered, provider-driven model to a student-centered, learner-driven model. This shift should not be technology driven, but the technology should be the value-added component to the future of pedagogy. Cybercolleges of the future will definitely be a component of mainstream education. This is not to say that traditional universities will no longer exist; however, they will become niche players in a diverse education arena.

# CREATING THE INFRASTRUCTURE

The infrastructure to support wide-spread online education involves changes for faculty, students, the curricula, and the institution. Central to the virtual university infrastructure is the implementation and support of a technologic tool set used by both faculty and students. This includes appropriate hardware, software, and connectivity. It is not sufficient to tell faculty to take their traditional lecture courses and put them on line. This would neither provide a good learning experience nor develop the changing workforce skills set. In addition, it would not be cost-effective.

Faculty need to shift their teaching styles and philosophies from that of a "sage on the stage" to that of a "guide on the side." Likewise, students need to alter their concept of the student role in order to take on the characteristics of a learner. Faculty and learners become partners in the process of education. The curriculum is student centered and learner driven as opposed to teacher centered and provider driven. Some faculty and students can adapt to this change, and others will struggle with this paradigm shift.

## Faculty Issues and Barriers

### Attitudes

For some faculty, changing their pedagogic orientation is arduous, if not impossible. They have too many years invested in the status quo and see few incentives in the current system for change, especially when this transition requires them to develop an ever-evolving set of technical skills to support their teaching activities. For the most part faculty need to develop a minimum set of technologic competencies to experience success in course delivery. Because many of these skills are new to them, their skill development must be supported. They must be afforded the time and resources to acquire basic skills and to become proficient in using those skills in their teaching. Individual faculty should be expected to independently develop their own electronic course materials, however. Generally, faculty do not have the time or the expertise to create a sustainable, scalable body of materials nor would that be a cost-effective use of their time.

### Structural Change and Support

External support for faculty without internal structural change will not lead to successful implementation of the incorporation of technology into teaching. At the University of Kansas School of Nursing, individual faculty or a team of faculty is coupled with educational or instructional technologists to successfully develop and implement Web-based instruction. Faculty are experts in content and learning outcomes, whereas the educational technologists are expert in technology hardware, software, and educational applications. Interactive learning experiences are designed and enhanced by technology. Faculty need basic skills to make good instructional design decisions as they develop, implement, and troubleshoot the course materials. The educational technologist provides the higher-level technical skills that include up-to-date applications.

This team approach allows faculty to participate in developing good learning examples that pique their interest and stimulate creativity. Once a few faculty experience this success in teaching, others will become interested. Faculty who use technology to teach find that they assume a multitude of roles as they interact with students. Faculty are *architects* as they design learning programs; *navigators* as they help advise students in their course of study; *instructors* when they lecture; *mentors* when they help students feel a sense of connectedness to the world; and *evaluators* and *certifiers* as they decide to grant grades or degrees (Massey and Zemsky, 1997).

### Reward System

The existing traditional reward system in academia also poses a barrier to change. The reward system in academia supports the status quo. Faculty are rewarded for bringing in external funding through research or program grants. What the system needs is to redefine evaluation and reward criteria to establish a major initiative that recognizes and compensates exceptional and innovative teaching that enhances productivity and contains cost. Without these incentives there is little motivation for change.

### The Committee System

Another roadblock to change is the academic environment, which endorses decision making by committee. Adoption of change by the collective faculty is a difficult and time-consuming process. Frequently the committee system tends to support the old way of doing things. This inability to collectively and efficiently make decisions often does not promote a climate for change.

## Student Issues and Barriers

Distance learners are people who, because of time, geographic, or other constraints, choose not to attend a traditional classroom. Financial constraints, family obligations, or work requirements may point to distance learning as an appropriate way to meet educational goals. Distance learners come from a wide variety of backgrounds and age groups. They turn to distance learning largely for convenience. These learners need to be highly motivated to succeed, serious about their educational and career goals, and self-motivated and disciplined enough to incorporate study time into busy daily lives.

Learners must have a basic technology skill set and access to appropriate technology hardware and software required for accessing course materials and assignments, but they also must accept other responsibilities. They must accept responsibility for the operation of their equipment. They must be willing to embrace new educational technologies and adapt to a new learning environment. They must be willing to assess their own competencies and to customize their own learning activities to accommodate their personal goals, learning styles, and abilities.

This new climate is learner franchised and individual driven; however, the teacher is still essential. Technology will not replace or devalue the human experience required in the educational process but will enhance the learning process by empowering students to have greater control over the acquisition of knowledge and skill. Students will learn more easily, enjoyably, and successfully. They will have the ability to learn on their own and at their own pace (Gates, 1996). Students who are not self-motivated and willing to assume responsibility and accountability for their own learning will not fare well in this revolutionized learning environment.

## Curricular Issues and Barriers

For the recent past, educators and employers have suggested that learning be redefined to instill concepts of critical thinking, enhanced communications, teamwork, interactive learning, experiential learning, and lifelong learning. This means we must rethink the traditional teacher-centered model of education with a primary focus on the classroom lecture as a means of transferring knowledge. This faculty-centered infrastructure is based on the abilities and interests of faculty who then build courses, curricula, teaching strategies, and assignments around those interests. The student is little more than a passive recipient of the teacher-defined processes and outcomes. This traditional model is expensive to maintain and is not capable of meeting the learning needs for citizens of the new millennium. It is too restrictive, too passive, and often inappropriate (Twigg, 1994). Students are treated as hostages rather than customers, told to take a course at a designated time, in a certain classroom, for a set fee, from an assigned professor.

Unbundling teaching from the traditional course and fee structure creates modular-like learning packages to better meet learners' needs for customized, flexible, and appropriately priced instruction. Such an arrangement is imperative for education to be individualized and customer focused. Only then will self-directed learners be free to choose not only what they want to learn but also when and how they want to learn it. Once education is not tied to traditional courses or programs of study within a single institution, the door is open for collaboration among institutions.

Twigg (1996) calls for the development of a National Learning Infrastructure (NLI) based on collaborative efforts among institutions. Driven by powerful social and economic needs, the NLI is well on its way to becoming a reality. The NLI will create the infrastructure necessary to connect institutions utilizing advanced telecommunication technology. The NLI is one of the fundamental building blocks behind the formation of the Western Governors Virtual University (WGU). WGU will offer accredited programs through numerous institutions, but it has no physical campus of its own. The question is: Will the higher education environment be prepared to take advantage of these opportunities?

## Institutional Issues and Barriers

The postsecondary education system in the United States is being challenged to be accountable for the competencies and successes of their graduates. Supporters of higher education are asking tough but fitting questions about accountability, appropriateness of curriculum, value versus costs, relevance of grades, and faculty workloads and performance indicators. The motives behind these questions are the escalating costs of higher education coupled with the public's concern about quality and access.

Increasingly institutions are being asked to educate more students without spending more dollars. Because approximately 80% of the cost of higher education is personnel, faculty productivity is seen as the problem, and technology-based education is frequently seen as the solution. Technology helped businesses to become more efficient; why would this not be the same for schools? Although colleges and universities would like to pour money into technologies, most are not in a position to do so. In addition, technology alone is not the answer.

The transformation to technology-based education takes time and commitment. The cultural climate to support the changes in faculty, students, and curricula as previously addressed must be actualized by the institution. Frequently tradition gets in the way of this radical culture change. It is not easy to change an institution or culture, especially one that is steeped in years of tradition.

Many institutions pride themselves that they are the oldest, most stable, and most unchanged institutions in the world (Pelton, 1996). What they are forgetting is that the world has changed and that to be part of it they need to join the information revolution to make education more relevant to societal needs and to the vision of a global economy. The time for change is at hand because new advanced technologies can revolutionize, as well as customize, education. Revolutionized tactics have the potential for capturing the growth market of nontraditional learners and increasing revenue streams. If revised teaching strategies are implemented, institutions will be able to do more with more.

## THE TECHNOLOGY TOOL SET: NOW AND THE FUTURE

Advanced technology offers the academic institutions new delivery options. Computers are a viable alternative because of their affordability, speed, and capacity.

### Problems

The amounts of information that can be sent over telephone lines or networks have increased dramatically in the last few years, and the amount of information and speed of transmitting it are projected to continue to increase. The World Wide Web, e-mail, listservs, and other tools are readily accessible and user friendly. With this expansion of available information and the ever-evolving technology tool set to access and disseminate information, it is imperative that teaching strategies be adapted to maximize the current technologies and prepare for the future. The traditional methods such as lecture and classroom discussions are too limited, by themselves, for today's world. When these strategies are appropriate, lecture and group discussions can be conducted on line but in a different way.

Today's advances in instructional technology are minimal compared with what the future has in store. The merging of video, telephone, virtual reality simulators, and computer technology will provide opportunities for innovative changes. These changes are foretold by the merging of industry giants. The cost of the future device (a combination of the computer, television, and telephone) will be drastically less expensive and more powerful than what exists today. The Telecommunications Act of 1996 provided the impetus for increased availability and affordability of services in rural and insular areas of our country. New technologies will be readily available in homes, libraries, schools, and businesses. Wireless communications will further expand availability to deliver anywhere, anytime access.

The Internet of the 1990s will be considered in its infancy compared with the future. The Next Generation Internet (NGI), currently under study by Aimes Research Corporation, will be a million times faster than home computer modems and a thousand times faster than current business lines. As video and audio capabilities improve, video and audio conferencing via the desktop computer and the Internet will become commonplace, reducing the need for large room-based video conferencing facilities. Content on the Internet will continue to expand exponentially, and security issues of the present will be resolved.

As the technologies improve, simulators and virtual reality will become critical components of education. As simulators become compellingly realistic and real clinical practice sites become scarce, we will enter the realm of virtual reality training for health care professionals. Much like today's airline pilots are expected to spend many hours in a flight simulator, future health care professionals will be expected to log in hours of practice on human simulators. This will give health professionals a chance to gain quality experiences and to develop skills that may not be available to them in real-world situations.

The challenge of higher education is to adapt teaching strategies to maximize these new technologies. As students and employers demand workplace-relevant education, more emphasis will shift to the application of new knowledge. The question is: Are institutions of higher education ready for this paradigm shift?

## TWO VISIONS OF THE FUTURE

Although there are many catalysts calling for change in higher education, the system struggles internally to relinquish the traditional pedagogy that has been in existence for nearly 200 years. Because of this strong dichotomy in forces, the future is difficult to predict. The following two scenarios offer alternative futures for the incorporation of information and telecommunications technology in higher education.

### Probable Future Scenario

As costs of higher education continue to increase and federal support for student loans and research funds decrease, the number of colleges and universities in the United States will decline. The cost of college education is prohibitive for many families, and the return on the investment in terms of jobs with a respectable income is insignificant. Universities have been reluctant to include technology in mainstream education because of fear of losing the human value in our education process. Those that have taken the virtual leap have done it sporadically. In addition, the failure of faculty to recognize the development of multimedia software by faculty as scholarship rather than entertainment is continuing to perpetuate traditional education.

Meanwhile corporations, such as General Electric, IBM, Motorola, and Microsoft, are offering associate and baccalaureate degrees through the use of technology and digital learning networks. These institutions provide fertile training grounds for acquisition of skills required in today's job market. Many students are seeing this as a more marketable alternative to the traditional education system; therefore enrollment in traditional universities is drastically declining.

Much to the delight of the traditional institutions, accreditors continue to scrutinize these corporate training programs. Although faculty are leaving academia for positions as educators in corporate training programs, there is still concern that these corporate institutions are too narrowly focused on job training; hence the depth and breadth of university education is being lost.

The colleges and universities that have survived are niche players in the higher education market. Mergers and acquisitions among colleges and universities are commonplace and are seen as mechanisms for survival. The consortia approach coupled with the use of telecommunications and information technologies generally offers universities economies of scale; however, some students and some parents continue to protest the use of technology as the primary learning tool. The competition for students is tremendous as institutions cast a wider net to recruit. Distance learning technologies are being used to cost effectively capture these new markets, including the global marketplace.

### Preferable Future Scenario

We have come to realize that the core principles of higher education, the creation and dissemination of knowledge and the socialization of individuals into the community of learning, are not confined only to the traditional classroom environment. The technology tool set produced to accommodate the information age has transformed higher education and enhanced the core principles of the university. Education in the information era is driven by business rather than government, and we have learned to combine the best of business and the best of the university to enhance outcomes and increase market share.

Traditional universities continue to exist but are fewer in number than in the past. These institutions cater to traditional students and use technology sparingly to augment the learning process devised in lecture, labs, and seminars. Generally speaking, these institutions are small in number, have a religious affiliation, and primarily focus on social sciences and the humanities. To keep the cost to consumers reasonable and affordable, many faculty have had to increase productivity by teaching more, at the expense of conducting their own research. Fortunately for these faculty seeking promotion, research and traditional publications have become less important, whereas teaching success and the development of digital teaching tools are viewed as more significant and are considered another form of scholarship. Of course tenure, a thing of the past, is no longer an option for anyone.

Other academic institutions have expanded their market to incorporate the nontraditional student. Some of these institutions have joined forces with corporations to deliver relevant onsite and online education to employees. Educating employees through the process of lifelong learning has become big business. Many institutions depend on this source of income to make up for major cutbacks in government funding.

Another major source of income for academic institutions is their alumni, specifically alumni who return to school for updating and refresher courses. To this extent major institutions are assuming risk by offering graduates a lifelong learning contract by which, for a designated fee, the institution guarantees to keep graduates current in their chosen field for the rest of their lives. Many alumni find this package very attractive. Quickly, universities found that there were many additional benefits to offering free or inexpensive access to their computer network for alumni. Networking alumni affords institutions an opportunity to tap graduates to assist with education of current students and bridges the gap between academia and business (University of Michigan, 1996).

Many faculty have incorporated technology into their repertoire of teaching strategies. Those who have mastered the technology and created courses using online information and multimedia technology have reaped the rewards. This is especially true when institutions have taken on the role of acting as a production company and distributor of the educational product created by faculty and featuring faculty as stars. The star system has increased competition among faculty, and a few superstars are demanding and getting exorbitant salaries and bonuses (University of Michigan, 1996). Faculty are rewarded for quality, innovative, cost-effective, and efficient education that increases the number of students enrolled.

## CONCLUSION

Today, nontraditional students are outnumbering traditional students. Technology has opened doors to education that were not possible in the past, for example, the opportunities for learners to interact with other cultures and learn firsthand about global economies. We are only beginning to see the potential of teaching with technologies. The future holds much promise in the discovery of new horizons for academia, if we can only let go of the shore.

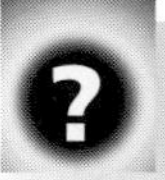

## *Discussion Exercises*

1. Imagine you are creating a virtual "school" of nursing. Describe your program, for example, entry requirements, structure of courses, clinical learning, graduation requirements, faculty, and administrative structure.
2. The chapter discusses traditional and nontraditional students. Identify some of the

problems inherent in meeting the needs of both groups of students. Suggest some strategies to resolve these problems.

3. The chapter proposes radical changes in higher education. How likely is the preferable future? Explain.

## References


Davis S, Botkin J: *The monster under the bed,* New York, 1994, Touchstone.

Dolence M, Norris D: *Transforming higher education: a vision of learning in the 21st century,* Ann Arbor, Mich, 1995, Society for College and University Planning.

Gates B: *The road ahead,* New York, 1996, Penguin USA.

Massy WF, Zemsky R: *Using information technology to enhance academic productivity,* (http://www.educom.edu/program/nlii/keydocs/massy.html), 1997.

Pelton JN: Cyberlearning vs the university: an irresistible force meets an immovable object, *Futurist,* p 17, November-December, 1996.

Telecommunications Act, Pub L No. 104-104, 110 stat 56, 1996.

Twigg C: *Academic productivity: the case for instructional software,* (htpp://www.educom.edu/program/nlii/keydocs/broadmoor.html), 1996.

Twigg C: The need for a national learning infrastructure, *EDUCOM Rev,* (http://www.educom.edu/program/nlii/keydocs/monograph.html), 1994.

University of Michigan: *Vision 2010: southeast quadrant scenario,* (http://www.si.umich.edu:80/V2010/scen-se.html), 1996

# 13 Faculty Practice

**Jane S. Norbeck**
**Diana L. Taylor**

*Leap and the net will appear.*

**Julia Cameron**
Artist

## EVOLUTION OF FACULTY PRACTICE

Key developments in the evolution of faculty practice serve as a bridge from the past to the present and the future. The need for faculty practice is linked to the divergence between education and service that arose in the 1940s when nursing education moved into educational institutions. Since that time an evolving dialogue regarding the relationship between education and service has occurred. The nursing literature in the 1970s and 1980s reflected the dominant theme or rationale for faculty practice, which was to maintain faculty members' clinical competency to support their teaching role. This limited goal of maintaining clinical competency was usually met through individualized arrangements for volunteer or salaried practice, and often only a small subset of faculty participated. The exception to this individualized approach occurred in a few schools of nursing that implemented highly structured models to link education and service, such as the unification and collaborative models described by Fagin (1985).

Faculty practice is not a new activity within schools of nursing; however, a qualitative shift in the purpose and scope of faculty practice emerged in the early 1990s that coincided with legislation extending prescriptive authority and reimbursement for advanced practice nursing. Table 13-1 summarizes attributes of faculty practice from the past and present and suggests qualities for the preferable future. It should be noted that the descriptions in this table are oversimplified to depict the relative emphasis that prevailed during each period; in reality overlap exists in many of these attributes across the periods.

**TABLE 13-1 Faculty Practice: Past, Present, and Future**

| Attributes | Past | Present/Probable Future | Preferable Future |
|---|---|---|---|
| **Practice Sites and Roles** | Faculty assume traditional roles in existing clinical agencies or hospitals on a salaried or volunteer basis. | Faculty participate in autonomous and interdependent roles in nurse-managed or nurse-owned practices that are similar in structure to existing practices in the health care system. | Faculty are part of an interdisciplinary team in creative, nontraditional models of service delivery developed to meet the full range of health-related needs of a population. |
| **Recipients of Services** | Recipients are clients within the agency or hospital. | The focus of many nursing centers and practices is underserved groups. | Recipients are defined by the populations served. |
| **Goals and Rationale** | Participating in clinical practice is a way for faculty to maintain their clinical competence. | In addition to maintaining clinical competence, practices contribute to (1) meeting multiple missions of the school (teaching, research), and (2) demonstrating and testing nursing models of care. | In addition to the goals of current practices, future practices will provide comprehensive outcome data of value to the health care delivery system and to the profession. |
| **Outcomes and Benefits** | Engagement in practice enhances the quality of clinical teaching for students. | Practices (1) contribute to the teaching and research missions by providing clinical placement sites, access to patients for research, and revenue for programs; and (2) provide nursing models of care to showcase and evaluate, while yielding clinical and cost outcome data in selected areas. | Scope of practices provide comprehensive clinical and cost outcome data on nursing roles and services to inform changes in the health care delivery system. Exemplary models of care enable validation of nursing interventions and identification of best practices. |

**TABLE 13-1 Faculty Practice: Past, Present, and Future—cont'd**

| Attributes | Past | Present/Probable Future | Preferable Future |
|---|---|---|---|
| **Technical Challenges** | Contracts for salary coverage or for joint appointments are negotiated. | Business plans and faculty practice plans are developed; payment for services through fee-for-service or through contracts is negotiated; and practices are converted to managed care. | Information systems with common databases that include input, process, and outcome variables relevant to nursing care are developed. |
| **Organizational Challenges** | | | |
| *Faculty Roles* | Except in a few models, faculty engage in practice as an additional activity. | A variety of models allows some integration of practice with teaching and/or research roles, but some role fragmentation persists. | Practice, teaching, and research in faculty roles are fully integrated. |
| *Promotion criteria* | Practice is unrelated to academic advancement. | Involvement in practice is increasingly expected and incorporated into academic advancement criteria in some settings. | The "scholarship of application" is included in criteria for academic advancement. |
| *Alignment of organizational structures of academia and practice* | Nursing service and education links at the level of administration, followed by joint appointments of faculty and clinicians. | Independent faculty practices exist with limited collaboration between service and education. New forms of faculty practice funding beyond federal grants stabilize faculty practice programs. Faculty practice plans formalize the relationship of clinical practice as both a revenue generating activity and a faculty expectation or responsibility. | Organizational support exists for faculty practice at the level of the individual faculty and faculty practice program. Faculty practice program funding is integrated into school/department budget. Diverse sources of funding stabilize these programs. |

## FACULTY PRACTICE MODELS: PRACTICE SITES AND ROLES

Recent models of faculty practice provide for a high level of engagement in practice with greater autonomy to design and control the practice than was possible in earlier models, which required accommodation to the demands of the large medical center operation or the clinical agency. These current models range from contracts to provide a specific nursing intervention (e.g., breast-feeding consultation) or specific services for a defined population (e.g., women's health services in a student health program) to the provision of primary care through a nursing center or within a managed care environment. The Faculty Practice Committee of the National Organization of Nurse Practitioner Faculties defined faculty practice broadly: "Faculty practice includes all aspects of the delivery of nursing service through the roles of clinician, educator, researcher, consultant, and administrator" (Potash and Taylor, 1993).

Regardless of how narrow or broad the definition of faculty practice, most schools of nursing will build or expand practice into education through a variety of faculty practice activities. Although modern faculty practice began with the unification model, in which nursing educators linked with hospital-based nurses (Barnard, 1983; Christman, 1982; Grace, 1981), future models of faculty practice will emerge, developed mostly by advanced practice nursing faculty.

These new models can be distinguished by *structural types* (nursing centers, joint appointments, faculty development), *faculty roles* (teacher, practitioner, administrator, consultant), *specialty practice* (community health, elder care, primary care, school health, midwifery services, anesthesia services, symptom management), or *administrative aspects* (volunteer model, collaborative arrangements, revenue-generating model, contractual model). Certainly some of these typologies will overlap in any one faculty practice (Taylor, 1996). The probable future involves the expansion of these current models implemented in a few leading institutions to widespread development of similar faculty practices in schools of nursing across the country.

### Faculty Practice Models for the Preferable Future

In addition to the expansion of autonomous practices with strong nursing leadership, models for the preferred future will be increasingly interdisciplinary in design, with multiple models of leadership based on expertise. These practices will transcend current approaches to health care by developing effective ways to respond to the full range of factors that affect health status, such as poverty, addiction, and violence.

### Nursing Centers

Nursing centers have had significant impact on the development of practice models in nursing. They have created opportunities for faculty to design nursing models of care that transcend the biomedical model of care to provide services to underserved groups. As such, these centers serve as a conceptual bridge between the past and the future because of their idealistic qualities.

In her chapter in the *Annual Review of Nursing Research,* Riesch (1992) defines nursing centers based on the results of a Delphi survey.

> Nursing centers are organizations that provide direct access to professional nurses who offer holistic client-centered health services for reimbursement. With the use of nursing models of health, professional nurses in nursing centers diagnose and treat human responses to potential and actual health problems. . . . Services are targeted to individuals and groups whose health needs are not being met (e.g., the poor, women, elderly, minorities) by current systems . . . .

Frenn and others (1996) document the positive outcomes from nursing centers related to student learning, client changes, changes in health status, client satisfaction, cost effectiveness, and quality of care. Future challenges for the success of nursing centers include securing stable funding; developing data sets that will be useful for the practice and for research; and outlining policy issues affecting nursing centers, such as prescriptive authority and reimbursement policies for nursing services.

Faculty practice programs of the future also will emphasize continuity of care across practice sites; increased multidisciplinary integration of practice, education, and research; improved access to early preventive care resulting in fewer hospitalizations; and increased focus on health promotion and education activities. Many schools of nursing have implemented one or more of these futures. At Columbia University School of Nursing, nurse practitioner faculty provide care for patients in both ambulatory and inpatient areas where they have been granted full hospital privileges in a major teaching hospital (Auerhahn, 1997).

## GOALS AND OUTCOMES OF FACULTY PRACTICE

In tracing faculty practice from the past through the present to the future, it can be seen that the dominant benefit or contribution of faculty practice evolved from the level of the individual faculty member in the past, to the institutional or school level in the present, and is moving toward the level of benefiting the health care delivery system and the nursing profession.

As noted earlier the main reason for participating in faculty practice in the past was to maintain the skills of the individual faculty member. Maintaining clinical competence enhances the effectiveness of clinical teaching which, in turn, benefits students. At the institutional level, as schools of nursing evaluate their investments in faculty practice, faculty practice is looked at not only as a vehicle to help faculty maintain clinical competence but also for its potential to make significant contributions to many aspects of the school's mission. Faculty practices are expected to provide clinical placement sites for student learning needs, opportunities for faculty and student research, arenas for faculty to maintain clinical competency and to integrate practice with education and research, and to generate revenue for the school (Norbeck, 1997).

### Goals and Rationale for the Preferable Future

Faculty practice goals for the preferable future should expand to include a major focus on benefits to the public through influencing policy and changing the health care delivery system. Outcome data from these practices also benefits the nursing profession as it seeks to advocate for nursing at all levels and settings. Specific endeavors to address these goals involve providing outcome data and demonstration models:

1. To make optimal use of professional nurses
2. To determine best practices along a continuum from testing specific interventions through evaluating systems of care
3. To address unmet health care needs, such as access to care for the uninsured, the provision of multidisciplinary care, and holistic approaches to care

Achievement of these future goals requires practices of greater scope than in the past. *Scope* does not necessarily mean size of practice; it refers to the capacity to develop answers of sufficient depth to influence policy and the health care delivery system. Such capacity can be gained through collaborative practices across schools of nursing and through establishing common databases for outcomes research.

### Outcomes and Benefits for the Preferable Future

Nursing faculty practices will build on nurses' strengths in health protection and health promotion, and faculty will become increasingly sophisticated in "selling" their services. In highly competitive managed care markets, faculty practices must emphasize services to specific target populations. For example, nurses have always been committed to caring for medically underserved groups, yet this dedication has had a negative impact by implying that nursing services are of value only to "second class" people. Increasingly, Medicaid eligible patients are required to choose physician-provided care by policy makers who insist that physician care is "first class" care, while rejecting the unique skills of advanced practice nurses. Marketing health care services for vulnerable populations as "intensive primary care nursing" uses the model of highly skilled, hospital-based intensive nursing care that negates the focus on second class care (Fiandt, 1997).

Edwards (1997) proposed a new model of evaluating nursing centers that will allow them to join the mainstream of providers while maintaining unique services and a community focus. Evaluation categories were derived from the requirements of regulating organizations, professional standards drawn from national accrediting bodies, rules and regulations of the Health Care Financing Administration, requirements of managed care organizations, policies and procedures of sponsoring organizations or institutions, professional standards, demands of the community, and the range of requirements of regulatory entities across the spectrum of health care delivery. This comprehensive evaluation plan assesses the nursing center in five areas:

1. Assessment and analysis of physical and environmental facilities
2. Organizational structure and governance
3. Client outcomes
4. Human resources
5. Financial processes

The future of nursing centers will depend on complete and comprehensive evaluation plans to ensure and continuously improve quality of services, to provide opportunity for health systems research and documentation of nurse practitioner practice, and to provide a database that will earn nursing credibility as members of managed care networks.

## TECHNICAL CHALLENGES IN THE EVOLUTION OF FACULTY PRACTICES

As shown in Table 13-1, just as the scope of faculty practice has developed, so has the need for a diversity of business and analytic skills expanded as well. In the past skills were needed to negotiate salary reimbursement for clinical hours at the individual level or joint appointments at the institutional level. As schools of nursing embarked on establishing autonomous practices, administrators needed skills to create comprehensive business plans, develop faculty practice plans for revenue sharing, and negotiate an ever-changing set of arrangements to gain reimbursement for clinical services. Nursing finally was granted entré into the fee-for-service environment just as that mechanism was being replaced by managed care and other capitated arrangements.

Presentations at the American Association of Colleges of Nursing (AACN) Faculty Practice Conferences focused on these new business skills (AACN, 1996). In addition, these annual conferences also include presentations on the emerging power of outcomes research for demonstrating the cost-effective value of nursing services.

### Technical Challenges for the Preferable Future

The goals for faculty practice in the preferred future will require another leap forward in technical skills, with emphasis on information systems, comprehensive clinical databases with common elements that can be shared across multiple sites, and the systematic inclusion of variables that are relevant to nursing care.

According to Palladino and Dower (1997), the absence of persuasive, large-scale databases in nursing faculty practices today is a failure not of technology but of collaboration. In the preferable future, building nursing knowledge from faculty practices will depend on the development of information systems that support school-wide missions, as well as the business of the faculty practice programs. Collaboration among the entire academic interests—research, education, practice, and administration—across multiple institutions could result in a "faculty practice data warehouse" managed by an independent association of nursing faculty practices (Palladino and Dower, 1997).

Little attention has been given to estimating the combined costs of faculty practice that integrate education and practice activities. The assumptions used by traditional cost accounting methods have provided imprecise approaches to understanding the costs of faculty practice. In the future new cost-finding methods that can analyze the processes of faculty practice will be applied. Storfjell (1997) describes one such cost-finding method, called *activity-based costing (ABC)*, and suggests its application to faculty practice cost analysis. According to Storfjell (1997), ABC can provide valuable information for faculty practices at the macro level (department or college) and within the faculty practice program by accurately determining costs of services and processes, targeting high-cost processes, and providing indicators for monitoring improvement.

## ORGANIZATIONAL CHALLENGES

In spite of the flourishing interest in faculty practice and persistent attempts to integrate practice with teaching and scholarly activities, practice has not always meshed easily with faculty roles. Practice contributes to scholarship and could or should promote the goals of academia and advancement within the academic system. On the other hand, role fragmentation and work overload result when faculty members attempt to address teaching and practice separately within the different social and bureaucratic structures of the school and health care delivery systems.

Presently, many faculty are expected to participate in faculty practice plans as a condition of employment and as part of their workload (Rudy and others, 1995) but with little attention paid to the match between faculty and academic organization. From the perspective of the faculty nurse as a consumer, Pesut and Misener (1997) have proposed a decision guide for prospective faculty practitioners that incorporates multiple logical levels of consideration (environments, behaviors, capabilities, values and beliefs, identity, and level of faculty-organizational match). For example, current environments are ripe with opportunity, and the organization needs a cadre of faculty who are motivated to engage in faculty practice (the behavior) and who have the capabilities necessary for doing so. But attending to the environment, behavior, and capability levels without attending to values, beliefs, identity, and mission can unbalance the system. In the preferable future faculty and administrators will use decision models like the one developed by Pesut and Misener that include expanded considerations of person and environment. Increased specificity in planning for faculty practice will align faculty nurses with the right organizations to maximize appropriate skilled matches and professional goals.

### Organizational Challenges in the Preferable Future

In the future faculty will be working in practice groups that will require a high degree of group adherence or commitment to group ideals, bylaws, or practice policies. Individual faculty and nursing faculty practice organizations will need to develop skills that support the development of group adherence. These skills are similar to community activism in which individuals form alliances for support, shared risk taking, and to achieve mutual goals (Fiandt, 1997). Group adherence assumes the acceptance of social responsibility and political activism for the benefit of shared group goals. Essentially, nursing faculty practice groups of the future will apply knowledge and skills of professional responsibility and community activism to the provision of care.

An expanded definition of scholarship will guide faculty practices of the future. Burns (1997) applies the conceptual framework of the Carnegie Foundation Report (Boyer, 1990) to the development of academic advancement criteria that reflects the activities of nursing faculty practitioners. The Boyer Report (1990) suggests that the current definition of academic scholarship is narrow, stunts the full potential of higher education, and has limited the commitment to service. Boyer recommends that scholarship be redefined into four domains—scholarship of discovery, scholarship of integration, scholarship of application, and scholarship of teaching—allowing broader criteria for academic advancement. Scholarship of application has been considered by Burns (1997) to be relevant to clinical practice by nursing faculty: To be considered scholarship, practice activities relate to one's "field of knowledge and relate to, and flow directly out of, this professional activity. Such service is serious, demanding work, requiring the rigor—and the accountability—traditionally associated with research activities" (Boyer, 1990). Burns (1997) proposes an academic advancement model that is based on such an expanded definition of scholarship.

The best approach to the future of practice-education integration that balances research, teaching, and service with practice activities will be to match faculty with organizational goals. If practice is not required of all faculty, viable options for attaining career goals for faculty who do wish to practice need to be offered and included in the academic workload. Faculty practice that requires faculty members to practice what they teach at a scholarly level can be encouraged without excessive workload or to the detriment of other components of nursing education.

In the future nursing faculty will collaborate to customize academic advancement criteria to include practice as a component. Wright (1993) suggests a set of general criteria to improve teaching and develop nursing research but to maintain expertise in nursing practice. Others believe that developing a tenure and nontenure, two-track system may encourage those not interested in doctoral study to pursue faculty practice and to provide appropriate criteria to reward expert practitioners. The typical hierarchy of research, teaching, and service is reversed in the practice-education track with nursing services, patient care, and competent practice-related skills receiving the highest criteria.

Most nursing faculty agree that faculty practice should not be another criteria that must be met in addition to the others. Some schools have revised their advancement criteria in an algorithmic approach: all faculty are required to teach, with faculty choosing either research *or* practice as the next criteria on which promotion and/or tenure decisions are based. The individual faculty member can decide which model fits best with their career goals.

deTornyay (1988), a former nursing school dean, suggests that each school should develop its own list of activities to be counted toward promotion and tenure, such as:

- Delivering nursing service in school-run clinics, school-operated day care centers, and private or group practices
- Providing consultation to various health care agencies or community organizations
- Designing new models for nursing care delivery
- Conducting demonstration projects
- Designing and presenting staff development programs
- Mentoring student projects or research
- Using nursing research findings to improve patient care

Also, because part of scholarship is the transmission of knowledge, credit could be given for developing computer programs that aid students' development of critical thinking or clinical judgement skills.

## FOR WHICH FUTURE SHOULD NURSING AIM?

In this chapter the attributes described for the present era are newly won accomplishments, and many schools of nursing have not implemented such practices yet. So the immediate future essentially involves expansion of pioneering these types of faculty practices to fuller implementation. This approach involves building on the successes that have been attained, identifying deficits in the existing implementation of practice models, and meeting the technical and organizational challenges inherent in present and future models.

Yet, nursing cannot rely exclusively on expanding on the present development of faculty practices. If it does not set its sights on the preferable future, the viability of present models is in jeopardy. This is because the capacity of the present faculty practice models only hints at the cost effectiveness of nursing, whereas the models of the future will provide comprehensive data about clinical and cost outcomes. In the absence of comprehensive data—that which cannot be dismissed as just a unique exception under special circumstances—the competition between nursing and medicine will escalate because of market pressures on medicine.

The faculty practice model projected for the preferable future is even more idealistic than the nursing centers that have been developed. Like nursing centers, future models will take the needs of the population as the starting point; however, health care needs will be defined even more holistically to incorporate the impact, for example, of poverty or violence, on health status. This enhanced scope requires the involvement of many disciplines beyond those that are directly associated with health care.

## STRATEGIES FOR SUCCESSFUL FACULTY PRACTICE

### Integration

Integration of the roles of educator, researcher, and practitioner is a persistent theme among many of the successful faculty practice models. A typical example may be an advanced practice nurse faculty member who provides nursing services to individuals, families, groups, or a community and who also supervises students and conducts clinical research at the practice site. The practitioner-teacher, either directly or indirectly through other clinical colleagues, provides nursing services; students assist with client care and clinical research. Thus one clinic site or service directed to a client population assists the faculty member with all three roles. The faculty member manages the practice, teaching, and research but may collaborate with other faculty colleagues to assist with duties and tasks.

Gresham-Kenton (1989) describes Luther Christman's implementation of successful clinical nurse specialist faculty practice in a unification model recommending an "economy of effort" approach. The model includes a series of questions used by nurse specialist faculty to maximize every clinical teaching situation. Balance among each area of academic missions (scholarly activity, teaching, practice, and service) will help avert faculty burnout and role conflict.

### Collaboration

Collaboration with nurses, faculty, and other practitioners is an important factor in helping the faculty practitioner develop support networks. For instance, a nurse practitioner faculty member who manages a teen mothers' program established a cooperative relationship with a psychiatric clinical nurse specialist faculty colleague to provide mental health services to selected teens, as well as to supervise student experiences in psychiatric assessment and management (Potash and Taylor, 1993). Collaboration also may facilitate direct payment for client services through group nursing contracts with third-party payers or billing through agencies or physician colleagues.

Creativity is another theme that is incorporated in successful faculty practice models. Advanced practice nurses are creating new ways to deal with familiar problems by embracing opportunities and exhibiting a willingness to pursue solutions rather than problems.

As faculty practice moves from a volunteer or model without reimbursement (to either the school of nursing or the individual faculty member), stable funding increasingly will become an important consideration for establishing new or expanded faculty practice ventures. Early faculty practices were non–revenue-generating or grant supported; reduced funding for nursing education will require new or expanded faculty practices to be revenue generating. Furthermore, academic salaries have lagged behind community salaries for advanced practice nurses, and faculty practice revenues are used for salary supplements to retain talented advanced practice nurses.

Administrators also believe that practice revenues should provide some support to the school of nursing general funds in the same way that research grants provide some financial support. Many schools of nursing and advanced practice nursing faculty are forming new organizational structures to allow competition in the current managed care market. The business of health care has forced nursing to integrate business principles into faculty practice. The challenge to future faculty practice development will be to balance high-revenue–generating practices with those that are essential to meet community needs regardless of funding.

## Organizational Support

Organizational support from administration, as well as from faculty governance and individual colleagues, is essential. Simple changes in advancement criteria to include faculty practice can be made by nursing faculty, usually without central university approval. Certain procedures must be considered, such as faculty bylaws, voting procedures, and the establishment of a faculty practice committee, to define faculty practice and establish practice-related policy. Depending on the size of the school or faculty, the faculty practice standing committee may be separately formed or be composed of all faculty. A recognized faculty practice committee provides quality assurance, professional guidance, and policy development for advanced practice nurses who practice as part of their faculty role. This professional and policy oversight will become more and more important with the establishment of managed care arrangements.

## Faculty Practice Plan

Faculty practice plans have been developed by a number of schools of nursing to provide guidance for financial and workload considerations. Although each state or institution has different requirements for the establishment of faculty practice plans, there are some general considerations to establishing a practice plan. First, a practice plan must be developed jointly between administration and faculty. Second, a practice plan should balance faculty practice philosophy with financial considerations. And third, financial incentives and revenue distribution should be included in a formal practice plan to promote faculty practice within the school of nursing. Although some schools of nursing include only revenue generation and distribution policy and procedures in their plan, other schools have elaborated on types of practice or on workload issues related to faculty practice. However practice-related workload is codified in a school, joint decision making among administrators and faculty about workload issues is crucial to the success of advanced practice nursing faculty practice. Although an average of 1 day per week of clinical practice has been a traditional expectation, new workload models should be considered that are dependent on each school's faculty practice program.

# CONCLUSION

Faculty practice has evolved from an integral component of education in hospital diploma programs in the first half of the twentieth century to distinctly separate from teaching activities in the latter part of the century. More recently faculty practice has emerged as an essential component of both undergraduate and graduate education, especially with the advent of nurse practitioner programs. Faculty practice offers schools of nursing opportunities to address unmet health care needs, to test specific interventions, to role model effective care, and to integrate practice with education and research. As a practice discipline, nursing education and its students' future patients will be well served by integrating faculty practice into programmatic endeavors.

Further consideration of faculty practice can be found in two publications from the National Organization of Nurse Practitioner Faculties, "Faculty Practice: Models & Methods" by Potash and Taylor (1993) and "Nursing Faculty Practice: A Practical Guide" by Marion (1997), as well as the proceedings of the Faculty Practice Conferences convened by the American Association of Colleges of Nursing (1996). The historic development of faculty practice is presented in detail by Broussard and others (1996) and Taylor (1996), and critical reviews of research on faculty practice have been published in the *Annual Review of Nursing Research* in two volumes approximately a decade apart (Chickadonz, 1987; Walker, 1995).

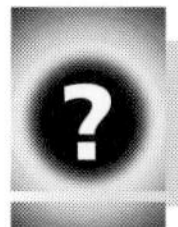

## *Discussion Exercises*

1. What are the major problems in organizing faculty practice in a school of nursing?
2. Using the problems listed in your answer to question 1, suggest a solution to each.
3. Describe the components of a successful faculty practice plan in a fictitious school of nursing.

## References


American Association of Colleges of Nursing: *The power of faculty practice,* proceedings of the AACN's 1995 and 1996 Faculty Practice Conferences, Washington, DC, 1996, The Association.

Auerhahn C: Columbia University School of Nursing faculty practice: a cross-site model. In Marion L, editor: *Nursing faculty practice: a practical guide,* Washington, DC, 1997, National Organization of Nurse Practitioner Faculties.

Barnard KE: *Structure to outcome: making it work,* Kansas City, Mo, 1983, American Academy of Nursing.

Boyer E: *Scholarship reconsidered: priorities for the professoriate,* Princeton, NJ, 1990, Carnegie Foundation for the Advancement of Teaching.

Broussard AB and others: The practice role in the academic nursing community, *J Nurs Educ* 35(2):82, 1996.

Burns C: Faculty clinical practice as a tenurable activity. In Marion L, editor: *Nursing faculty practice: a practical guide,* Washington, DC, 1997, National Organization of Nurse Practitioner Faculties.

Chickadonz GH: Faculty practice, *Annu Rev Nurs Res,* 5:137, 1987.

Christman L: The unification model. In Marriner A, editor: *Contemporary nursing management,* St. Louis, 1982, Mosby.

deTornyay R: What constitutes scholarly activities? *J Nurs Educ* 27(6):245, 1988.

Edwards J: Evaluating practice in nurse managed centers. In Marion L, editor: *Nursing faculty practice: a practical guide,* Washington, DC, 1997, National Organization of Nurse Practitioner Faculties.

Fagin CM: Institutionalizing practice: historical and future perspectives. In Barnard KE, Smith GR, editors: *Faculty practice in action,* Kansas City, Mo, 1985, American Academy of Nursing.

Fiandt K: Strategies for overcoming barriers to faculty practice. In Marion L, editor: *Nursing faculty practice: a practical guide,* Washington, DC, 1997, National Organization of Nurse Practitioner Faculties.

Frenn M and others: Symposium on nursing centers: past, present and future, *J Nurs Educ* 35(2):54, 1996.

Grace HK: Unification, re-unification: reconciliation or collaboration—bridging the education-service gap. In McCloskey JC, Grace HK, editors: *Current issues in nursing,* Boston, 1981, Blackwell Scientific.

Gresham-Kenton ML: The CNS in collaborative relationships between nursing service and nursing education: joint appointments. In Hamrick AB, Spross J, editors: *The clinical nurse specialist in theory and practice,* Philadelphia, 1989, WB Saunders.

Marion L, editor: Nursing faculty practice: a practical guide, Washington, DC, 1997, National Organization of Nurse Practitioner Faculties.

Norbeck JS: The value of faculty practice: a dean's perspective. In Marion L, editor: *Nursing faculty practice: a practical guide,* Washington, DC, 1997, National Organization of Nurse Practitioner Faculties.

Palladino M, Dower D: Nursing faculty practice: a collaborative model for information management. In Marion L, editors: *Nursing faculty practice: a practical guide,* Washington, DC 1997, National Organization of Nurse Practitioner Faculties.

Pesut D, Misener T: A decision guide for prospective faculty practitioners. In Marion L, editor: *Nursing faculty practice: a practical guide,* Washington, DC, 1997, National Organization of Nurse Practitioner Faculties.

Potash M, Taylor D: *Nursing faculty practice: models and methods,* Washington, DC, 1993, National Organization of Nurse Practitioner Faculties.

Riesch SK: Nursing centers, *Annu Rev Nurs Res* 10:145, 1992.

Rudy E and others: Faculty practice: creating a new culture, *J Prof Nurs 11*(2):78, 1995.

Storfjell J: The cost of faculty practice—the missing link. In Marion L, editor: *Nursing faculty practice: a practical guide,* Washington, DC, 1997, National Organization of Nurse Practitioner Faculties.

Taylor DL: Faculty practice: uniting advanced nursing practice and education. In Hamric AB and others, editors: *Advanced nursing practice,* Philadelphia, 1996, WB Saunders.

Walker PH: Faculty practice: interest, issues, and impact, *Annu Rev Nurs Res 13:*217, 1995.

Wright DJ: Faculty practice: criterion for academic advancement, *Nurs Health Care 14*(1):18, 1993.

# 14 Continuing Education

**Alice Kuramoto**

*The times they are a chang-in!*

**Bob Dylan**

What images do you visualize when you think of a continuing education conference? Do you think of a room of 50 to 100 nurses sitting classroom style in a dimly lit hotel meeting room listening to the keynote speaker? Picture it. The speaker is using beautiful color slides produced from PowerPoint software. The conference lasts 1 to 2 days and includes a series of plenary speakers and maybe a few concurrent sessions in the afternoon. Most of the audience sits as passive learners in the meeting room. The only time for active socialization with others is during breaks and at mealtimes. If the conference is a national one, the meeting location is usually in a large metropolitan city or at a conference resort during the midst of winter to attract nurses from the colder regions of the country. The sponsor of the continuing nursing education conference is a school or college of nursing, a hospital, a professional association, or an independent provider.

This is the scenario of a continuing education conference as it exists today. Will this scenario change in the future? Who will be providing the conference? Who will be participating? How will continuing education be delivered to participants? Will continuing education programs be similar to what we know today?

## WHAT IS CONTINUING EDUCATION?

Continuing education is defined as those professional learning experiences designed to enrich the nurse's contributions to quality health care and his or her pursuit of professional career goals (American Nurses Association, 1994). The purpose of continuing education is to build on educational and experiential bases to enhance practice, education, administration, research, or theory development to maintain and improve the health of the public. Continuing nursing education's ultimate goal is to enhance professional growth and to ensure safe and competent nursing care by improving nursing practice.

Staff development, which includes orientation and in-service in the workplace, overlaps with continuing education. Staff development focuses on learning activities that facilitate the nurse's job-related performance (see Chapter 15).

Continuing education has been used as a mechanism for quality control and to address competency issues. Learning needs to be lifelong and continuous to keep current with new knowledge and techniques (Huber, 1996). Society demands it. There is a legal mandate to practice at current standards, and in some states continuing education requirements are mandatory for relicensure. Nurses attend continuing education programs for a variety of reasons: meeting relicensure requirements for mandatory continuing education hours; meeting certification or recertification requirements; and updating knowledge and clinical skills. Thus, with the rapid changes in health care and technologic advances, there will continue to be a demand for continuing education in the future.

## THE PROBABLE FUTURE

The scenario for the probable future for continuing education will be a very competitive market with thousands of continuing education sponsors of continuing nursing and interdisciplinary education programs. There will be a rapid growth of entrepreneurial companies sponsoring continuing education conferences, repeated in cities across the country. Conferences still will be held at major hotels because such venues give participants a change from their work environment and home setting. Lecture format will still exist, with case studies increasingly used for group interactions. Most programs will be 1- or 2-day short-term courses. Fees will be very expensive to cover the high speaker costs, meeting room facilities, and the advanced audio/visual technology. Administrators will still attend these courses, but the number of staff nurses able to pay for their own continuing education courses will decline.

Nursing schools will face increasing financial pressures, so support for continuing education departments may be reduced or even eliminated, resulting in a budgetary crisis for continuing nursing education programs in academic settings. In addition, decreased enrollments, limited administrative commitment, fewer personnel, reduced support from participants' employers, and increased competition from other continuing education providers will affect academic continuing education programs. Some will not survive.

It will be imperative for continuing nursing educators to critically assess their current situations in academic settings and develop a new paradigm for survival. This can be accomplished by (1) seeking new sources of revenue other than primary dependence on registration/tuition fees, (2) developing new programming directions, and (3) reengineering a different organizational structure.

### New Sources of Revenue

There will be more pressure on the continuing education unit to seek out grants and contracts for major revenue support, compared with the old paradigm of depending on registration fees and nursing or campus revenue support. In the future continuing nursing education departments will depend less on state funds, campus funds, and school funds because of declining financial resources at the university level. Other funding sources and/or collaboration with other departments within the nursing school or other continuing education units on campus may be necessary for the future viability of all continuing education units in an academic setting. Partnerships and collaborations with other providers of continuing education will occur. Professional nursing associations, college providers, and hospital educational departments can merge resources for sponsoring selective regional or national conferences. Continuing education departments will work collaboratively with other universities, hospitals, and businesses and share resources in programming efforts. This has the added benefits of decreasing competitiveness among continuing education providers and decreasing duplication of programming

Few employers will be paying for continuing education held outside their agency. Instead, professional development funds will be used to educate their employees at their own work site. Collegiate continuing education departments will provide professional development programs for their own faculty and staff. Financial resources for faculty development will be available on campuses for updating faculty's teaching skills in using computers in distance learning and other technologic advancements in the classroom, as well as clinical skills.

## Developing New Programming Directions

A profitable future for continuing nursing education departments will occur if innovative programming and creative sources of funding are in place. Telephone and computer companies, for example, will be potential sources of funding for distance education programming. Increased use of telecommunication also will stimulate increased federal and state funding to develop and expand distance education courses.

The future in health care education emphasizes the importance of interdisciplinary education, so collaborative courses with continuing medical education and allied health education will be the norm. Interdisciplinary audiences will attend programs that present the best-quality courses. Typically, continuing medical education courses have charged higher fees for their courses than continuing nursing education courses have. In the future, course fees for interdisciplinary conferences will need to be reasonably priced for all health care providers.

## Reengineering a Different Organizational Structure

Academic nursing continuing education programs traditionally have resided within nursing schools' organizational structure. Financial pressures will require reexamination of this structure. Movement from decentralization to centralization is expected to reduce operating costs and maximize staff resources.

Consolidating and merging continuing education departments, which has already occurred in hospital education departments, will occur in academia. The primary reason is economic. For example, two weak departments that cannot survive alone could be strengthened by working together and sharing similar resources (e.g., publicity, meeting arrangements, registration). Nursing, medical, and allied health continuing education departments will merge within health science units of large teaching hospitals. This will be a positive change when planning and implementing interdisciplinary courses.

If nursing continuing education departments do not merge with other units on campuses, these departments may work collaboratively with competitor schools of nursing, especially in large metropolitan areas. For example, a consortium among four schools of nursing could be established to share in planning, marketing, implementing, and evaluating joint programs. Each school in the consortium would share financially in the profit or loss of program revenue.

Competition for the continuing education dollar will increase with more independent entrepreneurs providing continuing professional education. Collaboration and partnership will be a viable alternative for continuing nursing education to compete with for-profit entrepreneurs. Such collaboration will eliminate duplication of courses offered, as well as provide a more efficient continuing education unit by sharing human resources, financial resources, and computer services.

## THE PREFERABLE FUTURE

Visualize the following scenario of the future. Nurses will complete computerized assessment tests in their homes, offices, or learning assessment centers, where they will instantly receive their test results via electronic communication. They will automatically receive a list of suggested educational opportunities to address their weaknesses, enhance their skills, or develop new skills. Nurses will complete designated learning activities to meet their educational needs, which will be automatically recorded in a computerized continuing education portfolio. Systematic, self-managed professional development will be expected of all practicing registered nurses, who will be required to document that their continuing education activities relate directly to their practice or that they provide knowledge and skills applicable to their work environment.

### Self-Managed Professional Development

Smutz and Queeney (1990) suggested a strategy for maximizing professional growth by moving continuing professional education from an informal process to a more formal one. In the past, continuing education was undertaken on an informal basis by reading, attending conferences, and consulting with colleagues. Smutz and Queeney predict that a more formal, coherent continuing professional education strategy will be essential for the future. The continuing education activity should remedy deficiencies, foster growth, and facilitate change for professional practitioners, as well as improve daily practice. Each professional would select continuing education activities that address identified learning needs and that, when viewed collectively, represent a coherent curriculum for learning through the professional's life cycle.

The update and competence frameworks that have guided continuing education have an explicit, short-term orientation and focus on only immediate problems. This piecemeal, episodic involvement in learning will not be adequate for the future. In the preferred future the professional nurse will move away from the relatively isolated learning activities to a self-managed professional development process. Instead of focusing on maintaining minimal competence, emphasis in the future will be on maximizing the individual's potential.

The major reasons for not attending continuing education programs in the past were the absence of available programs, lack of time, and high cost. These barriers to continuing education will not be a problem in the preferable future because continuing education programs will be more accessible via computerized programming individualized to the participant, distance education technology, home study, virtual settings, and a variety of locations and program topics.

### Distance Education Technology

Nurses will no longer need to travel long distances to attend conferences. Instead there will be educational programming conducted 24 hours of the day via the Internet, similar to cable television programming. The Web TV network will provide Internet access to people without computers but with television access to an online network. Internet courses via the computer and Web TV will bring educational conferences to every nurse's living room or work place.

Virtual universities will offer a variety of topics, which also will be available to nurses around the world. A program will be available via the Internet that could be downloaded and printed for later use. Live on-site conferences will still take place at the hotels or campus facilities, but there will be more opportunities for a greater number of participants to interact with the speaker via desktop video conferencing at a designated time, somewhat similar to "pay for view" TV now available for special cable television events. Participants will pay for what they want to hear rather than paying the entire conference costs, thus making it more affordable.

Desktop video conferencing will be commonplace and cheaper to broadcast than satellite video teleconferencing. Video cameras will be built into computer systems so individuals can be viewed from their computers and see other participants as well. Picture telephones also will be an option for teleconferencing.

The challenge in the preferable future will not be access to programming but, rather, information overload. Many universities and independent providers will be competing for the same global market of participants. Marketing courses will be challenging because direct mailing of individual brochures will be obsolete; most conference brochures will be available through electronic delivery.

The continuing education director in the nursing school will play an integral role in effectively using distance education technology with adult learners and in recruiting prospective adult students into the undergraduate and graduate programs within the university. In addition, the director will be viewed as an expert in facilitating learning, developing programs, modeling principles of adult learning, and evaluating learning.

## Locations Will Change

Meeting locations will be at sites convenient to learners, such as in shopping malls, coffee houses, grocery stores, automobiles, and at their own homes. Some universities have already moved their continuing education classrooms from campus locations to downtown facilities or shopping malls. Alternative meeting room facilities attract adult learners because of easy accessibility from the freeway, more convenient parking, and more options for dining. Continuing education courses will be located anywhere there is a computer or a telephone. It could be on the beach in Hawaii, on a cruise ship, or at a mountaintop ski resort. Just as nursing clinics have moved into community neighborhoods and places where clients live, educational settings for learning will be where learners spend their time.

An increased number of independent study or home study programs will be available to nurses in audio and video CD-ROM, the Internet, and digital videocassette. Because the amount of time we spend commuting via automobiles or the rapid transit system will probably increase in the future, the nurse can use the time in transit by listening, reading, or viewing a continuing education program. Wireless telecommunication delivery systems will be the norm, so there will be no need to sit in an electronic classroom. Internet courses designed for independent learning will allow more flexibility for the learner to choose a course topic and choose the time and location for taking the course.

## Program Content Will Change

Currently, continuing education programming appears to be a smorgasbord of unrelated programs with a menu that is constantly changing in accordance with ephemeral tastes and fads (Kuramoto, 1992). The preferable future will have university-based continuing education departments offering specialty courses based on logical sequencing of courses leading toward a certificate or degree. Continuing educators will need to continuously look at the market and deliver courses that focus on the needs and goals of learners and ensure quality outcomes. Educators must be flexible and willing to make changes (Nowicki, 1996). New program topics will be developed by university continuing education departments when hospital staff development programs cannot offer these courses. The curriculum will require prerequisites for enrollment and will be in a specialty field, such as parish nursing, forensic nursing, case management, home health, ergonomics, or nursing informatics. These courses will have academic and continuing education credit offered by an academic institution. The delivery format will be through telecommunication technology for group and faculty consultations, with theory and practice components incorporated as needed.

The preferable future will encourage integration and utilization of research knowledge into nursing practice. Clinical topics at continuing education conferences will include more application and dissemination of research knowledge into the clinical work of nurses. There will be more joint research appointments of academic faculty in practice agencies where outcomes will be tested and evaluated. These partnerships will encourage an increasing number of collaborative research projects in hospitals and community settings.

There will be a shift in length of programs from a 1- or 2-day course to a 1-week institute or a 3-month curriculum. With the trend toward certification in a specialty field, there will be increased demand for more certification review courses and update courses for advanced practice nurses. Nurses will be expected to pay for a larger proportion of their own continuing education and professional development rather than depending solely on the employer's financial support.

Faculty from colleges and schools of nursing will be expected to obtain certification in their clinical nursing specialty. University-based continuing education programs will sponsor courses for faculty development in regional centers to assist faculty toward the goal of certification. With a shift in defining "scholarship" broadly to include "practice," faculty members will document evidence of their own professional development and competency in a clinical specialty field.

Post–masters certificate programs and special continuing education programs designed for nurses in different countries will be successful and profitable for the university-based continuing education programs. There will be more international faculty and student exchanges for short-term internships in different countries. Course work will be accomplished via Internet courses, followed by 2- to 4-week field experiences in a foreign country. Academic credit or continuing education credits will be acquired.

## CONCLUSION

The key factors for successful continuing education in the future will be collaboration, partnership, and integration among professional associations, regulatory agencies, higher education institutions, and employers. The sponsor or provider of continuing education must be focused on preparing the individual for lifelong learning, providing learning resources, and evaluating the overall outcomes. Lifelong learning will become a part of the pre-professional and professional curricula, as well as the continuing education operation.

The preferable future will bring a firmer financial base for continuing education sponsors who are able to provide current, usable content in a format convenient for participants. Consolidation and merging of continuing nursing education units into an interdisciplinary continuing education for the health professions will be the trend, which will produce positive outcomes for the practicing health professional. A delivery system of continuing education that promotes interdisciplinary interaction could be a powerful force in improving the quality of patient/client care.

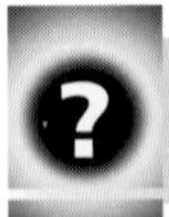

### *Discussion Exercises*

1. What are the pros and cons of maintaining an independent continuing education division versus an integrated division within the college or university?
2. Name three attributes you consider important for an administrator of a continuing education venture in a preferable future.

3. The preferable future described in the chapter suggests lifelong learning as a key component. What will be required of the learner in this model? How can schools of nursing prepare students to be lifelong learners? Be specific.

## References

American Nurses Association: *Standards for nursing professional development: continuing education and staff development,* Washington, DC, 1994, The Association.

Huber D: *Leadership and nursing care management,* Philadelphia, 1996, WB Saunders.

Kuramoto A: Present and future challenges for continuing nursing education. In *Challenge today: preparing for tomorrow, (conference proceedings)*, p 14, Calgary, Alberta, Canada, 1992.

Nowicki C: 21 predictions for the future of hospital staff development, *J Continuing Educ Nurs* 27:259, 1996.

Smutz WD, Queeney DS: Professionals as learners: a strategy for maximizing professional growth. In Cervero R and others: editors: *Visions for the future of continuing professional education,* Athens, Ga, 1990, Georgia Center for Continuing Education.

# 15 Staff Development

**Karen Kelly**

*If you think education is expensive, try ignorance.*

**Derek Bok**
President, Harvard University

There was once a time in health care organizations (then known primarily as *hospitals*) when there was a nursing education department (or nursing in-service department). There was also a training and development (T&D) office that was probably part of what was then referred to as the *personnel department*. The nursing educators and the T&D staff rarely spoke to one another except in the cafeteria, if at all. They each tended to their own domains: nursing education provided orientation and in-service education for those who worked for nursing; T&D took care of general hospital orientation and hospitalwide mandatory education (not related to clinical activities) and provided in-services to everyone outside of nursing. But rarely the twain should meet. Within progressive hospitals, nurses who worked outside the nursing department (in a few limited areas like risk management, information systems, and utilization review) would likely be invited to participate in nursing education programs. Sometimes they might be overlooked in educational programs, although not intentionally.

Then the winds of change swept through health care; nursing education and T&D departments were thrown into states of disequilibrium. Beginning with the advent of prospective payment (DRGs) and continuing into the present era of managed care, education in health care organizations has undergone tremendous change. In some organizations cost-cutting measures resulted in the elimination of both nursing education and T&D departments. The limited educational programs for nursing staff were developed and presented by administrators, managers, any surviving clinical specialists, and expert staff. For a few organizations, the two separate departments continued to coexist, consulting and collaborating with one another frequently and effectively. Still other organizations centralized all educational functions into a single department that might report through nursing (now patient care services) or personnel (now human resources). The nursing educators and the trainers worked side by side, or nursing education may have taken over most of the responsibilities of the training department. Educational programs, from general orientation to JCAHO-mandated in-service programs to clinical education, were developed and implemented by the new staff development department that served all organizational personnel.

In today's downsized, rightsized, redesigned, reengineered health care organizations, the need for staff development services is probably greater than ever. However, experience indicates that in any era of change and reform, one of the first cost-cutting measures implemented is too often the elimination of or draconian reduction of staff development personnel. Demands for the staff to develop new competencies, both cognitive and technologic, however, makes the staff development role essential, not optional (Shinn, 1994).

# THE FUTURE OF STAFF DEVELOPMENT

## Assumptions

There are some common assumptions that will underlie both the probable and the preferred futures for staff development. Change will continue to reshape health care. New venues for health care delivery, new roles for current health care providers, and, possibly, new categories of health care providers will confront our future. Staff development programs, as well as continuing education programs and formal academic programs, will be essential in supporting the current health care workforce in these future roles and in preparing new members for entry into the health care organizations of the future.

## Forces Shaping the Future

Shugars and others (1991) identified five forces shaping the future of health care into the next century. Each of these forces will influence the future of staff development/staff education.

1. Cost containment
2. A diverse and aging population
3. Continued growth of science and technology
4. Expanding empowerment of health care consumers
5. Focus on ethical concerns

## Demands Shaping the Future

### Cost Containment

The demands of cost containment will shape the practice of all health care providers. Changes in reimbursement, continually decreasing lengths of stay, changes in skill mix, and altered nursing and medical practice patterns, among other outcomes of cost containment, will create a continuing need to educate and reeducate the staff of health care organizations to implement and support cost-containment efforts.

### Aging Consumers

As the baby boomer generation ages, their need for services will place new demands on the health care delivery system. The health care system will have to respond to the largest aging population and will have to respond to them differently than in any prior generation. The sheer numbers of older adults will make historic demands on the health care delivery system.

Additionally, the aging baby boomer population will demand more from the health care delivery system in the way of access, quality, and affordability, just as this generation does currently as consumers of other products and services. The health care workforce, professional and nonprofessional, will have to respond to these demands for services in new ways. Their need for ongoing education will be intensified by these unprecedented numbers and demands for increased services. In addition, an increasingly diverse patient population and health care workforce will demand educational support to meet the needs of the patient population and to ensure an adequately prepared workforce.

The increasing empowerment of health care consumers has already created an emphasis on customer service and patient satisfaction in health care. As consumers' expectations for high-quality, low-cost health care grow, there is continued need for refocusing those in the health care workforce on improving communication and other customer service skills.

### Science and Technology

The explosion of scientific knowledge and technology also will expand the need for staff development efforts to ensure a workforce able to apply new knowledge and use cutting-edge technology. Changes in technology and scientific knowledge will likely create new roles for existing health care professions and may even create new professions. Those in the workforce will need to be knowledgeable about these new roles and professions to ensure their appropriate utilization. New venues for health care delivery also will result from these changes, which will require lifelong learning through staff development, continuing education, and formal academ-ic education.

### Ethical Challenges

The explosion of scientific knowledge and expanding technology will create even greater ethical dilemmas related to end-of-life decision making, genetic engineering, organ transplant and replacement, and other issues. These issues will influence the practice of health care professionals and the work of nonprofessionals within the health care delivery system, again creating the demand for continuing staff development efforts to empower health care professionals and nonprofessionals to deal with difficult ethical dilemmas.

In addition, all the changes in the health care delivery system will demand that clinicians be prepared to educate their patients and families to navigate the changing system, to empower patients and families to make informed health care decisions, to deal with new ethical issues, and to promote the health of their patients (Bailey and others, 1995). Clinicians will need ongoing education to prepare them to manage the new challenges that a turbulent health care delivery system will present to them and their patients. The impact and interaction of these and other forces not yet dreamed of will create demand for and shape the very nature of staff development services into the next century.

## STAFF DEVELOPMENT, CONTINUING EDUCATION, AND FORMAL EDUCATION

Cost cutting seems frequently to result in cutbacks in funding for education within health care organizations. Positions are cut from staff development departments, monies to fund travel and fees for outside conferences and workshops and to reimburse for college tuition are reduced, and training hours to provide paid education time for staff are slashed in the operating budget. Although this may be a short-sighted approach to managing the future of health care delivery, such cuts do not always reflect a devaluing of education but simply present an expedient way to make difficult budget decisions.

The differentiation of formal (or academic) education of the health care workforce from staff development education is generally simple. Formal education is sponsored by a college or university, which may be a subsidiary of a large health care organization, leads to the granting of college credit, and may lead to the award of an academic degree; staff development is an educational function of the employing health care organization that promotes the ability of staff to function effectively and efficiently within the organization. Staff development reflects the responsibility of the employer to prepare the workforce to function within that particular organization.

The line of demarcation between continuing education and staff development may not always be so clear. Staff development departments may offer continuing education programs that are accredited by state boards of nursing or by state nurses' associations and other groups approved by the American Nurses Credentialing Center, for example. A program on new technologies for intravenous therapy may be offered by a staff development department as a continuing education program for both nurses within that health care organization and nurses in the community. However, an educational program that focuses on the new intravenous pumps purchased for inpatient units, for example, and is offered to enable nurses to develop technical competency in the use the new equipment is a staff development program.

## THE PROBABLE FUTURE OF STAFF DEVELOPMENT

If current trends continue, the probable future of staff development looks very much like the models of staff development resources of today. One central theme for staff development in either a probable or preferred future is the implementation of research findings into daily practice to expand research-based nursing practice. Educators must keep abreast of the current research related to their clinical areas of responsibility so they can translate these findings into practical applications for nursing staff at the bedside and in other patient care settings (Gullen, 1995; Mottola, 1996).

Today's economic climate and the probable future will no longer support an in-house staff researcher—a doctorally prepared nurse researcher who facilitates the application of research findings into practice, encourages staff-initiated research projects, and conducts clinical and/or administrative studies to improve care and care delivery systems (Schutzenhofer, 1991). The future could bring, however, more collaborative efforts between health care organizations and schools of nursing to meet the research facilitation needs. The staff development educator must play an active role in bringing research findings to clinical practice in the future to continue the effort to make clinical practice research based and to keep nursing practice on the cutting edge.

Some staff development services will likely continue to be decentralized. In this decentralized model, staff development educators will report through the front line or middle managers of clinical departments and provide for the staff development needs of a particular group of nursing staff members on a unit or in a multiunit department. Although they report to different managers, ideally these staff developers work together in a coalition, sharing their individual talents and resources, to ensure that the diverse needs of the staff are being met. This sharing of skills and ideas is essential to the success of a decentralized staff development service. No one educator can address all the needs of a patient care department. Furthermore, staff development needs are likely to be similar along many dimensions across departments. Planning and implementing programs in isolation from other educators is a misuse of human, fiscal, and physical resources.

### The Staff Development Educator

The staff development educator in this probable future is also likely to juggle multiple roles. The educator may be the department's advanced practice nurse, either a clinical nurse specialist or nurse practitioner. The educator also will likely be involved in performance improvement, policy development, and in the clinical care and discharge planning for patients with complex needs. Some of the essential functions of staff developers (Sheridan, 1995) may not be addressed as the decentralized staff development educator tries to balance and maintain both clinical and educational roles. Leadership training and management development may be left out of the overall educational plan, along with career counseling for the organization's staff, as educators focus on orientation, in-service, and continuing education programming, along with the other foci noted previously.

Even in organizations that maintain a centralized staff development department, the demands on educators to fulfill many roles and assume responsibility for many functions will grow. Even these educators are likely to fulfill both clinical and educational roles. A centralized department allows for the more efficient and effective provision of services; intradepartmental collaboration minimizes duplication of effort and the specialization of staff in developing and implementing programs across the organization.

The probable future will likely find the use of lower credentialed educators growing. In an effort to cut the costs of providing education, persons with less than a graduate degree in nursing may be used as the primary educators, instead of in adjunct roles. Preferably, highly skilled clinical staff without advanced degrees can be used in a "train the trainer" model in which these clinical staff are trained by the staff development educator to provide programs for their clinical colleagues (Kirsivali-Farmer, 1994).

## Collaboration and Cooperation

The need for educational consortia and other interorganizational collaboration will be an integral part of this probable future. As organizations minimize their educational resources, educational needs will not diminish. Health care organizations will need to work cooperatively, and, ideally, in collaboration with schools of nursing to meet their common educational needs.

Sammut (1994) describes one model for a consortium in which five hospitals joined together to provide critical care nursing courses because it was not cost effective for each hospital to educate one or two nurses at a time. In rural and other underserved regions, partnerships between health care organizations and local colleges can meet the needs for staff education through technology such as audio conferences, interactive video, prerecorded video courses, interactive computer learning materials, and other high-tech methods (Penney and others, 1996). The use of technology, as described in Chapter 12, will be essential as staff development educators expand their services beyond the staff of acute care settings to encompass staff employed by integrated health care organizations that include long-term care, home care, sub-acute settings, ambulatory care, and community health.

# STAFF DEVELOPMENT'S PREFERRED FUTURE

## Organization

The staff development department in the preferred future will ideally demonstrate the best of both decentralized and centralized organizational models. Because the staff development department will have moved beyond just educating into planning, implementing, and evaluating all educational programs for integrated health care organizations, the department will be centralized under a single department head to ensure the comprehensive delivery of services. However, educators will provide point of service programming for their assigned areas, working with nursing and a variety of multidisciplinary groups of employees in the organization in a variety of settings outside the acute care area.

## Interdisciplinary Roles

Sheridan (1995) notes that staff development educators will assume a broader scope of responsibility as their focus moves beyond nursing and becomes interdisciplinary. Educators will become consultants within the acute care setting, across departments, and beyond traditional nursing care units (Sheridan, 1995). As hospitals continue to expand their reach beyond the acute care setting into new venues, including the community, and across organizations as multihospital systems expand, educators will expand their scope of responsibility to assist clinical and technical experts from other disciplines and occupations to develop and implement their own educational programs.

In addition, staff development educators routinely will assume responsibility for general educational programs, such as employee orientation, mandatory safety and infection control education, and other general programs, such as customer service skills, that cut across all departments. Staff development educators will assume more responsibility for developing, implementing, and marketing health and wellness education programs for the community, targeting those segments of the population being recruited by the health care organization.

### Research

The staff development department will not simply educate nurses about existing research but will do even more to integrate research findings into practice. Every staff development department will either have its own doctorally prepared nurse researcher to facilitate studies and to conduct his or her own research or will collaborate with an affiliated school of nursing to conduct research. Several collaborative models are possible. A nurse researcher may have a joint appointment in the school of nursing and the health care organization. The health care organization may buy the services of one or more faculty to facilitate research or may utilize clinical faculty to assist with research.

In an outcomes-oriented health care environment, staff development educators emphasize evaluation of programming and outcomes measures (Sheridan, 1995). These outcomes measures will also relate to changes in clinical practice, especially research-based clinical practice promoted by staff development educators and performance improvement measures.

Most staff development educators will be prepared at least at the graduate level in a clinical nursing specialty. Expert clinicians prepared at the baccalaureate level will be used to supplement the efforts of the regular staff in creative professional development models.

### Visibility, Viability, and Validity

Avillion's (1994) three "Vs" (visibility, viability, and validity) are applicable to staff development's preferred future. The staff development department in a preferred future must have high *visibility:* offering programming on all shifts, planning programs for both the professional and lay communities, and participating in interdisciplinary organizational committees. The *viable* department will have moved far from the in-service department image to a professional development image. Meaningful outcomes must be measured related to both educational programs and improvements in clinical practice. The focus of the department must be broad, including functions such as newsletters for the staff and the community, career counseling, and recruitment and retention programs. The department will demonstrate its *validity* by using needs assessment to drive programs and services, by meetings goals and deadlines, and by demonstrating how continuing education and staff development helps achieve positive personal and organizational outcomes.

## CONCLUSION

In a rapidly changing health care environment, the need for education will not just continue but will expand. The difference between the probable future and the preferred future will largely depend on the priorities of health care organizations: Is staff development viewed as a necessary drain on human and fiscal resources or an essential investment in the quality of an organization's staff and the quality of care provided by the staff? Or not.

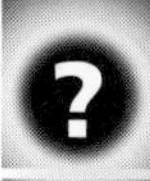

### *Discussion Exercises*

1. You are the CEO of a large, multihospital health care organization. You have been advised to eliminate your staff development department as a cost-cutting measure. Persuade your staff that such an action is ill advised.
2. The utilization of nursing research findings into practice occurs too infrequently. Explain how the staff development department can help staff put research into practice.
3. Differences between the probable and preferred futures are described in the chapter. Delineate strategies to achieve the preferred future for staff development.

## References

Avillion AE: Political savvy in staff development: building an indispensable department, *J Continuing Educ Nurs* 25:152, 1994.

Bailey K and others: The nurse as educator, *J Nurs Staff Dev* 11:205, 1995.

Gullen SE: The role of staff development in creating a research-based practice environment, *J Nurs Staff Dev* 11:170, 1995.

Kirsivali-Farmer K: Staff development sessions: a strategy to facilitate nursing staff education with limited teaching resources, *J Nurs Staff Dev* 10:214, 1994.

Mottola CA: Research utilization and the continuing/staff development educator, *J Continuing Educ Nurs* 27:168, 1996.

Penney NE and others. Partners in distance learning: project outreach, *J Nurs Adm* 26(7/8):27, 1996.

Sammut NA: Critical care education: a consortium approach, *J Nurs Staff Dev* 10:219, 1994.

Schutzenhofer K: Scholarly pursuit in the clinical setting: an obligation of professional nursing, *J Prof Nurs* 7:10, 1991.

Sheridan DR: The role of the staff developer: the last decade, the next decade, *Nurs Staff Dev Insider* p 1, September/October, 1995.

Shinn LJ: Health care reform: implications for competencies in staff development and continuing education, *J Nurs Staff Dev* 10: 164, 1994.

Shugars D and others, editors: *Health America: practitioners for 2005: an agenda for action for U.S. health professional schools: a report of the Pew Health Profession Commission,* Durham, NC, 1991, Pew Health Professions Commission.

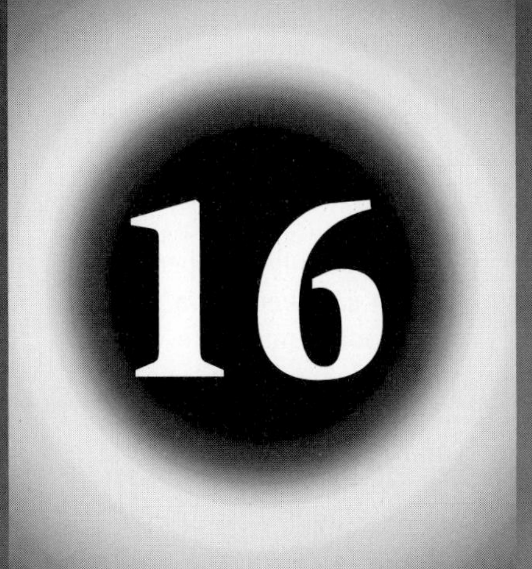

# 16 Challenges for Nursing in Higher Education

**Eleanor J. Sullivan**
**Daniel J. Pesut**

*The pessimist complains about the wind; the optimist expects it to change; the realist adjusts the sail.*

**William Arthur Ward**

What do futurists say about trends that are likely to influence the future of higher education? Consider trends forecasted by Marvin Cetron (1994) that will contribute to an American Renaissance by the year 2000. As you reflect on each consider what the consequences of this trend are for nursing curricula, faculty, and students in higher education and the public at large.

## TRENDS

The public and state legislatures will increasingly demand assessment of student achievements and will hold schools and universities accountable.

State, local, and private agencies will play a greater role in education and training by offering more internships, apprenticeships, preemployment training, and adult education.

More businesses will form partnerships with schools and offer job training.

Demand for lifelong education and training services will increase.

The new information-based model for the organization, a nonhierarchic, organic system able to respond quickly to environmental changes, fosters greater occupational flexibility and autonomy.

Computer-supported approaches to learning will improve educational techniques and make it possible to learn more in a given period. The ultimate consequence may be a one-sixth reduction in learning time overall.

By 2001 nearly all college textbooks will come with computer disks to aid in learning.

By 2001 there will not be enough adolescents to sustain the current numbers of colleges and universities. Colleges will close their doors, merge with other schools in a federation, reduce faculty size and class offerings, and seek more adult students.

Private commercial ventures will establish themselves as the proprietors of large electronic databases, eventually replacing the university library.

Students will adopt the scholar's mode of learning—by consulting books, journals, and primary sources.

The home electronic work study center will be the centerpiece of the fully integrated, information house.

Expert systems will issue reports and recommendations and actions based on data gathered electronically, without human intervention.

Personal wellness, prevention, and self-help will be the watchwords for a more health conscious population.

## HIGHER EDUCATION AT A CROSSROAD

Smith (1990) notes academics are too involved with presentism, specialization, knowledge for its own sake, relativism, academic fundamentalism, grantism, formalism, bureaucratic obtuseness, coldness of heart, and impoverishment of spirit. Smith pleads for revitalizing the spirit of higher education and for the academy to seek and engage the future with a focus on the unity of life and the creation of knowledge that aspires to wisdom that serves larger ends, reinforces moral character, advances academic entrepreneurship, and is responsive to service-based systems.

## DÉJÀ VU: MANAGED CARE AND MANAGED EDUCATION

Higher education's situation is similar to the health care industry's position a few years ago. Costs climbed but the industry paid scant attention, justifying the expense as necessary to keep the nation healthy. Fee for service provided high incomes for physicians and administrators and health care workers in short supply for specialty critical areas of care. Health care became a political issue. People used corporations, state legislatures, and Congress to demand and create change. Civic leadership replaced civic participation (Reed, 1996). Managed care forced health care providers to alter their practices.

Cost containment is becoming a way of life in health care. The values and dramatic shifts that have occurred in the health care industry are now being applied to higher education. Political pressure is mounting. People ask, Why are costs going up? How is quality measured? How can professors have lifetime jobs with few demands and little accountability? (Netherton, 1996)

Higher education is at a crossroads. It is facing unparalleled challenges—political, economic, sociologic, and technologic. Higher education's escalating costs with few restrictions or accountability has prompted public concern (Brand, 1993; Sullivan, 1997). The cost of a postsecondary education has climbed faster than the economy; however, graduates often are unable to find a job in the field for which they are prepared while some industry's needs go begging because few potential employees are prepared for the positions needed (Wagner, 1996). Students complain about irrelevant courses, filled classes, inflexible schedules, and classes taught by disinterested graduate students. Billions are expended on research, and yet society's most recalcitrant problems (e.g., crime, addiction, homelessness) go unresolved. Reasonably, the public wants to know how its money is being spent, and what the value-added benefits of higher education offer.

## MAINTAINING THE STATUS QUO

Let us assume current trends continue. What can we expect for the future of higher education? If nothing is done to change the course of today's events, higher education will experience additional and more severe problems. There are several factors that contribute to the maintenance of the status quo. Most of these factors involve values and beliefs held by those in key positions. Several other factors relate to material and human resources and politics. If nothing changes, the following scenario is likely to emerge.

## The University as Place Bound

Crumbling buildings will fuel the demand for more and better-equipped facilities on campuses. Those wanting to maintain the status quo will refuse to consider alternative instructional methods or extended course schedules that permit use of classrooms throughout the day, evening, and weekends. Existing buildings, equipment, and laboratories will deteriorate on some campuses, while wealthier universities will construct elaborate new facilities. Two tiers of universities will exist: the "haves" and the "have nots." Eventually place-bound learning sites will not survive the competitive cyber-space learning revolution.

## Student Demographics and Skill Mix

Enrollments in postsecondary education will rise for all minority groups, but the greatest growth will be in the number of Asian-American students. The rate of growth in the number of Hispanic and women students will surpass the number of men enrolled in college. The fastest growing group of students, however, will be those age 35 and older. They will make up half of the student population. Many colleges and universities will fail to create environments conducive to these students' needs. Consequently, student demands will intensify. Racial and cultural tensions will escalate as minority populations swell the ranks of college students. Women and older students, with existing responsibilities, will demand relevant courses, applicable skills, and value for their time and money. Colleges that remain entrenched in archaic teaching methods and rigid semester-driven schedules will see increasing student unrest.

## Financing and Resources

Tuition and fees will continue their upward swing, reducing the number of middle and lower income students who attend college. Although more than half of all Americans acquire postsecondary education in the 1990s (Trachtenberg, 1994), this percentage will drop as costs increase. In addition, students who choose to go to college will pay more of their own educational expenses and, for those without their own or their parents' resources, college debts will escalate. Higher debt, combined with the inability of many graduates to obtain jobs in their fields, will raise loan default rates.

## Public Scrutiny

Higher education's reputation will continue to suffer. Colleges that remain mired in the traditions of the past, refuse to respond to the needs of society, or grapple with the difficult issues facing higher education will increasingly suffer both financial problems and diminishing public regard. Scrutiny of resource use will head the list of accountability problems faced by the higher education community. Students, their parents, and industry will put increasing pressure on colleges and universities to demonstrate their educational effectiveness. Documenting program effectiveness by measuring graduate performance (e.g., testing) and future success (e.g., follow up with graduates) will be required. Also, colleges will be compelled to offer programs aligned with the job market, which will be the major criteria for program and university funding.

Resource utilization, faculty productivity, and student outcomes will be scrutinized, and performance standards will be well established. The relevancy and timeliness of programs and courses will come under increasing scrutiny. As a result of budget-cutting measures, some colleges, departments, and programs will close or merge with others. Faculty and student unrest will escalate as problems intensify. State legislatures, students, and parents will have the greatest concern and the most vested interest; however, alumni, donors, and the public will, in varying degrees, also be concerned with regard to how universities use their resources. Oversight of university budgets will become more and more stringent. The corporate world will put increasing pressure on higher education to produce graduates for industries' needs. Corporate leaders will be increasingly critical of retaining poorly performing faculty and will be likely to lead efforts to examine instructional productivity, especially at state-supported schools.

University governance will pass into the hands of professional administrators much as health care management today often is assigned to nonclinical managers. Programs of study and courses will be managed with a "bottom line" orientation. Teachers will be pressured to make their courses, their programs, and their college "user friendly" (read: popular), and their compliance will be measured by increasingly important student evaluations. Teachers who are not popular or who demand too much from students will be dismissed. Faculty morale will plummet and academic administrators' jobs will be eliminated. In an effort to fund depleting university coffers, fund-raising efforts will intensify with increasing competition among departments and universities for the largesse of donors with the biggest purses. Similarly, competition for scarce state and federal resources also will intensify.

### Administration and Governance

College presidents, deans, department chairs, and even faculty will be selected not only for their teaching and scholarship but also for their fund-raising ability. Faculty, who have the time to do research, will be urged to study popular, newsworthy topics. Enhancing and maintaining the university's reputation will be so critical and important that controversial professors, especially those without tenure, will be dismissed. Tenure and the value of academic freedom in a democratic society will be dismissed by those not involved in higher education and even by some in higher education, such as administrators struggling with unreasonable faculty demands.

Various retirement incentives will be used to reduce faculty ranks. Tenure will be reserved for faculty stars, top researchers, or people well known in their field; annual and multiyear contracts will be the norm for junior faculty, with few attaining professorial rank or tenure.

Because of changing trends in the external environment, time-honored college traditions will change. The university-centered model of old will be transformed into the information-based, student-centered model of the twenty-first century. Universal access, accountability, relevance, and cost-effectiveness will emerge for universities that have a future. Consider the following preferred future scenarios in terms of curricula, students, and faculty.

## PREFERRED FUTURE SCENARIO

### The University Community: Global Access

The university of tomorrow will no longer be place bound. Learning will occur in students' homes, at their offices or factories, in their cars, and at their computers. Shared teleconferencing arrangements among universities will conserve scarce resources and make faculty expertise accessible to a wider range of students and in a variety of settings (e.g., computerized virtual reality). Use-at-home videos, CD ROM disks, audiotapes, and classes over the Internet will help students work at their own pace and schedules.

Institutions will more clearly define their mission vis-à-vis teaching and research, with many institutions targeting teaching as their primary mission. Instructional excellence will be fostered, promoted, and recognized by the public. Students will choose such institutions for their learning environments, especially for undergraduate education.

Other institutions will focus on graduate instruction and research. These institutions will commit resources to establishing sustained programs in a few selected areas (e.g., molecular biology, geriatric research) and recruit faculty and students to these areas. Tomorrow's successful university, regardless of its mission, will be a loosely organized community of scholars who may be at times geographically dispersed but committed to furthering knowledge through science, scholarship, and teaching.

Campus facilities will be used days and evenings, weekdays and weekends, and during traditional college breaks. In fact, the semester system as we know it today will be restructured into short courses (e.g., 2- or 4-week intensives) or year-long individualized study. Science laboratories, visual art studios, and traditional classrooms will be used for activities that require such facilities. Individual learning environments and simulated practice areas will allow students to make use of realistic, efficient technologies (e.g., at their workplace).

The greatest change, however, will occur in courses taught on line (Connors and others, 1996). Neither faculty nor students will be required to be at a specific campus location at a specific time. Internet technology makes it possible to teach courses to students miles away and many time zones apart because students and faculty interact when their schedules permit. State, and even country, borders disappear. The growth of courses and entire programs offered via the Internet will revolutionize education in the twenty-first century.

Geographic areas will become both more and less important in planning. The availability of programs needed in certain regions will influence decisions about programs that need direct contact with an instructor (e.g., nurse practitioner in rural areas). For other programs and courses, however, technology will eliminate regional boundaries. For example, two-way teleconferencing makes it possible to teach real-time courses to widely dispersed audiences. Expensive equipment and facilities are required, though, for video teleconferencing. Teaching courses over the Internet, however, obviates those needs. A computer, a modem, and Internet access is all a student needs to participate in these courses (see Chapter 12).

Systems of accountability will be established and acceptable to both internal and external constituents. Reduced reliance on state and federal funding, as well as tuition and fees, will result from well-planned cost-containment strategies. Because universities will no longer attempt to be all things to all people, each will design its mission to respond to the needs of the community, differentiating itself from other institutions and maximizing its strengths (i.e., faculty areas of expertise). Teaching will be the focus of some campuses, whereas others will emphasize research productivity. Preparing future graduates for marketplace needs and civic leadership will be emphasized. Lifelong learning environments will be the norm. New student markets, innovative teaching methods, additional revenue streams, and invigorated and productive faculty will revitalize the university community, which will enjoy a reciprocal and positive relationship with its constituents and the public.

## Student Demographics and Skill Mix

Demographics will continue to alter the face of the student body. Working adults, single parents, and people pursuing second careers require flexible schedules and relevant, applicable courses. Lifelong learning will be pursued for information, work-related classes, degrees desired (although advanced degrees will become less valuable, and acquiring information will become more important), and enrichment. Age diversity on campus and those enrolled in classes will increase. Not only will traditional age college graduates return to school for second degrees or graduate study, but also more high school graduates (or dropouts) who do not go directly to college will take classes and often complete degrees in starts and stops. Increasing numbers of older workers will return for additional courses for second, or even third, careers. Retirees will pursue long-held dreams of a college education.

Ethnic and racial diversity will be fostered in culturally sensitive environments. Support services for nontraditional students (e.g., child care, off-hours learning labs) will be offered in addition to flexible scheduling to meet working students' needs. Increases in the racial and ethnic minority populations will challenge colleges to provide culturally receptive environments and maintain equitable opportunities for all. Students who choose nursing will be a more diverse, well-educated population. On the average, they will be older people with second degrees who are planning to pursue an advanced practice master's degree program. Successful students will be computer literate, self-directed, and goal oriented. Many will have grown up with health education software and will be aware of the many health-related programs available. Students will complain that they do not get enough telecognitive time to enhance their clinical knowledge base (Bezold and others, 1993).

## Curricula and Courses

Future curricula are likely to be influenced by federations of accrediting agencies. Standard curriculum based on national consensus will be the foundation for teaching and learning, so variations in curriculum will diminish. Standard fundamental nursing practice and principles will be accessed on the World Wide Web. Virtual nursing centers on the Web will be the learning and research tools used by both faculty and students. Access to these centers will be available to subscribers who pay fees. Funds once allocated for learning resources in an individual school or college now will support subscribers' services to Internet resources.

A few major regional schools of nursing will serve as magnet fundamental programs. These schools will form a federation for fundamentals preparation. Curricula and courses will be offered over telecommunications, Internet, and satellite. Packaged software programs with Web connections will provide self-paced tutorials for student learning. Differences in advanced curricula and research training will be provided by a federation of graduate schools that will have pooled resources and purchased satellite time.

Doctoral education in nursing will be offered by satellite. There will be a core set of doctoral and nursing theory courses offered by the top 25 nursing programs in the world. Research emphases in these programs will not be duplicated. Students who wish to study in one of the main nursing research emphasis areas will connect or travel to work with the community of scholars located at the campuses or sites for that program of research emphases. For example:

The University of California San Francisco is the leader in symptom management research.

The University of Washington excels in women's health.

Wayne State University will maintain its reputation in transcultural nursing research.

The Chicago-based federation of University of Illinois, Loyola, and Rush is the center for psychoneuroimmulogical, genetic, and ethical research.

The University of Kansas is known for its work in fatigue management for the chronically ill.

Already technology makes it possible for a degree to be earned without the student ever setting foot on campus. Internet courses can be offered worldwide, especially in graduate programs; voice mail and e-mail make communication feasible regardless of time differences and individual schedules. Teleconferencing enables real-time audio and video interaction with teachers and students in different locales. The use of this technologic learning will continue to expand in the future. Simulators and computer models will allow almost-real interventions and interactions. The educational clinical laboratory may look more like a CNN television studio than a hospital or clinic. Textbooks, journal articles, and professor-led lectures will be supplemented by these technologic opportunities just as in entertainment, television augmented movies and radio, several decades ago. Textbooks and electronics will be interactive.

Clinical skills will be developed through 24-hour telecommunications courses that combine cognitive, behavioral, and interactive experiences in the delivery of around-the-clock education and training. Clinical practice opportunities will involve work study and a variety of cooperative education arrangements (see Chapter 9). Student nurses will work with individuals, families, and communities, using telephone and computer communications to assess patient conditions, monitor chronic conditions, encourage health promotion, and conduct wellness checks.

Telehealth will be a required fundamentals course. Students will gain clinical experience working with individuals and families using this two-way communication system. Course work in informatics and health education will replace courses in nutrition and anatomy and physiology because these prerequisites will be required before students enter nursing education programs and can be easily learned through interactive software programs.

Because genetics is dramatically transformed health and medical care, students will learn and master categories of diseases that can be predicted and managed through genetic code, prediction, and treatment technology (Bezold and others, 1993) (see Chapter 10).

## Faculty: Knowledge Brokers

Faculty of the future will be independent contractors. Variety among faculty backgrounds and assignments will increase. Faculty will be recruited from the ranks of professional and corporate leaders who will offer their expertise on a full- or part-time basis, from their homes, offices, or in person. Some senior faculty will be recruited without requiring that they make a permanent physical move to the new campus. They will teach via the Internet, will make periodic visits to campus, and will interact with colleagues via e-mail and telephone conferencing (individual teleconferencing is promised for the future) from their home or business offices.

After schools of nursing downsize and/or close, many faculty will choose early retirement. Others will begin to retool based on the demands of the technologically driven educational environment. Of those who remain, independent contracting will be the preferred mode of employment. Faculty will contract with one or more federations, HMOs, businesses, or educator agencies. Services faculty will provide include development of health education/nursing practice software programs and design of education modules that employ use of World Wide Web resources. Some faculty will manage health-related Internet service organizations. Private consultation to groups and communities on health policy analyses and health promotion activities will still be a major part of the independent work performed by faculty. Some faculty will become brokers for clinical services.

Health advocacy will emerge as a new area of entrepreneurial activity for health care providers. Many faculty will serve as online peer reviewers for online publications. Faculty affiliated with one of the 25 doctoral nursing research centers will convene groups of students nationwide to conduct multisite research.

Two areas will promise opportunities for faculty interested in retooling: health education interactive software development and use of genetics to predict and manage illness (as opposed to the current system to diagnose and treat). Postdoctoral education in nursing will bring nurses' knowledge, skills, and abilities to these rapidly emerging developments.

## Administration and Governance

Innovative systems of administration and governance will be employed in the university of tomorrow. Rigid, hierarchical divisions will become permeable as multidisciplinary programs develop in response to workplace demands (e.g., information specialist in nursing, which combines information technology with clinical practice). New organizational structures will emerge, eliminating many internal units such as departments, schools, and colleges. Dean and department chair positions may disappear (Plater, 1995).

A modified form of self-governance will emerge on university campuses, with clearer delineation between faculty and administrative authority and responsibility. For example, faculty will continue to decide curricular issues, but administration will decide resource limitations and manage the budget. Professional staff (e.g., administrative assistants, student advisors, computer technicians) will increasingly handle more routine tasks not requiring faculty expertise. Efficiency will become routine.

Higher education will grapple with protecting academic freedom as it scrutinizes faculty tenure. Although tenure will be reserved for those few faculty whose future contributions have the most potential value to the university, safeguards for faculty to pursue controversial topics in the classroom and in the laboratory will be established for all faculty. (Due process law has nearly eliminated the original justification for tenure.) Innovative arrangements for faculty contracts will be devised. These will include longer tenure track schedules (e.g., 10 years), multiyear contracts, alternating full- and part-time work, reciprocal arrangements with business (using employees to teach and teachers to work for the business), rotating learning and teaching schedules (similar to periodic sabbaticals but used to update knowledge and skills), and many others.

### Public Trust and Respect

The successful university of tomorrow will recognize that it exists to serve society. Educational programs will be designed to meet the needs of the community, the nation, and the world, with universities specializing in particular areas. Programs will be designed in response to workforce requirements and the need to prepare graduates for work and for productive citizenship (e.g., community service). Critical and creative thinking, rather than acquisition of information, will define the goal of higher education.

Degree-granting programs will be important, but equally valuable will be a variety of continuing education programs. Some of these will be offered as contracts with businesses and nonprofit organizations for training; some will be short courses taught by permanent faculty or contracted from outside the university; some will be individual offerings for local citizens. In addition to community good will, these programmatic efforts will result in increased revenue for the university.

## RESPONDING TO THE FUTURE

How does one respond to the future? What will the future of higher education mean for nursing faculty, students, administrators, and the general public? How can individuals shape that future? Much of what happens depends on one's responses to emerging trends. Using trend-based information to develop personal and professional plans supports proactive individuals who can take advantage of evolving opportunities. Faculty who consider future trends as decision variables that demand engagement and involvement are in a position to foster excellence in higher education.

Responding to the future is a matter of awareness, choice, and action. In his book, *Managing at the Speed of Change* (1992), Daryl Conner reminds us that the Chinese symbol for crisis means death, danger, *and* opportunity. Conner characterizes response to change as reactive or proactive. Responses occur along a continuum of resilience (Box 16-1).

Reactive individuals prefer to maintain the status quo, a response that leads to stagnation. Such individuals retreat from change and seek security in a highly managed order. Reactive individuals generally respond in a protect-and-defend mode because change is seen as threatening and dangerous. Some consequences of reactive behavior, as shown in Box 16-2, are fear, anger, frustration, disappointment, guilt, loneliness, and feeling overwhelmed (Robbins, 1991).

## Box 16-1
### *Resilience Continuum*

| Low ←<br>D Type (Danger Oriented) | → High<br>O Type (Opportunity Oriented) |
|---|---|
| **Ability To Be Positive** | |
| Interprets the world as binary and sequential. | Interprets the world as multifaceted and overlapping. |
| Expects future to be orderly and predictable. | Expects future to be filled with constantly shifting variables. |
| Interprets unmet expectations as personal vendettas or conspiracies. | Views disruptions as the natural result of a changing world. |
| Spends time resolving many contradictions. | Spends time understanding many paradoxes. |
| Sees major change as uncomfortable and a problem to avoid. | Also sees major change as uncomfortable but views it as often presenting opportunities to exploit. |
| Feels that most challenges are unfair and serve no purpose. | Believes there are usually lessons to be learned from challenges. |
| Sees life as generally punishing. | Sees life as generally rewarding. |
| **Ability To Be Focused** | |
| Lacks an overarching purpose or vision and/or the ability to stay focused on its achievement. | Maintains a strong purpose or vision that serves both as a source of meaning and as a guidance system to reestablish perspectives following significant disruption. |
| Engages in too many diverse change projects that collectively drain assimilation resources. | Consolidates what appear to be several unrelated change projects into a single effort with a central theme. |
| Cannot establish and/or update priorities during change. | Sets and renegotiates priorities during change. |
| Fails to effectively manage multiple tasks and demands that occur at the same time. | Manages many simultaneous tasks and demands successfully. |
| Cannot compartmentalize tasks and pressures, so one stress point spills over into other areas. | Skilled at compartmentalizing so that stress in one area does not carry over to other projects or parts of one's life. |
| Fails to ask others for help when it is needed. | Recognizes when to ask others for help. |
| Is prone to knee-jerk reactions. | Engages action only after careful planning. |
| **Ability To Be Proactive** | |
| Unable to recognize impending or potential change situations. | Determines when a change is inevitable, necessary, or advantageous. |
| Rigidly adheres to old operating style when facing the unexpected. | Reframes changing situations, improvises new approaches, and maneuvers to gain an advantage. |

*Continued*

## Box 16-1
### *Resilience Continuum—cont'd*

| Low ←<br>D Type (Danger Oriented)—cont'd | → High<br>O Type (Opportunity Oriented)—cont'd |
|---|---|
| Does not take risks when consequences are difficult to determine or are clearly negative. | Takes risks in spite of potentially negative consequences. |
| Can repeat the same kind of change without significant learning taking place. | Draws important lessons from change-related experiences that are then applied to similar situations. |
| Reacts to disruption by blaming, attacking, and CYA activity. | Responds to disruption by investing energy in problem solving and teamwork. |
| Unable to influence others or resolve conflicts effectively. | Able to influence others and resolve conflicts. |
| **Ability To Be Flexible** | |
| Approaches change as a mysterious event. | Believes change is a manageable process. |
| Has a low tolerance for ambiguity as evidenced by poor performance in unstructured or uncertain work environments. | Has a high tolerance for ambiguity. |
| Needs a long recovery time after adversity or disappointment. | Needs only a short time to recover after adversity or disappointment. |
| Feels victimized during change. | Feels empowered during change. |
| Engages in changes that are beyond personal or organizational capabilities. | Recognizes own strengths and weaknesses and knows when to accept internal or external limits. |
| Fails to break from established way of seeing things. | Challenges and when necessary modifies own assumptions or frame of reference. |
| Does not develop and maintain nurturing relationships that can be used for support. | Relies on nurturing relationships for support. |
| Lacks patience, understanding, and humor in the face of change. | Displays patience, understanding, and humor when dealing with change. |
| **Ability To Be Organized** | |
| Becomes lost when faced with confusing information. | Identifies the underlying themes embedded in confusing situations. |

Modified from Connor DR: *Managing at the speed of change,* New York, 1992, Villard Books.

Common defense mechanisms used by reactive individuals who Conner (1992) refers to as *reactive individuals type D* (danger oriented) include denial, distortion, and delusion.

Proactive individuals, on the other hand, see creative opportunities embedded in change, seeking and acting on possibilities inherent in change. They have a strong life vision and meaning, which guides them through change. They have learned the art of reflection. They are able to compartmentalize stress, challenge their own assumptions, reframe situations and events, rely on relationships, look for balance, and know where to ask for help. Connor (1992) calls them *type O* (opportunity oriented) *individuals.*

Reactive responses to change provide clues for action to respond in a more proactive, re-

### Box 16-2
### *Signals of Reactive Response*

1. Discomfort
2. Fear
3. Hurt
4. Anger
5. Frustration
6. Disappointment
7. Guilt
8. Inadequacy
9. Overload, overwhelm
10. Loneliness

From Robbins A: *Awaken the giant within,* New York, 1991, Simon & Schuster.

### Box 16-3
### *Emotions of Power*

1. Love and warmth
2. Appreciation and gratitude
3. Curiosity
4. Excitement and passion
5. Determination
6. Flexibility
7. Confidence
8. Cheerfulness
9. Vitality
10. Contribution

From Robbins A: *Awaken the giant within,* New York, 1991, Simon & Schuster.

### Box 16-4
### *Nineteen Questions About the Future*

1. Do faculty have a clear and collective point of view about how the future will be or could be different?
2. Do faculty see themselves as revolutionaries, or are they content with the status quo?
3. Does the school or university have a clear and collective agenda for building core competencies and for involving the student, faculty, and community interface?
4. Are top administrators allocating as much time and intellectual energy to the potential market as to current competitive markets?
5. Is the organization exercising any influence over the industry/education evolution?
6. Do all faculty share an aspiration for the enterprise and possess a clear sense of the legacy they are working to build?
7. Is there a significant amount of stretch in that aspiration; does it exceed current resources by a substantial amount?
8. Has senior leadership operationalized that aspiration into a clear set of corporate or school challenges?
9. Is it clear to everyone in the organization how his or her individual contribution links into the overall aspiration?
10. Have leaders clearly identified current practices and subjected those practices to close scrutiny?
11. Are economic threats clear to all?
12. Do employees at all levels possess a deep sense of urgency about the challenge of sustaining success?
13. Does the school's opportunity horizon extend sufficiently far beyond the boundaries of existing markets?
14. Is there an explicit process for identifying and exploiting opportunities that lie between or transcend individual educational/business units?
15. Are there a sufficient number of ongoing experiments to ensure that the organization learns faster than rivals about the precise location of tomorrow's opportunities?
16. Have all the possible opportunities for resource leverage been exploited fully?
17. Does the organization have the capacity for global recognition?
18. Are senior leaders confident they will leave a legacy to future members that exceeds the legacy they themselves inherited?
19. Are you having fun competing for the future?

Modified from Hamal G, Prahalad CK: *Competing for the future: nineteen questions about the future,* Boston, 1994, Harvard Business School Press.

silient way. Box 16-3 illustrates the 10 emotions of power used by proactive individuals to sustain proactivity (Robbins, 1991).

It is not easy to determine if faculty are danger or opportunity oriented. The presence or absence of action signals and emotions of power (see Boxes 16-2 and 16-3) may provide a sense of the faculty responses that are operative in your organization.

Type O students and faculty:

Display a sense of security and self-assurance based on life as complex but filled with opportunity; they are positive.
Have clear vision of what they want; they are focused.
Demonstrate a special resilience when responding to uncertainty; they are flexible.
Develop structures to manage ambiguity; they are organized.
Engage change rather than defend against it; they are proactive.

Will you be a part of maintaining the status quo or facilitating progress? Do you considered yourself a danger- or opportunity-oriented individual? Questions that can help people anticipate and thrive in the future follow. Reflect on the answers. Consider both the dangers and opportunities offered in Box 16-4. Your future and the future of your organization depends on it.

## CONCLUSION

Progressive universities will flourish in the coming decades and enhance higher education's reputation. Relationships with state legislative leaders, Congressional representatives, and decision makers in state and federal agencies (e.g., state department of health, National Institutes of Health) will be positive and reciprocal and will improve the nation's future. Students will have access to educational opportunities that prepare them for life and work, and the business world will have employees and entrepreneurs able to foster economic growth and productivity. Colleges and universities that take advantage of the changes will be successful; those that do not will fail.

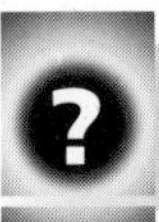

## *Discussion Exercises*

1. You are dean of a university school of nursing. Given the trends discussed in the chapter, what steps will you take to create a preferred future for (1) your school, (2) your university, and (3) your profession?
2. Take a position in favor of or opposed to tenure. Defend your position.
3. Your career plans include becoming a faculty member in a university. How will you prepare for this role in light of the changing academic environment?

## References

Bezold C and others: *2020 visions: health care information standards and technologies,* Rockville, Md, 1993, USPC.

Brand M: The challenge to change: reforming higher education, *Educ Rec* 74(2):7, 1993.

Cetron M: *An American renaissance in the year 2000: seventy-four trends that will affect America's future and yours,* Bethesda, Md, 1994, World Future Society.

Conner DR: *Managing at the speed of change,* New York, 1992, Vallard Books.

Connors HR and others: Kansas nurses surf web for master's degrees, *Reflections* 22(2):16, 1996.

Hamal G, Prahalad CK: *Competing for the future,* Boston, 1994, Harvard Business School Press.

Netherton R: How the public sees higher education (and) how higher education is responding, *Currents* 22(5):10, 1996.

Plater WM: Future work: faculty time in the 21st century, *Change* 27(3):22, 1995.

Reed T: A new understanding of "followers" as leaders: emerging theory of civic leadership, *J Leadership Stud* 3(1):95, 1996.

Robbins A: *Awaken the giant within,* New York, 1991, Simon & Schuster.

Smith P: *Killing the spirit,* New York, 1990, Viking Publishing.

Sullivan EJ: A changing higher education environment, *J Prof Nurs* 13(3):143, 1997.

Trachtenberg SJ: Doing more (really!) with less (really!): the cultural-economic revolution now upon us, *J Tertiary Educ Adm* 16(1):9, 1994.

Wagner A: Financing higher education: new approaches, new issues, *Higher Educ Manage* 8(1):7, 1996.

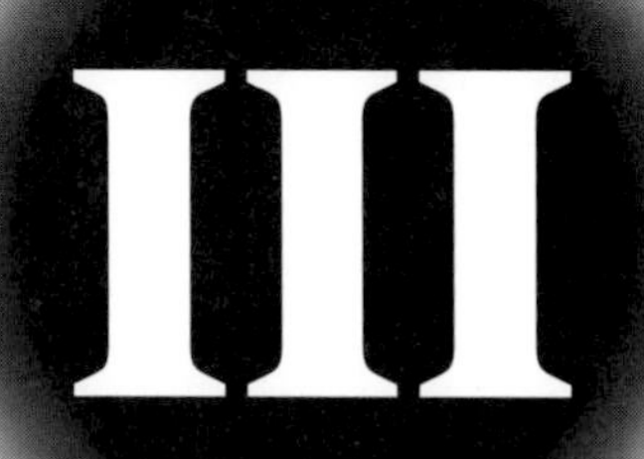

# III

# Administration in the Future

# 17 Planning for Tomorrow's Health Care System

**Maryann F. Fralic**

*So little of what could happen does happen.*

**Salvador Dali**

Seldom has there been a time of such rapid and monumental evolution in the health care industry, yet we are now in the midst of such a time. Several very fundamental shifts are occurring. First, there has been an aggressive move from unmanaged or loosely managed health care systems to tightly managed systems. During such times, all rules change. Many of the measurements, methods, systems, and rewards that were successful in the former system no longer apply, and incentives shift completely. In traditional systems the delivery of patient care was a source of great revenue. This is illustrated very clearly by the growth of the hospital sector and the emphasis toward utilization of high-cost services. Hospitals were in the enviable position of receiving high levels of revenue, limited only by the amount of activity that could be generated. High technology was developing at warp speed, and utilization of this technology was highly profitable. More admissions, more diagnostic tests, more procedures, and more surgeries created strong revenue streams. Prestige and power were judged by the number of inpatient beds that hospitals operated. Then everything changed.

The reasons for this change are well established and widely dispersed throughout in popular and professional literature. But the results are unmistakable. In the old system the delivery of patient care was sheer revenue. In the new system, with capitated prenegotiated payment rates coupled with the growing requirement for the management of health across lifetimes, the delivery of traditional modes of patient care is clearly expensive. This is why some have quipped that "an empty bed is a happy bed," aptly describing that yesterday's asset has become tomorrow's liability for hospitals. This example typifies the dramatic shift in health care, when managed care is also managed cost. Futhermore, managing cost requires moving the locus of care away from expensive high-technology sectors.

So the inexorable transition continues, from institutionally based to community-based care and from a focus on illness to a focus on prevention and wellness.

Another fundamental shift has been the transition from a preponderance of single health care institutions to integrated health care delivery systems. This change is particularly profound. In the past several years there appears to have been an inexorable rush into networks, alliances, mergers, affiliations, and acquisitions. The rate and nature of activity mimic that of the corporate world. In addition, the influence, and in some areas the dominance, of for-profit health care corporations has been interjected. This is a phenomenon that is both new and uncomfortable for many in the health care field. And yet, for-profit health care organizations are becoming mainstreamed, and desensitization to the profit status has begun. The concept of shareholders in health care is one that is both startling and unsavory to many, yet is the current and future reality. We begin to see an amalgamation of structures, systems, ownership status, and governance within these newly emerging organizations. All of these changes describe a very different future that will require careful and thoughtful planning.

Peter Drucker (1998), in his many writings on the topic of management, states that effective strategic planning does not rely on crystal-ball gazing and speculation. He does not see it as "mystery." Rather, he states that effective planners consistently and thoughtfully look at what has happened, and then make best judgements about what those events will mean for the future.

Following Drucker's logic, every signpost for the future of health care is known. Every indicator is there. Many major events have occurred, and some have emerged as trends that are being replicated in the field, clearly pointing to tomorrow's realities. It is now up to us to figure out what it means for our areas of responsibility.

With such significant change occurring and the evolution process far from complete, it is important to examine several factors, including the new integrated delivery systems, the new work of nursing, and the new work of nursing administration.

## THE NEW INTEGRATED DELIVERY SYSTEMS

Current health care literature is replete with discussion about integrated delivery systems (IDSs), the emerging, predominant model for tomorrow's health care. The many new approaches to organizing and delivering care could not have been imagined only yesterday. It is difficult to determine exactly what these new systems are and to judge their effectiveness because the concept is relatively new, somewhat amorphous, and changing daily. Informational resources on the topic are now being developed.

### Sharing Information on the World Wide Web

A new Web site (http:///www.kurtsalmon.com/idshome.htm#jourstop, Hamilton/KSA) is "dedicated to exploring the common issues facing organizations seeking to become Integrated Health Care Delivery Systems." These systems are defined on the Web site as, "A system of healthcare providers organized to provide comprehensive, coordinated health-care services to defined geographic regions."

As an example of emerging information, the Web site notes the following:

> To be effective, capitation requires restricted, contracted systems, now called Integrated Delivery Systems (IDSs). A fully integrated system has the following four characteristics:
>
> 1. Owns or contracts for a comprehensive set of services-physicians, etc. for its defined population
> 2. Contracts directly with buyers—employers, individuals, governmental entities and their beneficiaries—to provide health care services

3. Pools the profits of each of the system's components (health plan, physicians, hospitals, etc.) for investment back into the system
4. Evaluates performance of each of the system's components based on their record of quality care and cost control

The Web site also identifies four stages of IDS development:

1. Visioning/direction
2. Organizing
3. Developing integrated processes
4. Creating value through clinical integration

Electronic communication methods such as this represent contemporary modalities for sharing important information in real time.

"One cannot deliver true value without true clinical integration. Value is added only when the organization delivers better clinical care because it is an integrated delivery system with integrated processes" (Hamilton/KSA). Value is commonly being defined as clinical, financial, and service quality. High performance in each area is expected and carefully measured in effective IDSs.

### Comprehensive Information Systems

One fundamental reality is that all successful integrated systems will have comprehensive information systems. It is very clear that health care systems will be increasingly data driven, based on facts and probabilities amassed from large populations, and will utilize the processes and outcomes derived from very large data sets. Therefore in tomorrow's health care organizations, computers become increasingly important, both as technology and as extenders of health care providers, an important concept forwarded by Hamilton/KSA. They state, "To enable communications, computers may be the most important 'extender' in the health care system." Interesting thoughts indeed as new systems form.

The emergence of IDSs presents many unprecedented and exciting opportunities for professional nurses, working in close collaboration with physician colleagues and other caregiver groups. To be effective, however, nurses must clearly understand this new world and new nursing work.

## THE NEW WORK OF NURSING

Tomorrow's health care environment can be characterized by the following:

Rules change almost daily.
Radical new care delivery models are developed.
Multisite/multimodal care delivery is available across time and place.
Radical new payment models characterized by risk assumption across lifetimes are developed.
Far fewer resources are available, and fewer are to come.
Precise quantification is expected.
Far more accountability is required for clinical and financial outcomes.

New systems of care demand new modes of practice and new modes of preparation for the professional nurse. As systems become more integrated, as care occurs across broad continuums, and as patients in the hospital and in the home are more acutely ill, new types of nursing practice must emerge. Also, with the requirement for achieving specific clinical and financial outcomes from care that is population based and data based, new requirements emerge.

### Team Care

It is becoming increasingly clear that no single professional group can meet patient needs in such complex, fast-paced, and demanding environments. More than ever, patient care will require teams of health care providers that are constructed to match the clinical needs of specific populations. It is no longer possible, for example, when faced with a 3- to 4-day length of stay for an open heart procedure in a hospital, to determine which professional is singularly responsible for the achieved outcomes. The clinical care process is so truncated, demanding, and interdependent that it is absolutely essential that a team of professionals plan to provide care. This is by no means the old "team nursing." It is anything but that. Instead it is a well-designed and constructed group of selected multidisciplinary professionals that together merge their skills and talents to organize and deliver care for groups of patients. These teams will come together as the patient's needs evolve.

## Nursing's Strengths

With dramatic changes occurring in the overall context of health care, many unprecedented opportunities for nursing follow. This is clearly illustrated by the fact that effective integrated health care systems have key attributes that blend well with nursing strengths. Some examples follow.

- The ability to coordinate care across time and place
- The ability to organize and link the processes of care
- The ability to focus and be effective in well care, not simply sick care
- The ability to achieve desired clinical outcomes
- The ability to function in an affordable cost-effective manner
- The ability to organize care utilizing multidisciplinary, multiskilled, nonhierarchic teams

Nursing's strength lies in each of these areas. First, the organization of processes across time and place is what properly prepared nurses do well. They link processes across sites and over a lifetime. They mesh this skill well with physicians who have strength in treating episodes of care. Also, nursing's strength in prevention and wellness has been well documented over time. That strength becomes ever more important in an environment that requires the management of the health of large populations across lifetimes. Effective nurses know how to assist people to maintain health, from prenatality through senescence. Nurses can integrate and carefully blend care delivery skills with those of other care team members. Nurses have the ability to organize teams of caregivers, meshing individual skills with the specific clinical care requirements of patient populations.

Given these existing strengths, a desired future for nursing must reflect increased competency in the determination and measurement of three areas of outcomes: clinical, financial, and service. More quantification capability and more depth in data management are required. A desired future will also reflect increased incorporation of knowledge from the fields of epidemiology and biostatistics, because effective management of large populations will be crucial.

## The New Nurse

The following are some of the characteristics of the new nurse:

- Care team manager, coordinator
- Care team member
- Delegator
- Interdisciplinary collaborator
- Standard setter
- Outcomes monitor
- Quality monitor
- Incorporates research and data into practice
- Practices multisite/multimodal care
- Resilient, responsive, resourceful

These new characteristics are essential to fit the "new work." The new work of the new nurse can be described as follows:

- Manages/coordinates care teams
- Manages a multiskilled work group
- Demonstrates clinical excellence
- Manages efficient and rapid throughput of patients
- Tracks and shares accountability for clinical outcomes
- Tracks and shares accountability for financial outcomes

Key words emerge. There will be new operating models, new financing mechanisms, new emphasis on data management and analytic skill, multidisciplinary/crossdisciplinary team-based practice, emphasis on delegatory skill, and the ability to effectively practice within integrated delivery systems that are both multisite and multimodal.

A core requirement of practice in these still-emerging environments is the ability to be both flexible and resilient. One is reminded of the "morphing" process as depicted by the metal man in the film "Terminator II." First he appeared in one form, then resurrected into another, and then quickly reshaped into still another, depending on what the needs of the moment were. Nurses also must adapt a morphing mentality, albeit much less dramatic. The essence is that this new nurse must be able to acquire quickly the skills and competencies that are essential for new practice environments. A *Wall Street Journal* column (Lancaster, 11/15/94) was headlined "You, and Only You, Must Stay in Charge of Your Employability." This is a new mandate for nursing today.

Any remnants of a paternalistic system that ensured employment over a lifetime are quickly disappearing. Organizations cannot be expected to be concerned about the survival of each individual, because the organization is focused on its own survival. Therefore there is a new responsibility to always have the essential knowledge, skills, and competencies for the new era. How do physicians and nurses link together for efficient practice around discrete patient populations? How effective is the nurse in a multidisciplinary care team? How much leadership can/should nurses exert? The emergence and positive strength of nursing can be a strong leadership force for tomorrow. This is essential if patients are to be well served in challenging new times.

### Technology and Practice

One cannot discuss the new nurse and the new work without acknowledging the preeminence of technology and its application to practice. People are beginning to discuss "the wired health care professional" with computer linkages to resources and information. The concept should not be new; we have experienced "the wired UPS man" for quite some time. Nurses, too, will become more mobile in their practice sites, no longer always practicing in a single location with defined geography. Nursing will become both digital and virtual. Technology in the hospital, in the home, in the clinics, and at all other sites will be quite sophisticated and will serve as very effective, coordinating mechanisms of care. We will confront the issue of telepresence versus actual presence of health professionals in many care sites.

### New Roles

Some prominent and natural nursing roles evolve from these future scenarios. Some roles are new; some will be performed in different ways. Each will be utilized in increasing numbers. For example:

- The nurse case manager/care manager/care coordinator
- Advanced practice nurses (nurse practitioners (NPs) and clinical nurse specialists (CNSs)
- Telenursing positions (triage nurses, remote, telephonic, electronic)
- Nurses with advanced skills in data analysis, measurement, and outcomes

One thing that is perfectly clear is tomorrow's nurses must be well educated and well prepared if they are to exert leadership to positively influence the new health care systems as they emerge.

## THE NEW WORK OF NURSING ADMINISTRATION

When the rate of change is traumatic, rapid, and incessant, those persons with the capacity to manage that change effectively will be successful. Those nursing leaders who can be stimulated and energized by change and who can view this health care environment as highly challenging will succeed.

## Preparing for the New World

Nurse executives must first prepare themselves for this new world. They must acquire new skills and competencies that fit the current context of health care. None of us has all of the skills that we need, because this has not been done before. All senior executives in health care organizations are busily acquiring the necessary knowledge and skills. Many nurse executives in practice today have learned their skills in a health care world that was characterized by cost-plus reimbursement and retrospective payment. This was the era of revenue center management. Today, very different skills are required to successfully manage cost centers. Our old skills frequently do not apply in new contexts. It is relatively easy and exciting to manage growth scenarios; it is much more difficult to handle cost center management, knowing exactly what and where costs are and then tying them to outcomes. This is the hallmark of contemporary executive skill.

## Cost, Quality, Access, and Service

We have moved from an era in which cost was irrelevant to one in which cost is dominant. Quality has equal importance. Cost and quality are mandates, and one cannot supersede the other. The requirement is that cost be competitive and that quality standards must be met or exceeded. This makes difficult executive work much more difficult.

The nurse executive of tomorrow will require far more financial and quantitative skill. The ability to measure inputs and outcomes will be a fundamental requirement. For many years we have measured processes or inputs of care. For example, every nursing office in every hospital is likely to contain closets full of records of nursing hours per patient day that were delivered; however, the question has not been asked to what end? That is, what was the impact or outcome of the investment in nursing hours? This determination requires far different skills. The value of nursing care is its contribution to the required clinical, financial, and service outcomes. The new systems of managed care through HMOs permit enrollment or disenrollment on an annual basis. This means that our organizations will be judged by their costs, their quality, the ease of access to care, and customer service. To be successful in a sustained way, our organizations must meet stringent standards in each area. Performance in each of these areas will be very carefully measured. Therefore we are entering an era of precision and measurement in the delivery of health care that has been heretofore unknown.

## Evaluation

Nurse executives must acquire the skills that permit the systematic evaluation of all processes that relate to the delivery of patient care. Fundamental to that skill is the ability to oversee the redesign of core processes and the creation of new models of patient care delivery. This has emerged as a cornerstone capability for contemporary nurse executive practice. It is absolutely predictable that if we do not design new care models that fit with today's requirements for cost and quality, we will work with those models created by others. Therefore there is an urgency to provide leadership for the initiatives that will result in improved clinical processes.

All models or systems of care delivery must achieve a desired patient outcome; contribute to staff satisfaction, staff retention, and productivity; and contribute to the financial integrity of the organization. Unless each of these requirements are met, new models will not be sustained. Inherent in this requirement is that without careful measurement systems in place, one cannot know if these objectives have been achieved. These measurement systems must be developed.

Also of interest is the reality that in capitated environments patient care will increasingly be contracted across patient populations and patient lifetimes. The site of care (where) is becoming increasingly irrelevant. Rather, the processes of care (what is done), the clinical outcomes of care (to what end), and the financial outcomes of care (at what cost) will be the compelling themes. Obviously, this requires new methods of management. This also reinforces the requirement to use research data as a basis for decision support for both clinical and administrative decisions. This becomes essential in tightly managed care environments. Therefore evaluation research is increasingly important as a quantitative, objective, and measurable depiction of outcomes.

## CONCLUSION

Nurse executives must respond quickly to these emerging environments with new skills and new competencies. Unless we do, we lose the ability to exert leadership in the design of tomorrow's patient care systems. But this is never easy in such uncertain and chaotic times. Rosabeth Moss-Kanter (1983) said it well when she observed that the ability to absorb uncertainty will be a core characteristic of contemporary leadership. It will be *the* core characteristic.

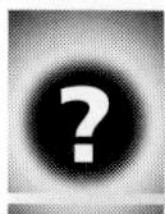

## *Discussion Exercises*

1. The shift to integrated delivery systems has radically changed health care. How has nursing changed in your community?
2. Why might nursing (collectively) and nurses (individually) not be able to adapt to the "new work of nursing" as described in this chapter? Include forces external to nursing, as well as internal factors.
3. How would you prepare to become an administrator in the new world of nursing work?

## References

Drucker P: The profession of management, Boston, 1998, Harvard Business School Press.
Hamilton/KSA: Web site address: *(http:///www.kurtsalmon.com/idshome.htm#jourstop)*.
Lancaster: H: You, and only you, must stay in charge of your employability, *Wall Street Journal*, November 15, 1994.
Moss-Kantor R: *The change masters,* New York, 1983, Simon & Schuster.

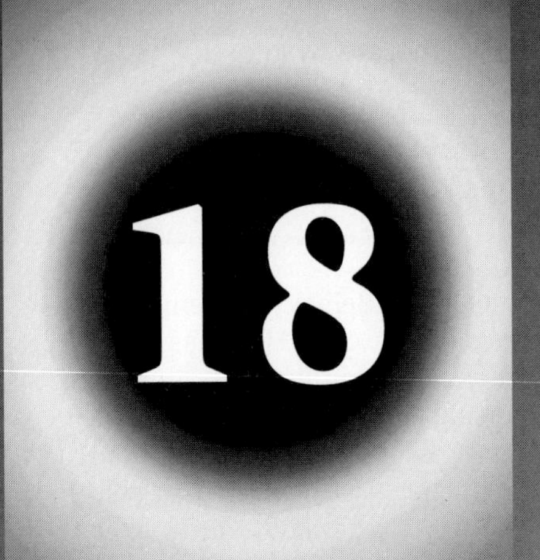

# 18 Governance: From the Boardroom to Patient Care

**Karlene Kerfoot**

*We have, I fear, confused power with greatness.*

**Stewart Udall**
Dartmouth College, 1965

## THE NURSE'S ROLES AND RESPONSIBILITIES

Organizational structures are changing rapidly in health care from the traditional models of independent facilities to large integrated networks of very diverse facilities and organizations. Merger-mania is running rampant in health care as organizations struggle to find the best partners to build their integrated networks. What will this mean for the future of nursing as we work to carve out roles and our governance structures in these rapidly changing structures?

We have two options. We can be the helpless victims of these processes, or we can be a codesigner for these new models of governance and organizational design. Our only hope to advocate for the right kind of patient care lies in our ability to understand governance structures and be influential in the future designs of these structures. Unfortunately, the role of architect in organizational design and governance has not been a consistent part of nursing's past. However, we have the opportunity to change that in the future if we so choose.

An understanding of our past and the traditional models of governance provides information to better design our preferred future. A short digression into our history is in order so we may use the past as a learning experience for what can and cannot happen in the future.

## GOVERNANCE STRUCTURES IN HEALTH CARE

An important concept in understanding the background of governance structures in health care is to remember the religious and militaristic roots of our origins. Before the advent of modern medicine, caring for the ill that was not done in families was the purview of religious organizations. Historically, these religious organizations were designed around an autocratic central control model; so was the kind of care that was provided by religious organizations. Nursing was born through the work of Florence Nightingale in a military setting in the Crimean War. The Nightingale schools of nursing that were established continued this highly controlled style of organization with directive, central control that was the norm of the time. With the proliferation of hospitals, which was stimulated by advances in medicine that created treatments and interventions for disease, this centralized, autocratic tradition continued (Figure 18.1). Frederick Taylor's influence on organizational design in the beginning of this century further solidified a bureaucratic style of governance in health care.

Therefore health care's roots became planted firmly in the command/control model of our military and religious structural roots. Although it might have been possible to command people to do prescribed work in the past, the evolution of the present-day culture into one of more participative interaction rather than the old industrial model in organizations demands a change in governance structures.

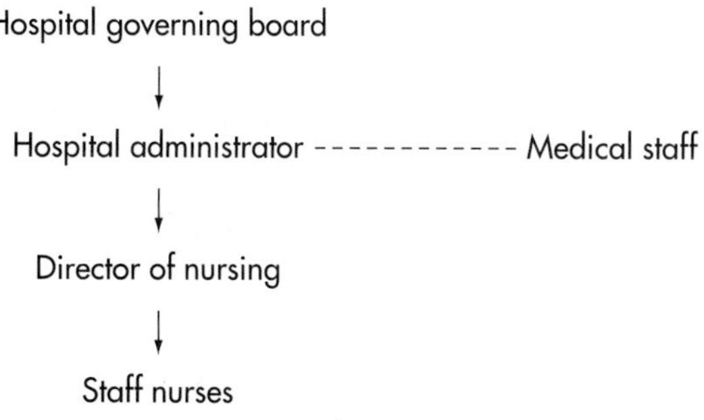


**Figure 18-1** Traditional hospital structure.

The history of nursing in the governance of health care is sparse because nurses have not been involved at the governance level for most of the history of health care. In the role of employee in most health care organizations, access to interaction at the top level of the organization has not been available. Nor has the profession of nursing had the empowerment that medicine and the law have had with their self-governed professional models.

In summary, the history of the involvement of nursing in governance in health care has been lacking because of the absence of extensive involvement in governance and our roots in centralized models. However, the past is just the past and does not have to be a predictor of the future unless we choose to make it one.

## A FUTURISTIC VIEW OF HEALTH CARE GOVERNANCE STRUCTURES

### New Paradigms

The mechanistic, industrial, widget-production–based mindset of organizations is gradually giving way to viewing the organization as living dynamism of ecologic activity. The Newtonian model of organizations that focuses on things rather than relationships is being put aside as organizations are increasingly viewed as holistic systems in which relationships and connections are seen as the key determinants of outcomes. Writers exploring the world of quantum physics, chaos theory, and biology are opening up new paradigms that force new ways of thinking about governance structures (Jantsch, 1980; Gleick, 1987; Wheatley, 1994). As the concepts from chaos theory are brought into the world of organizational dynamics and design, new governance structures must be considered for the future. A brief review of some of these concepts follows.

Leland Kaiser, a health care futurist, believes that the best organizational model for the future of health care is that of natural systems (Kaiser, 1996). He predicts the organizations of the future will parallel biologic ones. Kaiser believes that health care must be the organizing framework around which the building of healthier communities and the revitalization of our society can begin.

The design of this new kind of organization would be bottom up with no unnecessary structure and with each layer subsuming the one beneath it. The concepts from this model include bottom-up authority replacing central authority and the encouragement of diversity, eccentricity, and even instability. Organizations are seen as process structures rather than machines in this model (Kaiser, 1996). Governance in this kind of model must therefore change from the command/control of centralized decision making to the holistic thinking of organizations as self-renewing learning organizations. The responsibility of renewal must be in the hands of the self-managed teams that make up this new model of organizations.

Studies of companies that survive over time show that the key to their survival is based on long-term priorities that involve (1) developing people to carry their mission into the years ahead, and (2) encouraging growth without endangering the long-term viability of the origination (DeGues, 1997). High tolerance for new ideas and eccentricities and high levels of interaction and learning between and among people have spelled success for these organizations. Therefore the governance structures of the future must provide an environment of tolerance for innovation and evolution through the development of a community of learning that unleashes the intellectual and spiritual power of people throughout the organization. Peter Senge refers to these kinds of organizations as *learning organizations* (Senge, 1990).

## Integrated Delivery Systems

With the advent of integrated delivery systems, the organization of health care has changed dramatically. Previously, it was necessary for governance structures to be concerned with only the purposes and objectives of a single unit or facility. Now with mergers, regional structures, and even national structures for the delivery of health care, structures are much more complex. As different units come together to build the integrated delivery system, the challenge is to create new forms of governance that stretch over very heterogeneous units such as an HMO, several hospitals, rehabilitation, home care, and prevention activities.

One way to conceptualize the kind of governance needed for these structures is to think of each unit as a module that must be plugged into and integrated effectively into the other modules in the network (Baldwin and Clark, 1997). Governance structures can be the kind of interface around which all activities can be organized throughout the organization. If these interfaces are not created through a governance structure, then decentralized activities that are occurring in each module with no relation to the other modules will create a dysfunctional system and result in high costs because of duplication and poor quality. To be effective, governance structures must be created across these boundaries. The most effective structures will be the ones that honor diversity and create interdependence within the modules of the organization and between the modules. These structures also must be flexible to quickly integrate the plugging in of a new module that becomes a part of the system.

To meet the kind of challenges just outlined above, Charles Handy (1997) has suggested that organizations of the future must see themselves as communities and individuals as citizens of these communities rather than employees or human resources. Individuals within this community are viewed as having responsibilities, as well as rights. He believes that the concept of the company as property of the shareholders who own it or of the board or affiliate organization (such as a church) is the wrong metaphor and structure for the future. He sees an affront to natural justice in the old models (see Figure 18-1), because the terms of ownership and the concept of the corporation and the people who work within it as property is an insult to the concept of democracy. These old forms do not give enough recognition to the fact that people, especially in the structures of the future, will be the greatest asset the organization has. Handy believes that free people will refuse to join the old style of organization or will exact a high price for the loss of their rights.

If the organization is conceptualized as community and that community is placed within the community in which the organization operates, we have an interesting picture of overlapping communities necessarily interfacing with each other. Leland Kaiser challenges health care organizations to go beyond the walls of the illness-oriented facility to get out into the community and take ownership of the factors in the community such as violence and crime that contribute to poor health. His challenge is for all of us to serve the community through models, such as parish nursing, and to support people in self-care activities that will improve wellness in the community (Kaiser, 1996).

## GOVERNANCE STRUCTURES FOR THE FUTURE

### Continuous Quality Improvement to Self-Managed Teams

Bottom-up governance structures must become more important in the future. Already the movement to self-managed teams has occurred in some areas of health care. The quality movement in health care, when it is done well, has helped to eliminate the stratification by developing multidisciplinary Continuous Quality Improvement (CQI) teams. As these teams evolve, they move from participatory to self-managed structures that actually investigate and implement changes as needed on their own. The challenge for these groups is to design the work that needs to be done based on the external environment and the needs of the community, patients, and families, as well as the unit-based facility work that these teams have traditionally been challenged to do.

Developing governance structures across the network of the health care organization will be a challenge for the future. The consumers of illness and wellness will reside in many physical locations but have the right to one standard of care that is not compromised by the variability of geographic location or health care practitioner. As these delivery systems become networked throughout with computer technology, much more of the work of governance across widely dispersed geographic areas will take place. With videoconferencing, chat rooms, and e-mail, councils can do the work of governing the practice of patient care across the continuum of care.

### Governing Councils

Toyota Automatic Looms Works pioneered companywide governing councils to bridge between their six main corporate divisions (of which Toyota Motor is one) in a system called the Cross-Function Control System (Dimancescu, 1992). A long-term management plan is the tangible expression of the corporate vision that guides the work of the councils. Coordinating councils can be the interfaces that bring various modular divisions together. For example, in the Memorial Healthcare System in Houston, Texas, care is coordinated over 10 inpatient facilities, ambulatory functions, and wellness activities with the use of coordinating councils. These councils coordinate the functional work across facilities in structures such as the emergency center, intensive care, medical surgical, and psychiatric councils. Other councils that are more service line based do work under structures such as the women's council and the cardiovascular council.

Structures for governance at the top level of the organization are predicted to consist of small boards at the system level and probably a series of boards that attend to the functions of the rest of the organization much as subsidiary boards oversee the work in complex corporations. Structures that allow the work of the teams and councils on the front lines to be valued at the subsidiary board level and considered for policy will be the challenge for the next few years. When this is done well, the opportunities for a high-performance organization are much enhanced.

# IMPLICATIONS FOR NURSING

## Is Nursing a Profession?

A relentless debate has focused on whether nursing is a profession or a semiprofession. With that debate ongoing, it is difficult to have consensus about the governance structures for nursing. For example, if it was determined that nursing was clearly a profession, then peer review of practice and governance systems similar to medical staff governance structures would be incorporated. We would educate our young in the concepts of professional, autonomous practice. We would be willing to take on the accountability and responsibility for the professional practice of nursing through personal accountability and through the implementation of systems that support a shared governance model of nursing practice.

Timothy Porter-O'Grady has conceptualized and helped implement professional practice in systems and the community. His recent publication, *Whole-Systems Shared Governance* (Porter-O'Grady and others, 1997) articulates this patient-centered, point-of-care model, with governance consisting of a patient care council, an operations council, a governance council, and a systems councils. To realize this vision of practice, several challenges are ahead for the profession.

## Preparing for the Future

The first challenge is educating and developing competency-based testing for students throughout the educational continuum about how to function in a professional practice environment. The second challenge is to educate and competency test managers in leadership positions about how to implement and support the kind of professional practice necessary for our future. The third challenge is to help health care organizations understand how to make the transition from traditional centralized models into shared governance models. The final challenge is to help nursing professionals prepare themselves to serve on governing boards in health care, as well as on boards outside health care.

# CONCLUSION

The care of our patients, their families, and our communities will be greatly enhanced by the development of front-line–based structures that can quickly address the needs of the community and the health care needs of the constituents of the integrated network. Governance structures that are close to the core processes of health care and are structured around the needs of the community and patients will be the best for the future. The perennial downsizing and right sizing of our health care organizations makes it imperative that our systems of governance be effective and efficient at the optimal level. Anything less will almost certainly have an eroding effect on the consumer's perception that the quality of health care is in a tailspin.

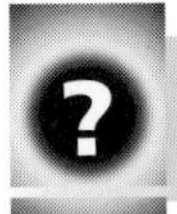

### *Discussion Exercises*

1. Select one of the models of the future described in the chapter and describe how the current health care system could be redesigned to fit the model. Be creative.
2. What changes are necessary in nursing to help it become a full-fledged profession?
3. Draw an organizational chart for a health care organization (fictitious or an actual organization), and critique it using concepts presented in the chapter.

## References


Baldwin C, Clark K: Managing in an age of modularity, *Harvard Business Rev 75*(1):84, 1997.

DeGues A: The living company, *Harvard Business Rev, 75*(2):51, 1997.

Dimancescu D: *The seamless enterprise,* New York, 1992, HarperCollins.

Gleick JC: *Making a new science,* New York, 1987, Viking.

Handy C: The citizen corporation, *Harvard Business Rev 75*(1):26, 1997.

Jantsch E: *The self-organizing universe,* Oxford, 1980, Pergamon Press.

Kaiser L: Health care in the 21st century, *Physician Executive* 22(1):12, 1996

Porter-O'Grady T and others: *Whole systems shared governance,* Gaithersburg, Md, 1997, Aspen.

Senge P: *The fifth discipline: the art and practice of the learning organization,* New York, 1990, Doubleday/Currency.

*Wheatley MJ: Leadership and the new science,* San Francisco, 1994, Berrett-Koehler.

# 19 Managing Across Disciplines

**Ann Marie T. Brooks**
**Toni Smith**

*The Question "Who ought to be boss?" is like asking "Who ought to be the tenor in the quartet?" Obviously, the man who can sing tenor.*

**Henry Ford**

Leaders in this dynamic health care environment face many new opportunities and challenges. Hospital-based leaders are creating care models that go beyond the walls of the hospital. They are restructuring and redesigning operational processes to improve efficiency and lower costs. They are also recruiting innovative thinkers and doers and creating innovative programs to retain highly qualified staff. Leaders in ambulatory or home care are also examining their programs, streamlining services and seeking to optimize resource use and improve outcomes.

For all leaders in health care, there is growing pressure to form new partnerships or become part of integrated networks to be better able to provide care across care settings. Reasons given include: It is a way to expand services; health care leaders fear that consumers will choose other plans or services that they currently do not offer; it is a method to capture a market niche or a prudent business decision. In addition, leaders are responding to the trend of investor-owned health care companies buying hospitals and other health care facilities and implementing business practices that substantially improve the health of the organization's bottom line. Although there is mixed reaction to this trend of for-profit expansions and resulting changes in organizational operating styles, data evaluating the effect on patients' outcomes and quality is not consistent or conclusive.

Community leaders have raised concerns about changes in ownership of hospitals and other partnering arrangements because they fear the impact that these new entities may have on the quality of life of their residents. In addition, the reliance of the community on hospitals and other health care facilities for employment and economic stability is important. However, the record number of mergers and joint ventures that have taken place in the last 10 years does indicate a trend toward a wide variety of new entities to strengthen market share, ensure long-term viability, and respond to changes in a dynamic health care environment.

Attention to fraud and abuse violations in health care has increased in this changing marketplace. The government has launched major initiatives related to improving the compliance of health care organizations with Medicare regulations. New requirements in federal and state regulations are aimed at providing more consistent monitoring and place new demands on providers and provider organizations. At the same time, organizations are working to strengthen their internal processes to avoid any potential for public disclosures that may jeopardize their image or standing within the community. Being known as "noncompliant" with Medicare regulations or other external requirements not only brings governmental repercussions but also may result in a negative image.

Managing across care settings outside the walls of hospitals is part of the new order in health care. What challenges the leader will face and how the leader will go about building teams, rewarding innovation, and promoting continuous learning and staying healthy in this dynamic environment are discussed in this chapter.

## THE IMAGE OF HEALTH CARE

Health care organizations and systems with innovative, patient-focused models of care that demonstrate a high degree of organizational effectiveness will receive world-class provider recognition and status. Greater prominence is being given to published ratings of providers of health care organizations. Payers, providers, and consumers are paying attention to these ratings that purport to measure quality through a variety of ways. The annual rating of the 100 best hospitals in the United States conducted by *U.S. News and World Report*, the Baldridge Award, and other public report cards such as Joint Commission on Accreditation of Healthcare Organizations (JCAHO) are examples of these surveys and published findings. Because of the widespread exposure and marketing of these data, health care organizations are working to create quality systems that will achieve recognition and accreditation. They are careful to avoid any unnecessary negative publicity that could create uncertainty and anxiety in the minds and hearts of the public and patients. In addition, negative findings from external accrediting and regulatory bodies may appear in newspapers and other media because of their newsworthy effect on the welfare and the quality of life of citizens within a community.

Professional associations representing disciplines or specialty groups are taking a more active role in helping their members maintain a positive image. Association members may provide consultation, sponsor forums, or serve on groups developing regulatory requirements or planning as part of their public commitment to their members to advance health care, uphold professional standards, and monitor patient safety.

It is not easy for the average patient or consumer to understand the implications of changes in health care, legislation, or the published information about diseases. Patients and their families report confusion about how the data affect them or how to use it in making health care decisions. The disclosure of health care information to the public does provide new opportunities for health care providers and/or health care organizations to assist consumers in seeking and obtaining the information necessary for informed decision making to improve their health status.

Nurses are in a unique position to promote information dissemination. Because of the direct and ongoing contact with patients, nurses are being hired by health care systems as information officers. In these new roles nurses are creating new methods to help patients and consumers gain access and understand information, evaluate its usefulness, and use it in their decision-making process. Nurses have always been involved in teaching, but the role of nurses and other health care providers in imparting information needed to maximize knowledge-based decision making and satisfaction is part of a commitment to quality patient care and outcomes.

## CHANGE

Because of the rapidity of change and the brief shelf life of solutions, leaders in health care are major stakeholders in mastering and leading change. They serve as champions for new thinking and creators of a new order of care delivery. Organizational designs in the future will be fluid and flexible and will foster collaborative relationships to achieve a common vision and the outcomes needed to compete and prosper within the market-driven health care environment. As new structures are put into place, the need to continue to apply sound management principles remains an imperative. New models will align incentives to foster and reward creativity of health care team members. Provision of care across the care continuum to specialized and culturally diverse populations will require a cadre of qualified health care practitioners with different backgrounds and skills working together in teams to treat illness, promote health, and evaluate outcomes. In addition, the team will blend the talents and skills of its members to continuously seek ways to improve care delivery and satisfaction of consumers and families.

Organizational leaders will be expected to manage operations across discipline boundaries, care settings, and institutions; to integrate and align incentives; to address cross-training issues; to foster productivity; and to balance multiple priorities required to meet changing patient and consumer needs. Although this may sound overwhelming, leaders will be required to translate the organization's vision into easily understood objectives. In conjunction with others, they will also manage the tangible and intangible assets of the organization in an energetic and productive way, remain sensitive to the morale of the employees, and keep an eye on the future.

### Interdisciplinary Leadership

During the past decade, nurses and physicians have taken on new roles that expand their responsibility for managing across systems, programs, and discipline boundaries. As more care delivery moves into community settings and new sites of care and models emerge, professional discipline boundaries will become less apparent and less important. Emphasis on competencies and care protocols will provide common frameworks to direct monitoring and evaluation of expected outcomes. Nurse executives are well prepared to assume expanded leadership roles and become trailblazers who design models of health care that are community based and innovative. They understand how to share accountability for managing populations and evaluating outcomes. The expertise and track records of nurse executives in managing clinical operations and partners with patients makes them ideal leaders for these challenging roles leading into the next century.

Interdisciplinary collaboration is not a new concept to health care leaders. It has long been a part of how nurses operate in health care. As part of the rich history of various disciplines working together, in the 1970s the National Commission on Joint Practice designed strategies that focused on physicians and nurses working together in genuine cooperative and collaborative relationships. During the past two decades many physicians and nurses have participated in national projects and studies aimed at enriching the practice environment and patient outcomes through innovative models of physician-nurse collaboration.

### Collaboration

As providers address quality and cost-effective care and prepare for the future, new approaches and thinking are needed. It is apparent that the effective utilization of diverse types and levels of professionals will be a critical factor in achievement of patient care outcomes. These models will depend heavily on the quality, efficiency, and cost-effectiveness of collaboration. Although health professionals proclaim verbally that they support collaboration, the actual understanding and commitment to its scope, breadth, and processes still appear limited. For some, interdisciplinary collaboration in health care means a nurse practitioner and primary care physician working together in joint practice, refers to an interdisciplinary practice team in a medical center that establishes care protocols, or denotes a single episode of conflict resolution that has been carried out involving nurses and physicians. Although these can be called selected examples of interdisciplinary collaboration processes, to state that the examples reflect the true essence of collaboration or the type of processes that ensure success in managing across disciplines would be misleading. In addition, the number of studies that measure the quality and effectiveness of collaborative practice models of physicians and nurses in acute and ambulatory settings is not bountiful.

Collaboration should be a process and behavior used as a basic operating principle by all health professionals. We know that the skill and commitment of physicians and nursing groups and other disciplines to work together to achieve common goals is critical to the success of health care delivery today. It will remain important in the new millennium. In the 1993 PEW Commission Report, O'Neil notes that the skills, attitudes, and values of the nation's 10 million health care workers have a fundamental impact on health care. The recommendations in this document engendered lively debate and discussion at institutions of higher learning for health care professional education and health care systems for several years. The PEW report readily acknowledged the importance of discipline practices on health care delivery outcomes and pointed to the substantial effect that they have in determining the quality, cost, and availability of health care services. For the nursing profession, with a base of 2.5 million registered nurses, this comes as no surprise. However, in the past, nursing has not necessarily used or had outcomes data available to demonstrate the cost effectiveness and impact of nursing care on quality. Aiken and others (1994) report that lower mortality rates occurred in hospitals where registered nurses had the ability to exercise clinical judgments at critical times in the management of patient care. She also noted that effective collaborative relationships with medical staff contributed to improved patient outcomes. Other researchers (Baggs and Schmitt, 1988) have consistently reported on improvements in patient outcomes, strengthened communication, and increased collegiality in effective collaborative practice models. Recognition of the importance of funding to evaluate the effect of collaboration on patient care outcomes is increasing and will be able to provide important data in future health care system development.

Unfortunately, the paucity of research on the effect of nursing on patient care outcomes continues to make it difficult to demonstrate what a valuable and cost-effective role nurses play in care settings and in patient satisfaction. Surveys on patient satisfaction usually report nursing care as either the first or second most important determinant of satisfaction in the patient experience.

The PEW report also recommended that the number of nursing and medical schools be reduced and emphasized the need for effective collaboration, mutual problem solving, and planning by all health professionals. At present, there has not been any major action taken in response to these recommendations. Nevertheless, the subsequent dialogue following the publication of the report supports the fundamental need to collaborate to overcome existing barriers and create cross-discipline competencies as part of a commitment to quality, cost efficiency, and customer satisfaction.

## ORGANIZATIONAL CHANGES

### Redesigning and Restructuring

Organizational redesign and restructuring of managing and services across a continuum of care requires crossing boundaries. Although cross-functional roles and reporting are not new, the widespread use, rationale, and acceptance of the trend to reassign is different today. In the past, organizations that supported cross-disciplinary reporting structures had designed them because of the strength or background of individual leaders, perceived efficiency, or tradition within the system. Now, as a result of redesign and a need for new processes, leaders acknowledge that flattening organizational structures can be growth producing and cost efficient and creates new opportunities for team building within the clinical enterprise and system. Whether these changes are due primarily to redesign or some other type of restructuring process, the leader in these roles is expected to exhibit a system perspective, serve as a productive and visible member of the senior executive team, and make timely and consumer-oriented decisions. At the same time, the leader is expected to be a role model, collaborate, foster team building, and exhibit flexibility in setting and achieving outcomes. The accountability for managing the work carried out by different professional groups across programs and care sites is aimed at eliminating the "silo" mentality, that is, separateness and isolation often fostered by traditional organizational, program, and discipline boundaries.

## Changing Role of the Chief Nurse

In the past most nurse executives and nurse managers were valued, recognized, and rewarded for their ability to control and allocate resources, maintain a positive image of the nurse, protect turf, and preserve the traditional stereotype of the nurse at the patient's bedside. Although the values of nursing remain intact, the vision, voice, and vitality of nursing has changed remarkably and will continue to change as the demand for care changes and the sites of care and care models undergo transformation. Command and control are no longer primary anchors for leaders in nursing or other departments. Reliance on these elements as an operating style usually results in major organizational and communication problems and creates tensions within the work environment. Cooperation and collaboration are expected if mutual problem solving and goal achievement is to occur.

The new health care environment offers many opportunities and challenges for the nurse executive. The role for nurses in leadership involves being a strategic planner, primary spokesperson for clinical practice, advocate for patient care, and manager of system patient care outcomes. As nurse executives broaden their span of influence and advocacy to include other disciplines, programs, and services, those in these evolving roles indicate satisfaction with their ability to influence across boundaries, speak with one voice for patient care, and represent a talented pool of health care professionals with specialized skills and abilities. In addition, they report pride in knowing that their expertise and skills and experiences in administrative and clinical care have prepared them to successfully lead across professional boundaries and programs.

### A Traditional Model

What we find today are organizational structures with nurses in various types of roles, in response to a changing and dynamic environment. Table 19-1 provides examples of current roles in hospital-based or integrated networks. Today, a large number of nurse executives continue to hold traditional positions in which the nurse executive maintains primary leadership for the nursing department. In this model, common titles include Director of Nursing or Vice President of Nursing Services. This leadership role is usually part of the management team within the organization. The position reports to the chief operating officer (COO) or chief executive officer (CEO). In most academic health centers this position usually appears on the same level as the medical director or chief of staff and in other organizations may be at the senior operational level.

### An Expanded Model

The nurse executive assumes operational responsibility for nursing and for other areas from the clinical or nonclinical operational side in an expanded model. The breadth of this responsibility varies across types of care settings or organizations. Examples of the areas of responsi-

**TABLE 19-1 Comparison of Organizational Structures**

| Traditional Model | Expanded Model | Corporate Model |
|---|---|---|
| **Title** | | |
| Vice President, Nursing | Vice President, Patient Care Services | Corporate Vice President, Clinical Operations |
| **Reporting to** | | |
| COO, CEO | Executive VP, COO or CEO | President or CEO of hospital or system |
| **Key aspects** | | |
| Line authority<br>Budgetary control<br>Directs operation | Line authority<br>Budgetary control<br>Accountability across disciplines/programs | System accountability<br>Limited budget control<br>No or limited line authority |
| **Scope** | | |
| Nursing focus<br>Interaction at department level | Collaborative focus<br>Consolidation<br>Facilitates team formation and interdisciplinary outcomes<br>Decreases redundancies<br>Decreases workload processes | Staff role<br>Outcomes focus/performance focus<br>Facilitates system thinking, action, and benchmarking<br>Balances decentralization and centralization<br>Fosters integration |
| **Responsibility** | | |
| Nursing department<br>Resources<br>Practice<br>Quality<br>Education<br>Recruitment/retention | Nursing plus other areas, which may include<br>Pharmacy<br>Respiratory therapy<br>Housekeeping<br>Dietary<br>Laboratory<br>Transportation<br>Physical therapy | Corporate level planning<br>Standard bearer for nursing and clinical services |
| **Member** | | |
| Management team | Executive management team<br>Board of trustees | Executive corporate team board of trustees/system board |

bility could include pharmacy, respiratory therapy, laboratory, physical therapy, and dietary. A frequently used title is Vice President for Patient Care Services. This leader in most cases is a member of the senior management team, and the reporting relationship is to the most senior executive position. This role is aimed at overcoming the duplication of roles within the organization or system. It is designed to support timely, integrated, and relevant decision making and foster shared accountabilities for outcomes.

### The Integrated Model

This model has become popular especially in evolving integrated systems or networks that are bringing together diverse types of care delivery organizational structures. Individuals being appointed to this role usually have a background of leadership in acute care and in some cases are learning as they establish these new roles. As they undergo this transition, they begin to acquire a new set of skills in influencing and advocating for change and forming alliances and leading in new ways based on different types of system drivers and stakeholders. Their colleagues are at the system level, and their exposure to community and external groups is at a higher level.

The nurse executive who manages across disciplines and beyond will need to lead in new ways. A new playbook is needed for designing work processes, managing human resources, and achieving outcomes to help navigate in different ways. Vestal (1997) notes that culture is the critical link between strategy and results in any system. The alignment of an organization's culture with its business strategy, work processes and roles, and its human resource strategies is critical to organizational success.

Nurse executives with strategic planning experience and success will be able to use it as they design and apply continuous learning strategies in building teams and bringing people together for a common goal. However, nurse executives who have been involved in planning primarily on the operational level that has limited experience in strategic planning can also be successful but will require additional educational training and ongoing mentoring as they lead the planning effort with others.

### The Evolving Model

The model for the future will be a hybrid of the current models. Depending on the system, purpose, and business arrangements, the nurse executive who manages across disciplines may be part of an executive team in one system, a chief operating officer in another, and a consultant in other components of the entity. Kerfoot (1997) uses the term "glue" as the element needed in organizations to keep all the various parts together. According to Kerfoot, leaders create the culture and manufacture the glue needed for successful synergy (Box 19-1).

Leaders who manage across disciplines should assume that the expectations for leadership competencies are universal. In Figure 19-1 the results from a survey done in 1987 and replicated in 1995 indicate that there are basic characteristics people value in their leaders. Treating people with respect and working with them based on a shared vision goes a long way in fostering a healthy and productive work environment and in retaining qualified staff. The nurse leader who manages across discipline and program boundaries will need to gain trust and establish credibility with individuals who may assume that nurses will receive priority based on their past management experience. It will be important for the leader to demonstrate commitment, expertise in leading, team building skills, and the ability to not favor any particular group. Box 19-2 identifies the specific behaviors that individuals perceive as important to their effectiveness.

## MANAGING ACROSS BOUNDARIES

### Creating the Environment

Leaders who manage across disciplines and other boundaries will be successful if their systems and organizations help reinforce the richness that results from working to blend talents,

**Box 19-1**
***Evolving Model***

Title: Executive Nurse
Reporting to: To be determined; may be the board or system leaders
Key aspects: Leading, building, networking, and mentoring
Scope: System development and expansion
Responsibility: System oversight and consultation
Member: Executive group

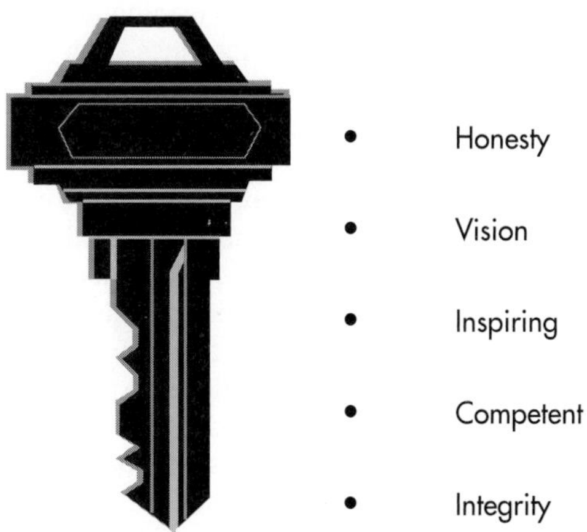


**Figure 19-1** Expectations of leaders (From Seligman, ME: *Learned optimism,* New York, 1991, Simon & Schuster).

skills, and abilities of various disciplines and other work groups. There can be long-term gains when leaders take actions that will provide visibility, support, and legitimacy for interdisciplinary learning, valuing, and shared accountability. In some organizations this is already taking place, and leaders will continue to expand this important and successful process. Where valuing collaboration has been more limited, leaders will need to become more active in role modeling, creating and aligning incentives and systems for valuing the partnership process approach. In a limited number of organizations, in which leaders are in transition and may be expanding parts of the system and redefining its mission, there will be a need for fundamental structural change and integration of the principles of interdisciplinary collaboration at all levels and components of the organization. Sample strategies to strengthen collaboration through practice, education, and research include the following:

1. Build cross-discipline competencies into performance systems
2. Establish interdisciplinary learning centers that include consumer input and provide incentives
3. Design interdisciplinary outcomes research initiatives to produce evidence-based outcomes
4. Align incentives and rewards to foster collaboration

**Box 19-2**
***Activities of Leaders***

What do admired leaders do?
- Empower and acknowledge contributions of others
- Make time for people
- Share the vision
- Open doors for opportunity
- Overcome personal hardships in their lives
- Admit mistakes that they made
- Advise others
- Solve problems creatively
- Teach well

To successfully manage change the leader will need to continuously seek new learning opportunities and behaviors that engender trust within the environment. Competencies to navigate the health care system in the new millennium include the following:

1. System thinking
2. Team building
3. Operational savvy
4. Risk taking
5. Humor
6. Creativity/innovation

## Preparing to Lead

There are many ways to prepare to lead in these new roles for managing across discipline and organizational boundaries. Qualifications related to education and experience are important and help to provide the underpinnings for success in managing and leading in a dynamic environment. In addition, the commitment to continuous learning is key to the continual replenishment of mind and spirit and organizational effectiveness.

As one looks outside of health care to others who have achieved success in bringing talented individuals together to achieve a common goal, several names immediately come to mind. One well-known individual who received the highest recognition in the field of sports in July 1997 is Don Shula, the former football coach of the Miami Dolphins. His induction into the Football Hall of Fame during his first year of eligibility plus his record-breaking achievements as the leader of a world-class sports team indicates that his skill in working with people and building systems deserves attention. In 1995 he coauthored a book with Ken Blanchard (leadership expert) entitled *Everyone's A Coach.* This book addresses the fundamental principles needed by all leaders involved in working with people. For nurse executives who manage across disciplines, it has special meaning because it emphasizes the outcomes of the team rather than organizational subgroups and reinforces the need to continually update the playbook. The acronym *COACH* is used as a way to describe the five secrets of coaching that are applicable to leading and managing any group. Box 19-3 describes each of the five secrets, and Box 19-4 offers sample questions to be asked to determine your ability in each of these areas of focus.

Although some may argue that these five secrets are too simplistic or do not contain anything new, it is important to acknowledge that Don Shula's track record of success, his recognition as a world-class leader of a world-class team within a world-class organization, and his status as a highly regarded leader inside and outside of sports are based on this process. Using his ideas and perspectives can add to our understanding and recognition of achieved outcomes. As Blanchard, a well-known author and expert in business points out, Shula's secrets are part of his fabric and a key ingredient to the success of his teams (Shula and Blanchard, 1995).

His principles are also useful in thinking about how the team's performance links to the fans and their satisfaction. Although the analogy may not be as easy as one would hope, there are certain similarities that can be drawn in thinking about the relationship and connectedness that the football coach, team, and players have to the public and the type of accountability that the health care leader and team has to patients, families, and the public.

Answer the sample questions in Box 19-4 to evaluate your skill in coaching your team to achieve goals. How do you rate yourself in preparing others? Are staff ready to meet the challenges of daily life? Can they adjust to a changing environment?

Use these sample questions to start a discussion with those you work with about continuous improvement. Using something that is outside their experience can help to break down boundaries, focus on outcomes, and generate new approaches to working together. Designing new ways to evaluate individual and team performance is critical to cooperation and collaboration and achievement of goals. There are many

### Box 19-3
### *COACH*
### *Five Secrets*

| | |
|---|---|
| **C**onviction driven | Effective leaders stand for something. |
| **O**verlearning | Effective leaders help their teams achieve practice perfection. |
| **A**udible ready | Effective leaders, and the people and teams they coach, are ready to change their game plan when the situation demands it. |
| **C**onsistency | Effective leaders are predictable in their response to performance. |
| **H**onesty based | Effective leaders have high integrity and are clear and straightforward in their interactions with others. |

From Shula D, Blanchard K: *Everyone's a coach,* New York, 1995, Harper Business.

**Box 19-4**
***Score Sheet—Sample Questions***

**Secret 1. Conviction driven**

1. Articulates a vision
   __ Strength __ Needs improvement
   What is your vision for your organization, department, or program?
   What convictions drive your vision?
2. Values respect more than popularity
   __ Strength __ Needs improvement
   How important is it for you to be liked?
   How do you share yourself with your team members?
   What do you want your team to remember you for?

**Secret 2. Overlearning**

1. Limits the number of player-development goals
   __ Strength __ Needs improvement
   How many things do you have your employees working on at any one time?
2. Reduces practice errors
   __ Strength __ Needs improvement
   How important are "practice errors" to you?
   How good are you at catching somebody doing things right?

ways to foster spirit and teamwork. It is up to the leader to bring new ideas and ways for others to be able to demonstrate capability and capacity to manage change and produce outcomes. Often in nursing and in health care we get stuck because we limit the problem-solving strategies that we use. Trying our new plays and relying on substitutes as a way to develop future leaders should be part of our game plan.

## CONCLUSION

Where are we going? Managing across disciplines is a professional and career opportunity for nurse executives. Nurses have always made a difference in patient care and have a strong track record in leading nurses and being champions of clinical thinking in health care organizations. Patient care and systems will benefit from nurses leading across discipline and organizational boundaries. Nurses are trailblazers of new thinking, processes, and outcomes. They understand and value excellence in patient care and know how to build teams and create the type of partnerships needed for excellence. The success of leading, coaching, and transforming will depend on the individual's ability to address workplace issues, recruit, retain, and promote talented, culturally diverse individuals and serve as a standard bearer and leader of excellence in clinical operations.

So, obviously when one considers the question of managing across disciplines asked by Henry Ford, the answer will be *the nurse*. It is up to us to make it happen.

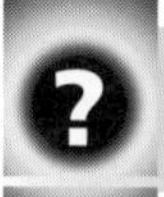

## *Discussion Exercises*

1. What system factors would prevent nurse executives from leading in expanded areas, such as across disciplines or across settings?
2. What professional and personal factors would prevent nurse executives from leading in expanded areas?
3. You are a nurse executive in a traditional role in a hospital that has just merged with a large, multisite health care system. What steps will you take to prepare to become part of the executive team of the system?

## References

Aiken LH and others: Lower Medicare mortality among a set of hospitals known for good nursing care, *Med Care* 32(8):771, 1994.

Baggs JG, Schmitt MH: Collaboration between nurses and physicians, *Image J Nurs Sch* 20:145, 1998.

Kerfoot K: Glue: the essence of leadership, *Nurs Econ* 15(2):100, 1997.

O'Neil EH: *Health professions education for the future: schools in service to the nation,* San Francisco, 1993, Pew Health Professions Commission, University of California at San Francisco Center for Health Professions.

Seligman ME: *Learned optimism,* New York, 1991, Simon & Schuster.

Shula D, Blanchard K: *Everyone's a coach,* New York, 1995, Harper Business.

Vestal KW: Organizational culture: the critical link between strategy and results, *Hosp Health Serv Adm* 42(3):339, 1997.

# 20 The Future of Collective Bargaining in Nursing

**Lea Acord**

*The organization can never be something the people are not.*

**H.S. Pritchett**

## THE PAST

For more than 50 years, registered nurses have effectively used the collective bargaining process to enhance their economic status and their working conditions in an effort to protect their practice and improve care to their patients. The growth of collective bargaining for nurses is tied directly to the history of the American Nurses Association (ANA). One of the original purposes for establishing ANA in 1896 was "to promote the usefulness and honor, the financial and other interests in the nursing profession" (ANA, 1896). Even though protecting the welfare of nurses was an early priority for ANA, it took 50 years for ANA to establish a formal, comprehensive economic and general welfare program including the representation of nurses in their places of employment through collective bargaining.

### The Beginning

The movement began with the California State Nurses Association (CSNA, later known as the California Nurses Association), under the direction of Shirley Titus, Executive Director. In the early 1940s appalling working conditions and extremely low wages were forcing many nurses to leave the profession or to choose other types of employment. Titus foresaw that if the nurses association didn't step in to remedy the situation, traditional labor unions would attempt to represent nurses. She appealed to the CSNA Board in 1942 to act as the collective bargaining agent for nurses in California. In January 1943 the CSNA Board voted to endorse collective bargaining for nurses and an aggressive program, including organizing, was launched (Ketter, 1996).

At the same time that the California association decided to organize and represent nurses, ANA commissioned a study of the working conditions of nurses around the country. The report of this study by Raymond Rich and Associates proclaimed: "Nursing cannot hope to maintain high standards of practice, attract qualified recruits, or retain the best nurses unless the profession does everything in its power to gain for nurses a decent measure of social and economic security." The report further stated that the representation of nurses by unions was inevitable. "The only choice is whether that representation would take place within or outside the profession." The consulting firm recommended that ANA assume responsibility for representing nurses (Rich and Associates, 1944).

At the ANA convention in 1946 a resolution was brought to the House of Delegates by the California Nurses Association that would change the nature of the profession and the organization forever. The resolution created a national economic security program and endorsed the 8-hour work day and 40-hour work week for all nurses. In addition, delegates called for the elimination of discrimination against minority groups. Primarily because of the successes of CSNA and the determination of Shirley Titus, the resolution was adopted unanimously by the ANA House of Delegates. It was not, however, without controversy. The endorsement of collective bargaining by the professional association triggered a great deal of debate, much of which has yet to be resolved even now, more than 50 years later.

## Representation

Much of the early work in collective bargaining by state nurses associations (SNAs) dealt with recognition of the associations as appropriate representatives of nurses. Until 1974 many nurses were denied legal protection of their right to organize and bargain collectively by the Taft-Hartley Act, which exempted private nonprofit hospitals from coverage under the National Labor Relations Act (NLRA). After considerable effort this exemption was finally removed in 1974. The protection of the NLRA, including collective bargaining rights, was thus extended to nonsupervisory employees of all health care facilities, including those private nonprofits previously excluded. This change in legislation affected about 495,000 RNs in 7000 health care institutions. After 1974 collective bargaining in hospitals grew dramatically. In the late 1960s only 9% of hospital workers were represented by labor unions. By 1977 that number exceeded 20% (Acord, 1982).

Representing nurses through the collective bargaining process was challenged legally as well as legislatively. In 1989 the National Labor Relations Board (NLRB) issued final rules regarding appropriate bargaining units in health care, including an exclusive bargaining unit for registered nurses. Appeals from the American Hospital Association delayed the implementation of this ruling for 2 years. Finally, in 1991 the U.S. Supreme Court upheld the NLRB's rule establishing appropriate units for collective bargaining in hospitals (Ketter, 1996). The unanimous decision of the Supreme Court in 1991 that allows for an all RN bargaining unit opened a new window of opportunity for increased unionization of registered nurses by all labor organizations.

## Definition of Supervisor

A second legal challenge occurred in 1994 when the U.S. Supreme Court ruled, in *NLRB v. Health Care and Retirement Corp.*, that three LPNs who worked at a nursing home and directed the work of others were supervisors and therefore not eligible for collective bargaining. For 20 years the NLRB had ruled that in the health care industry nurses who direct the work of others are doing so "in the interest of the patient" and not "in the interest of the employer," thus exempting them from the definition of a supervisor under the law.

The potential effects of the 1994 Supreme Court ruling on all nurses were profound. Some employers immediately tried to use the decision as a way to keep from bargaining with nurses in their agency. One such hospital, Providence Hospital in Anchorage, Alaska, claimed that registered nurses were ineligible because, as charge nurses, they directed the work of others and were therefore supervisors.

The NLRB was asked to rule in light of the recent Supreme Court decision on the supervisory status of charge nurses as defined by the National Labor Relations Act. The Board made two distinctions that assisted in their ultimate ruling that charge nurses were not, by virtue of their title, considered supervisors. The first distinction had to do with the issue of judgment. The Board ruled that all nurses exercise judgment as part of their professional practice and this does not distinguish nurses as supervisors. The second distinction had to do with the general authority of charge nurses. The Board noted that there were institutional limits on the general authority of the charge nurse and that decisions made by nurses are part of the professional responsibility of all nurses, not just that of charge nurses. The implications of the Board's decision are that RNs who work as professional, nonsupervisory employees have the right to organize for collective bargaining purposes and to engage in other concerted activity (Ketter, 1996).

### Economic and General Welfare Programs

Since 1946 ANA has helped its state nurses association members establish and implement economic and general welfare programs. The vast majority of registered nurses still practice their profession as institutional employees; for this reason, collective bargaining is a key component of many state nurses association programs. In the early days attention was focused on improving salaries, fringe benefits, and working conditions. ANA promoted the 40-hour work week with time and a half for overtime; cost of living salary increases; paid vacations and sick leave; and financial protection in sickness, old age, and death.

As time passed the state nurses associations also started to use collective bargaining to address professional practice issues. Contracts began to incorporate language on health and safety issues, appropriate staffing levels, salary scales with incentives for advanced training and credentials, nursing roles, and many other professional issues. Although contracts negotiated by state nurses associations vary according to the needs of the nurses being represented, control and protection of nursing practice, in addition to the economic advantages, is the ultimate goal of all SNA contracts.

### Today

More than 300,000 RNs in the United States (15% of the total registered nurse population) belong to unions. Through its state nurses associations ANA is still the labor organization representing the largest number of nurses. The issue of collective bargaining still causes conflict among the SNAs. In 1995 the California Nurses Association, with a membership of approximately 22,000 nurses, 85% of whom were under contract, elected to disaffiliate with the American Nurses Association because of conflicts between resource allocations to support the activities of ANA as a professional association and resources to support the activities of ANA as a labor organization.

## THE PRESENT

Major changes are influencing the effectiveness of the American Nurses Association and other labor organizations in representing registered nurses through collective bargaining. These changes fall into three critical areas: (1) changes in health care, (2) changes in higher education with an emphasis on nursing education, and (3) changes in the American labor movement.

### Changes in Health Care

In 1946 the U.S. Congress passed the Hill-Burton Act, which established a minimum standard of health care based on a ratio of 5 hospital beds per 1000 population. By adhering to the Act, the United States developed a good, though increasingly costly, health system. As costs escalated and reimbursement declined, ratios have fallen below the Hill-Burton standards. Hospitals have downsized and merged, and care has moved out of hospitals and into communities.

### Downsizing

During the 1990s 10 states closed down 10% or more of their hospital beds. Massachusetts eliminated nearly 25%, and Illinois eliminated more than 20% of their hospital beds (Freeman, 1997). Many rural areas have been left without hospitals, requiring patients to travel long distances to obtain care. Hospital mergers and acquisitions are transforming remaining medical centers into immense intensive care units and 1-day surgicenters.

These changes have had a profound effect on the nursing workforce. Starting in the early 1990s the percentage of RNs employed in hospitals began to decline while the growth in nonhospital employment rose. However, earnings for RNs stagnated and there has been no growth in the inflation-adjusted wages of RNs since 1991 (Buerhaus and Staiger, 1996). Hospitals are cutting costs by laying off nurses and replacing them with less skilled and less experienced workers. Aiken (1994) noted that the ratio of registered nurses to unlicensed assistive personnel has decreased in recent years. As a result, nurses are reporting higher levels of stress because fewer employees are expected to do more work. Job expectations are higher, and the use of sick leave has increased because nurses feel exhausted and unsatisfied (Richardson, 1997).

As hospitals have become smaller and more focused, many have been acquired by large and lucrative managed care systems of integrated care that combine primary, specialty, and hospital services. Because of the potential for financial gain, these systems often use powerful economic influences to inhibit attempts by workers to unionize.

Ironically, although some believe the need for the kind of protection afforded through collective bargaining agreements has become even greater, it has become harder to achieve with decreased numbers of nurses working in hospitals that have become part of larger systems. Huge profits of these multihospital systems are used against attempts by labor organizations to organize the workforce.

### Dispersed Worksites

A second trend in health care that has implications for unionization is the lack of geographic proximity of nurses working for the same system employer. As health care moves to the community, nurses are disseminated throughout the system, both inside and outside the hospital, with little chance for interaction with other nurses. Unions count on a critical mass or core of nurses who can speak for the interests of all the nurses being represented. In many organizations there is no longer a core that represents all nurses. Instead, nurses work in a variety of positions—both supervisory and nonsupervisory—which makes it difficult to determine a community of interest, much less an appropriate bargaining unit.

### Patient-Centered Care

A third trend in health care relates to the increasingly interdisciplinary nature of care. Even the term "nursing care" is becoming outdated as care shifts from that rendered by a particular provider to care given to the client that can be supplied by any number of providers. Nurses work closely with others to support such patient-centered care. This trend erodes the exclusivity of nurses.

## Changes in Nursing Education

### Higher Education

Similar to the changes in health care, higher education in the United States also is experiencing profound change. State and federal support of higher education is diminishing. Also, students are older, more diverse, and more likely to be enrolled on a part-time basis. A more flexible learning environment is required. Lifelong learning is an expectation for graduates in all fields. Although the major setting for learning is still on the campus, more and more learning is taking place off-site as distance education becomes more accessible. Institutions are networking to deliver programs designed by teams of faculty with diverse talents but common interests (see Chapter 16).

## Nursing Education

Nursing education is not immune to changes taking place in higher education. In addition, nursing faculty are responding to the changes in health care by revising curricula to address the new health care environment and by differentiating associate degrees from baccalaureate degrees. In 1995 approximately two thirds of new RN graduates were prepared in 2-year associate degree programs, which prepare nurses for hospital-based patient care (U.S. Department of Labor, 1996). Curricula of associate degree programs reflect this practice. The education of students in baccalaureate and higher degree programs focuses on case management and primary care, as well as acute care, and prepares students for more autonomous practice, reflecting the migration of health care out of the institutional setting.

In terms of collective bargaining, this means that registered nurses are being divided not only in the workplace but also in the educational setting. To add to this confusion, the trend in LPN education is to offer an associate degree. Thus far, only North Dakota has standardized nursing education by educating and employing two levels of nurses only—the professional nurse with a baccalaureate degree in nursing and the licensed practical nurse with an associate degree in nursing.

## Changes in the American Labor Movement

Workers throughout the United States have effectively used the collective bargaining process to improve their economic status. The increase in the standard of living for Americans in general can also be attributed to the economic and political climate fostered by the growth of collective bargaining. Workers' rights to organize and bargain collectively with their employers has been legally established in most democratic countries and is also cited in the Declaration of Human Rights approved by the General Assembly of the United Nations on December 10, 1948.

The labor movement in the United States has shifted in the last few years. Although the mission of collective bargaining has always been to improve the economic status and better the lives of working families, the AFL-CIO recently stated: "To accomplish this mission we will build and change the American labor movement" (AFL-CIO, 1996). The document goes on to say that the way this organization will change is through enhanced organizing efforts, strengthening their political agenda, and transforming the role of the union "from an organization that focuses on a member's contract to one that gives workers a say in all the decisions that affect our working lives."

In November 1995 the Bureau of Labor Statistics (BLS), U.S. Department of Labor, released its latest employment projections by industry and occupation for the period 1994 to 2005. "Health Services" is listed among the 10 industries with the fastest projected job growth, and "Registered Nurses" ranks fifth in the top 10 occupations with the largest projected job growth. The new AFL-CIO leadership and an increased commitment to organizing workers mean health care employees, and specifically registered nurses, will become prime targets for organizing. Vast resources have already been poured into this effort, and the trend is likely to continue.

Unions that represent registered nurses as part of the AFL-CIO include the National Union of Hospital and Health Care Employees of Retail, Wholesale, and Department Store Union; the American Federation of Government Employees; the American Federation of State, County, and Municipal Employees; and the American Federation of Teachers. In addition, the Service Employees Union International (SEIU) is a separate union that is continuing to aggressively organize health care workers, including nurses. SEIU currently represents about 450,000 health care workers.

# THE FUTURE

## Probable Short-Term Future

What is likely to happen to health care, the nursing profession, and the representation of nurses through collective bargaining? Although there are many unknowns, it is not difficult to determine a probable scenario for the immediate future. In the short term, the outlook is bleak as the health care system continues to spiral downward. The staffing ratio of unlicensed and inadequately trained personnel will continue to increase even though employers are finding the turnover rate of these workers high. The small number of professional nurses working in the few hospitals that are left in the United States will remain frustrated by their inability to provide appropriate care.

Controlling costs will endure as the driving force in health care as for-profit integrated systems continue to proliferate; profits will multiply exponentially. In addition, for-profit organizations will pour vast resources into combating the organizing efforts of nurses because the nursing workforce will be ripe to organize for collective bargaining. Unfortunately, with the small number of nurses in any one place to be organized for collective bargaining, unions will look very closely at the investment of time and money to launch an organizing campaign. Those unions with few resources will not survive or will choose to dilute the exclusivity of RN-bargaining units in favor of a more lucrative unknown combination of employee groups.

Hospital cutbacks of nurses will cause a severe nationwide reduction in the quality of patient care and an increase in hospital mortality and morbidity. As staffing levels erode, patients will not receive the care required for the healing process to occur in the hospital, and they will be prematurely discharged without the necessary help for optimal healing at home. Soon, the quality of the health care system will reach an all-time low.

## Preferable Long-Term Future

If nurses band together and work with consumers and other health care providers, the above scenario will last only a few years. A public outcry unequaled in force and unparalleled in persistence will demand that health care be accessible, affordable, and appropriate. Nurses will once again become the mainstay of better-managed hospitals and health care centers and will hold positions of authority, as well as provide care. In partnership with nurses, consumers will take more responsibility for their health as prevention and healthy lifestyles become a way of life. Nurses will continue to not only be the largest health care provider but also the glue that holds the health care system together because of their focus on holistic care of the client and their ability to help consumers manage their own health and find appropriate resources when needed.

Managed care will go through a major transition as the client becomes the core of the health care system rather than the system being the center to which clients must adapt. Although integrated health care systems will still be in place, some systems will become so large that the government will step in to break up the monopolies and encouraging competition.

Standardization of nursing education will occur. Technical nurses with 2-year educations and associate degree credentials will take a prominent place in the new integrated health care system. Professional nurses with at least a baccalaureate degree in nursing will be prepared to take on a variety of roles both inside and outside the traditional hospital setting.

Collective bargaining will continue to play a prominent role in the protection of practice, especially for technical nurses. ANA will be the labor organization of choice as nonsupervisory nurses realize that the professional association is the most appropriate union to address the issues of most concern to nurses—protecting their practice and improving care to their patients. Through their SNAs the American Nurses Association will be creative in their organizing efforts and organize networks of nurses working in integrated systems. In addition, ANA will continue workplace advocacy programs that will allow nurses to protect and preserve caregiving and expand nursing's influence in the health care system.

In a presentation on the economics of practice at the 1982 convention of the American Nurses Association, Catherine Welch, Executive Director of the New York State Nurses Association, stated: "The organization that controls collective bargaining will control every vital aspect of the profession. If control is not through the professional association, the American Nurses Association, nurses will not be dominated by their employers, but by other unions" (American Nurses Association, 1982).

## CONCLUSION

Collective bargaining in nursing has paralleled the American labor movement in the twentieth century. More recently, as massive changes in health care have occurred, changes in nurses' employment have altered the traditional relationship between nurses' representatives and their employers. The controversy regarding the appropriate representation for nurses and whether nurses should be represented by collective bargaining units has not abated. For a preferable future nurses should join consumers in demanding quality nursing care. The professional association is the appropriate representative for nurses.

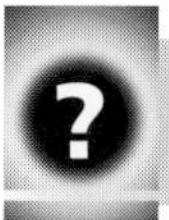

## *Discussion Exercises*

1. Why do you think the labor movement, in nursing and in industry, was successful in the early part of the twentieth century? Are the conditions that necessitated unionization still true?
2. Professional purposes versus collective bargaining goals have been debated since ANA began representing nurses. Explain the controversy.
3. What is your view on collective bargaining for nurses? Defend your perspective.

## References

Acord L: Protection of nursing practice through collective bargaining, *Int Nurs Rev,* p 150, September/October, 1982.

AFL-CIO: *1997 Program summary,* December 18, 1996.

Aiken L: Transformation of the nursing workforce, *Nurs Outlook* 43(5), 1995.

American Nurses Association: *Bylaws,* 1896, The Association.

American Nurses Association: *Economic and General Welfare Commission Report to the House of Delegates,* 1982 Convention, The Association.

Buerhaus P, Staiger D: Managed care and the nurse workforce, *JAMA Am* 11:1487, 1996.

Freeman R: Managed care's scorched earth medical and hospital policy, *Revolution Nurs Empowerment,* p 34, Spring, 1997.

Ketter J: *A seat at the table: 50 years of progress,* 1996, American Nurses Association.

*NLRB v. Health Care and Retirement Corp,* 94 CDOS 3649, 1994.

Rich and Associates: *Report to ANA board of directors,* 1944.

Richardson T: Total quality management programs UNA update, *Revolution J Nurs Empowerment,* p 26, Spring, 1997.

U.S. Department of Labor, Bureau of Labor Statistics: *Employment and wages: annual averages,* Washington, DC, November, 1996, The Department.

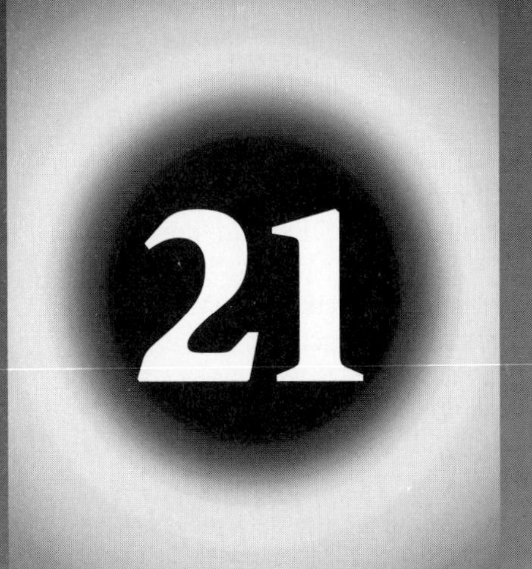

# 21 Managing an Academic Program in Nursing

**Eleanor J. Sullivan**
**Rachel Z. Booth**

*To rule is easy, to govern difficult.*

**Goethe**

Higher education, like health care of a few years ago, is facing enormous change. Similar to the forces that changed health care, external and internal threats, along with massive technologic change, are permanently altering higher education (Keller, 1995; Sullivan, 1997). Nursing education, as part of both higher education and health care, is encountering change from both systems (see Chapter 16). The challenge for the nurse executive in the nation's colleges and universities has never been greater.

## THE NURSE EXECUTIVE'S ROLE

Whether the nursing education unit is a school, college, division, or department, its chief executive officer is called a dean, director, head, or chair; whether the parent college or university is large or small or public or private, the responsibilities of the nurse executive are largely the same. The nurse executive is responsible for the internal operation of the education unit and for interacting with the external environment. What characterizes dynamic organizations, however, is a focus on futuristic and strong leadership. This leadership energizes the faculty and staff to recognize challenges as opportunities to accomplish the school's goals and to affect the future in a positive fashion.

The internal and external environments consist of individuals and groups who are better informed, more knowledgeable, and highly ambitious and who have a passion to be involved in the decisions of the organization. Unlike the hierarchic and rigid structures of the past, the future will demand fewer levels of administration or management; greater dependence on group dialogue and decision making; and infrastructures that are flexible, fluid, and positioned to change on short notice and in a short time. Organizations of the future will be in constant motion to maintain a viable, competitive edge in the marketplace. The nursing education unit will be the center of this action and will need a highly competent nurse leader who can deal effectively with ambiguity and chaos, take risks, loosen controls, remove barriers, and partner with both internal and external constituencies.

## Internal Role

Although administrative or managerial activities must be performed, the characteristics of the workforce and the environment require an executive who is a strategic thinker, a visionary, and a people person with a high level of confidence and trust in the ability of others. The nurse executive inspires the faculty and staff to invest in the organization, creates rewards for faculty and staff contributions, and creates processes that allow the organization to change in minimal time, with minimal deliberation, and with minimal obstacles.

The academic executive is responsible for ensuring that the educational program in nursing is offered in a competent, timely, and cost-effective manner. To accomplish this, the executive secures and allocates financial resources, administers a recruitment process, employs and monitors faculty and staff (often through other individuals, such as associate deans, coordinators, or directors), and configures the academic unit into workable groups. The executive is responsible for monitoring the integrity of the curriculum and ensuring that students are appropriately recruited, selected, educated, and graduated. Ensuring that the program meets state and voluntary accreditation requirements also is the responsibility of the educational administrator.

### Financial Resources

Securing financial resources is an important responsibility and one that cannot be delegated, although others can assist with the technical aspects of budget preparation, disbursements, and monitoring. Securing resources is largely a component of the external role and includes the operational budget, philanthropic activities, research awards, and other sources of funding.

Once the budget has been approved and funding is assured, the executive ensures that money is spent to accomplish the school's goals. The one error that inexperienced executives often make is conserving financial resources at the expense of accomplishing the school's goals. For example, if the school is trying to recruit outstanding students but produces a poorly designed and inexpensive recruitment brochure, few top-notch students will be attracted to the program. The key to budgetary success is to determine goals, prioritize them, and allocate funds to achieve these goals, all within the context of the academic unit's vision and mission. Monitoring budget allocations and the achievement of goals during the fiscal year ensures that funding is used appropriately.

### Faculty

Executives accomplish their work through others (Sullivan and Decker, 1997), and faculty members and staff are the people who make educational executives successful (or unsuccessful). Executives inherit faculty (unless they are starting a new program), who often are long-term, tenured employees, as well as hire new faculty who are either beginning or experienced scientists and clinicians. The potential conflict between established faculty and beginning researchers is inevitable, although all are valuable to the organization and important to the success of the program. Long-term faculty often are experienced educators and clinicians who are able to teach students with ease. In addition, they have a sustained record of commitment to the program and the "institutional memory" that is often valuable to avoid well-known "land mines".

Recently-graduated faculty have research skills, curiosity, and enthusiasm, whereas seasoned scientists and clinicians come with a wealth of knowledge and experience from a variety of other institutions and health care organizations. Nonetheless, the academic executive must be able to assure tenured faculty that satisfying opportunities exist for them, while stimulating new faculty to develop their careers in research, teaching, and service. An organizational infrastructure must be devised to assist the faculty in achieving both individual and organizational goals, regardless of the length of time they have been employed at the institution.

## Organizational Infrastructure

The academic nurse executive must organize faculty, staff, and other administrators into a working coherent whole with freedom to move between and among other groups as needed to accomplish the mission of the academic unit. What makes the organization of an academic unit unique, however, is the governance structure of faculty.

Higher education has operated on a shared governance model since the beginning of its existence and long before the concept became popular in corporate circles. Faculty elect representatives to committees, councils, or senates that have unlimited opportunities to apply considerable creativity and expertise to the development, implementation, and evaluation of program offerings, curriculum, courses, student programs, and research pursuits. On the other hand, this creativity and expertise can be silenced and stifled as a result of a lack of understanding of the recipricocity between faculty governance and administration.

Everyone loses when faculty develop an adversarial relationship with administration, have difficulty making decisions, and assume a "bunker mentality" yet view themselves as the guardians of academic quality. It is the executive's job to clearly delineate which responsibilities belong to administration (e.g., budgetary, legal liability, political connections) and which are faculty responsibilities (e.g., curriculum, admission, progression, graduation policies), as well as where the two overlap (e.g., program offerings that have both curricular and budgetary components). This delineation must be communicated clearly and often.

To function successfully the academic unit must be organized into a system that supports and facilitates the work to be done by the faculty and staff. In small colleges the nursing unit may be a department and the structure may be more informal than in large schools of nursing. The department chair may have one or two faculty who assist with administration, whereas large schools may be divided into departments, programs, or divisions.

Educational, clinical, and research activities may be divided in various ways. Some schools, for example, have research directors with staff responsibilities, whereas others have associate deans for research who have line responsibilities. (The difference between staff and line responsibilities is that staff facilitate the faculty's work but do not supervise faculty, whereas line administrators have responsibility for faculty and staff and are held accountable for that responsibility). In large schools the dean may have one or two associate deans who are able to represent the school in the dean's absence and several administrators who make up an executive committee or cabinet to advise the dean about day-to-day operations and major decisions.

The organizational infrastructure has one purpose: to accomplish the unit's goals in the most effective and efficient manner. The organizational infrastructure should be systems oriented and organized with an appropriate understanding of lines of communication, authority, responsibility, and accountability. The dean has a systems view of what must be accomplished; however, faculty may have a more limited, focused view of someone who represents them to administration (George and Coudret, 1986).

It is the academic executive's job to make sure that each individual given responsibility has the authority needed to accomplish the assigned tasks (e.g., the research associate dean has input into faculty assignments that include research objectives), assumes responsibility for the job (e.g., to see that faculty *A* submits a research grant), and is accountable for the outcome (e.g., the research dean's annual evaluation is based on faculty accomplishing their research objectives). The academic executive is responsible ultimately for all of the activities and initiatives within the unit and is held accountable for the outcomes of the faculty and staff's work, as well as for the students' accomplishments.

A college or school of nursing may be organized into departments according to research interests (e.g., health promotion) or educational offerings (e.g., nursing of infants and children), or the two may overlap depending on the structure of the curriculum and faculty research programs. However, departmental lines may assume a rigidity and separateness that creates artificial barriers and precludes an organization from being adaptable to rapid and innovative change. Likewise, these lines may interfere with research and teaching alliances that are essential in today's environment.

A matrix structure may be appropriate for some organizations, whereby faculty report to one individual for educational assignments and supervision and to another for research development and evaluation. The matrix structure requires excellent coordination, communication, and flexibility between the two administrators. Schools also may be organized according to program levels, with an associate or assistant dean (or director) who is responsible for the baccalaureate program(s) and one who is assigned to supervise the graduate program(s). The important point to remember in whatever structure is chosen is that there must be flexibility and the ability to change rapidly to accommodate new initiatives.

Subordinate administrators may be full time in administration, but more often they have faculty responsibilities as well. Role conflict is often inevitable as they try to juggle both jobs. In addition, subordinate administrators are often the link between faculty and dean and, as such, may be caught in the middle of controversy and conflict.

The degree of hierarchy and control maintained by the executive is a function of the size and structure of the organization, capability of subordinate administrators, length of time subordinates have been in the position, and the experience and comfort level of the executive. Hierarchic levels should be kept at a minimum to place more responsibility closer to where decisions should be made at the operational level. Faculty are knowledge workers and should not require the traditional form of "supervision"; however, if the faculty culture is one of dependency, the executive must develop strategies to reduce the dependency and increase the mastery of decision making, team work, and goal accomplishment. Considerable variation in structures exist, and they also may be altered as time and conditions change.

## Students

Higher education exists to meet society's needs for its future citizens and to educate students to become such citizens, a fact that is sometimes forgotten by academicians and administrators alike. The "business" of higher education is to ensure a high quality of education for students. Research and service exists to enrich and enhance the educational process, as well as to improve the whole of society. Once a program is designed to meet market needs and a qualified faculty is prepared to teach, student qualifications, abilities, and motivation determine a school's success. Students can be the best advertisement and best advocates for the school, or their performance after graduation can result in a mediocre reputation. Selecting the students most likely to succeed, offering them the best education possible, and treating them with respect will go a long way in enhancing the school's future. There should be a reciprocity of pride between the faculty and students and a commitment of both groups to achieve excellence in the academic enterprise.

Every interaction with students and their families and friends provides an opportunity to either enhance the school's reputation or harm it. For example, actively seeking the assistance of leaders in the various ethnic communities to recruit qualified minority applicants not only helps in the recruitment of such students but also helps enhance the school's reputation in the community, which can have long-lasting and sustained effects on the school's future (e.g., funding from the state legislature).

Generally the academic executive works through staff (e.g., recruiters, advisors, faculty, office staff) to affect student recruitment, selection, education, and graduation. Relying on appropriate individuals for information, the executive additionally must monitor student performance and be alert to individual student problems at the earliest stage to intervene when necessary. Dealt with swiftly and successfully, many problems remain small and are more easily resolved.

### Staff

Often invisible in academic organizations, the office and support staff affect the functioning of the academic unit and its success and reputation. The first person a potential student or donor encounters is a staff member, whether on the phone, by mail, or in person. That encounter sets the tone and creates an image for all other (or no other) interactions with the school. Think of a business that you contacted. Was the person courteous and helpful? Distracted, uninformed, or rude? Did he or she offer to get information for you or tell you, "It isn't my fault?" Did you want to go back or did you find some other place for your business?

Academia has been slow to learn customer-oriented service (as was health care). Competition resulting from a rapidly growing cadre of courses and programs offered via the Internet, as well as creative programming and customer-friendly services of rival schools, promises to cause many institutions to improve services to students (Sullivan, 1997). Front-line staff are key to these efforts.

Nursing education programs may have a variety of staff depending on the size of the unit and the services provided by the parent university. For example, a college of nursing in a large university may have its own development staff responsible for fund-raising, alumni staff to coordinate alumni activities, a person responsible for public relations, or a special events coordinator. A financial officer is usually part of the administrative team, and the dean may have a cadre of office staff (e.g., administrative assistant, secretary, receptionist). Generally, deans are involved only in directly hiring and supervising staff who report to them. In contrast, the chair of a department of nursing in a small college may hire and supervise the office staff, which may have only a single secretary who serves both the department chair and the faculty, with the college providing all other services centrally.

### Programs and Curriculum

The academic executive has varying levels of involvement in the educational program and curriculum, depending on the size of the unit and the organizational structure (e.g., an academic associate dean responsible for the curriculum). Regardless who is delegated the responsibility to manage specific programs (e.g., director of nurse practitioner program) or the curriculum (e.g., curriculum coordinator), it is the executive who is ultimately responsible for the quality, quantity, and timeliness of programs and for ensuring that they are offered according to publicized materials (i.e., college catalog).

## External Role

Except for single-purpose institutions, the nursing unit is one component of a larger college or university. Some nursing schools are an integral part of a health sciences university or medical center. Others may be in a comprehensive university or a community college. Still others are located in small, liberal arts colleges. The nurse executive's involvement in and participation with constituents and administrators in the parent institution is crucial to the nursing unit's success.

The academic executive also is involved in and seeks partnerships in the larger nursing practice community. In a university medical center, the school of nursing and nursing service may be integrated at varying levels. More often the school has reciprocal relationships with a variety of health care organizations. These relationships have come under increasing strain in today's managed care environment, and schools are finding it more and more difficult to obtain adequate clinical opportunities for student experiences (see Chapter 9). Reciprocal relationships with nursing practice and the larger health care community are essential for the academic executive and the school to keep current about practice and health care, respond to the needs of employers, and initiate activities to further nursing education and research. Partnering with practice colleagues facilitates the availability of clinical sites for students needing clinical experience, for faculty needing practice sites, and for faculty recruiting subjects for research.

## Securing Funding

One of the academic nurse executive's major, and most essential, roles is securing funding for the nursing unit. In public colleges and universities the majority of funding is appropriated from state tax dollars for the most part, although some universities now refer to themselves as state assisted rather than state supported because they receive so much of their funding from sources outside of state appropriations (e.g., grants, endowments).

The nursing executive seldom deals directly with the state legislature but rather submits a proposed budget to the administrator above the dean (e.g., provost, vice president, vice chancellor), who in turn submits a budget from a larger designated unit (e.g., health sciences center) to the university's chief administrator. The president (or chancellor) presents the university budget to the governing board, who requests funding from the legislature. The governing board receives the state's appropriation and assigns it to the university (or all state universities in some states). University administrators then assign portions to its component schools, institutes, and divisions. The resulting appropriation may mirror the original budget the dean submitted, but often it is less. The nurse executive's challenge is to accomplish the next year's (some universities operate on biennial budgets) activities with less than optimal funding. As higher education is increasingly criticized for lack of responsiveness and frivolous expenditures, an even greater reduction in state appropriations can be expected.

As expenses continue to rise and traditional sources of revenues continue to decline, the executive must seek other sources of financial support. Philanthropic gifts are crucial to the long-term survival and thriving of a nursing education unit. To employ a development officer to identify prospects, assist in establishing relationships with those prospects, and solicit gifts for the school or college is a must for nursing. Endowed chairs, professorships, scholarships, fellowships, and funds for faculty development and research endeavors add to a school or college's ability to excel in its mission. The nurse executive's role is pivotal in the development of prospects and solicitation of gifts.

If the institution's mission includes research, the nurse executive has a key responsibility in either creating or maintaining an infrastructure for faculty to be successful in competing for extramural research funding. Mechanisms should be in place for interdisciplinary and collaborative research to occur among disciplines within the campus and with other sites. Space, equipment, supplies, professional staff, consultants, funds to conduct pilot studies, and faculty development are all ingredients for establishing or maintaining a successful research program in the nursing education unit.

## Other External Constituents

Alumni, donors, governing boards, legislators, and state agencies (e.g., state board of nursing, health department, medical board) are all external constituents of the academic executive in nursing. Relationships must be developed, nurtured, and utilized appropriately. Many instances arise when the executive must be able to garner support and gain assistance in solving a problem. Alumni and donors are indispensable in securing funding for a new school of nursing building, for example.

## Interface With the Public

The academic nurse executive is a public person whose every activity represents the school of nursing and the university. Every interaction, offhand remark, or observation reflects on the college and on nursing. Even one's choice of vehicle affects others' perception. For example, does your impression of a person differ if the person drives a four-wheel Land Rover or a Lincoln Town Car? The degree of public persona varies by the local culture and the size of the city where the school resides (small towns are notorious for knowing what everyone is doing).

In addition to personal encounters, the executive interacts with the public through the media and by involvement in community organizations. Each meeting is an opportunity to present nursing and academia in a positive and competent light. Media encounters vary, however, depending on the issue. Reports of misconduct or crime, for example, are especially difficult and require the counsel of university administrators. Many other issues often can be discussed from a positive point of view, or another side of the issue can be presented. Declining enrollments, for example, can be seen as a failure of nursing education to attract quality applicants or a refinement in the health care system to use nurses' skills better.

Community organizations present many opportunities for the academic executive to foster the nursing school's positive image. Nonprofit organizations can benefit from the executive's experience in nursing and academia and provide satisfaction in serving the community. Monetary contributions carry a message of commitment and involvement as well.

### Role in the Profession

As a visible leader in the profession, the academic nurse executive has an important role to play in the nursing profession. The collective expertise and wisdom of such leaders is necessary to respond to immediate problems in the profession and to help craft the future of nursing.

A variety of organizations are available for support. The primary one is the American Association of Colleges of Nursing, to which most nursing schools belong. The executive nurse is the institution's representative. Meetings provide opportunities to acquire current information on higher education, health care, and nursing; to strategize with colleagues about threats and opportunities; and to discuss problems and issues both formally and informally with colleagues. Participation in this organization is invaluable to the administrator's development and success, and networking with colleagues is a vital benefit as the environment increases in complexity.

Other professional organizations may capture the nurse executive's enthusiasm. The American Nurses Association, the American Academy of Nursing, the National League for Nursing, and Sigma Theta Tau International are all worthwhile choices. One's clinical specialty area or research field may be especially inviting. Also, the nurse executive may be able to represent nursing in other health care organizations, such as the American Hospital Association or the Association of Academic Health Centers. Participation is limited only by time, energy, and other commitments.

## THE FUTURE FOR ACADEMIC EXECUTIVES IN NURSING

If current trends in health care and higher education continue, the future for academic executives in nursing is exciting and will require a higher level of problem solving, strategizing, and systems negotiation. As governing boards of colleges and universities face the public demand for increasing accountability, appropriations will increasingly be tied to performance. Academic executives will be forced to identify priorities, target funding for those priorities, and reduce expenditures. Faculty will be expected to generate revenues to support their salary and to be competitive for extramural funding to support research and teaching initiatives.

Nurse executives will face the added burden of changes in health care that reconfigure nurses' roles and trigger curriculum changes. Applicant pools, quality and quantity, traditionally have been used as a measurement of the academic executive's success. In the future, entire programs may be closed or consolidation of disciplines may occur to achieve efficiency. Better informed and more knowledgeable students will demand flexibility in learning strategies and a high-quality educational experience, including competent faculty who possess the knowledge and skills expected of a master teacher and clinician. Quality of the educational experience will become as paramount in higher education as it has become in health care delivery. The competitive edge will emerge from the academic institution that provides the highest-quality education at the lowest cost.

In a preferred future the executive will be an active participant in solving the problems facing higher education and health care, although, admittedly, the executive will be only one member of the team in these complex situations. The nurse executive will participate in making the difficult, but necessary, cost-cutting decisions and program reductions, while assisting the university to develop responsible accountability systems for faculty, students, and administrators. A system to encourage faculty productivity will be implemented, and outcomes measures will drive the system. Collaboration among university units will increase (albeit by necessity), and the process of strategic planning and evaluation to monitor performance and maintain a focus on the achievement of goals and priorities will be ongoing.

These university-wide strategies will carry over into the nursing unit. The effective executive will organize the faculty and staff into a coherent and workable group; create a vision of a preferable future; initiate strategic planning to identify viable goals; connect resources to priorities; secure the commitment of internal and external constituents; and implement streamlined, cutting-edge programs of education and research. A system of accountability for faculty, staff, students, and administrators will be developed, accepted, and implemented. A productive and energized faculty will offer valuable input into system decision making.

Arrangements for faculty employment and assignments will be creative and varied. Some faculty work will be contracted to health care organizations (e.g., pediatric nurse will teach nursing of children) on a time-limited basis, such as an 8-week rotation, whereas others, such as a nurse practitioner, will work for the school 1 day a week, supervising students at the employing clinic. Still other faculty will be employed for specific teaching, clinical, or research assignments and will be hired on contracts from 1 to 5 years. Some faculty, with potential to secure sustained external funding, will enter the traditional tenure-track positions. Tenure will be granted sparingly to those who have proven research records and grant-funding competencies. As a result, contracts will be the major method of employment for most nursing faculty.

Faculty time will be monitored and productivity will be measured (Plater, 1995). Faculty will be expected to contribute a full measure to the university's goals and to contribute substantially to the direct generation of revenues for salary support. Unproductive faculty, even those with tenure, will find it increasingly difficult to remain in the university (social pressure will mount), and either their productivity will improve or they will leave.

A variety of mechanisms will be used to enhance the school's funding. Faculty will practice in nurse-managed clinics or contracts with health care organizations will provide opportunities for faculty to maintain currency in clinical skills, offer student experiences, and generate needed revenue. Contracts for continuing education and specialized training for business, industry, health care organizations, and schools, for example, will contribute additional revenue and promote the faculty's and school's reputation. Large endowments will be created to sustain the nursing education unit into perpetuity.

Other health care, offered in a free clinic and without compensation, will provide opportunities to contribute to the larger good; set an example of generosity of spirit for students, faculty, and the community; and enhance the community's perception of nursing. Revenues for providing care to these groups will be available to the providers of care from various public and private sources. The nursing school will enjoy a positive image in the community and receive enhanced local support, including funding. The executive will be known as a respected contributor to the good of the community from the school's activities and from participation in community organizations and on boards.

Virtual teaching-learning opportunities will be available worldwide. Students will be enrolled in courses that may be offered between countries, and universities will offer greater flexibility in accepting transfer credits from other universities. The speed of communicating will be greatly increased as technology continues to develop. Regulatory mechanisms will be relaxed to allow license and certification requirements to span states and countries. Likewise, deregulation of telecommunications will occur worldwide.

## CONCLUSION

The traditional nursing education unit of the future may be smaller and funding may be reduced, but the streamlined, productive organization will still be able to function and accomplish its goals. Academic executive leadership will be a satisfying career choice and valued as a career trajectory. In addition to a formal degree program, preparation for the leadership role will be established or kept updated via short courses offered by universities and professional associations, as well as structured mentoring experiences. Nurse executives will be recruited to head corporations, health care systems, and universities. Talented and capable nurses will be encouraged to pursue leadership opportunities at all levels of the organization, and competition will be keen for open deanships. A positive future for nursing education will be ensured.

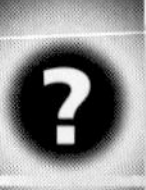

### *Discussion Exercises*

1. If you were an academic administrator with the numerous roles described in the chapter, what strategies would you use to be successful?
2. Answer the following questions as if you were an academic administrator. Be specific.
   a. What is your biggest problem?
   b. What is most rewarding about your job?
   c. If you had it to do over, would you accept your position again?
   d. What advice would you give to others who are interest in academic administration?
3. You intend to be a dean someday. What steps will you take to prepare for this role?

### References


George SA, Coudret NA: Dynamics and dilemmas of the associate and assistant dean role, *J Prof Nurs 2:* 173, 1986.

Keller G: Managing in tomorrow's academic environment, *New Dir Institutional Res 85:* 59, 1995.

Plater WM: Future work: faculty time in the 21st century, *Change* 27(3):22, 1995

Sullivan EJ: A changing higher education environment, *J Prof Nurs 13*(3):143, 1997.

Sullivan EJ, Decker PJ: *Effective leadership and management in nursing, ed 4,* Menlo Park, Calif, 1997, Addison-Wesley Longman.

# IV

# Accountability, Quality, and Control

# 22 Accountability and Quality

**Marjorie Beyers**

*Don't compromise yourself.*
*You are all you've got.*

**Janis Joplin**

## DEFINITION OF NURSING

> Nursing is primarily helping people (sick or well) in the performance of those activities contributing to health or its recovery (or to a peaceful death) that they would perform unaided if they had the necessary strength, will, or knowledge. It is likewise the unique contribution of nursing to help people to be independent of such assistance as soon as possible (Henderson and Nite, 1978).
>
> The professional nurse will be one who recognizes and understands the fundamental (health) needs of a person, sick or well, and who knows how these needs can best be met. She will possess a body of scientific nursing knowledge which is based upon and keeps pace with general scientific advancement, and she will be able to apply this knowledge in meeting the nursing needs of a person and a community. She must possess that kind of discriminative judgment which will enable her to recognize those activities which fall within the area of professional nursing and those activities which have been identified with the fields of other professional or nonprofessional groups (Brown, 1948).

Nursing, like all professions, is accountable for its practice. The reputation of a profession is based in part on how its members individually and as a profession attend to this vital issue. This chapter discusses how nursing's accountability will be affected as patient care and the health care environment continue to change.

## ACCOUNTABILITY

Accountability is a complex concept because it takes place both on a personal level, and in the context in which one is practicing. The word *accountability* itself seems straightforward, especially when everyone involved is clear about the nature and scope of the accountability. Enacting accountability in daily practice, however, is a different story. Accountability is subject to perceptions and is an expression of values and beliefs.

Accountability is interpreted differently by different people. Some people draw lines around their accountability, which is evidenced by statements such as, "That is not my job," or "I must do this because I am accountable for it." It is important to make accountability clear and to prevent misperceptions and misunderstandings. Clear accountability also helps people rationalize their actions, for example, "I did everything that I was supposed to do," or "Even though the outcome was not what we wanted, I did all that I could." When accountability is clear, nurses know if they are doing a good job.

In direct contrast to those who circumscribe their accountability, some people reach out to take on accountability. These people are not restrained by rules or habit. They do not set limits but rather step in. "Well, someone had to do it, and I knew how," or "Can you imagine what would have happened if I had not stepped into that situation?"

## What Is Accountability?

How does accountability become so complex? The definition of accountability in *Bailey's 16th Century Dictionary* is that accountability can be assigned, accepted, or absorbed. Assignments of accountability usually take place within relationships, such as the employer and employee, senior and junior staff, or authority and novice. Traditional management literature considers accountability within the context of delegation. Although accountability can be delegated, the ultimate accountability is retained by the delegator. This is the basis for supervision and oversight of those to whom accountability has been delegated.

Even though accountability is delegated, it must be accepted. One has the option of saying, "Yes, I will do that," or "I cannot take on this job." The reasons for not accepting accountability are varied and may include factors such as time limitations, lack of skill, or unwillingness. The wise person does not accept accountability without thought about how it will be carried out. Some people have an affinity for being accountable; these are the individuals who reach out and take on accountability.

The sixteenth century definition of accountability can be easily adapted to current practice, which suggests that accountability is a constant over time. Thus one could posit that as long as there is a nursing profession, there will be nursing accountability. Throughout the centuries, accountability has proved to be complex because it is both very personal and interdependent within the context of all of one's behaviors.

## Nursing's Accountability

To make accountability more understandable, it is useful to identify the domains of nursing's accountability. A professional nurse is accountable to the following:

Personal integrity
Public good
Service of and by the profession
Leadership

*Personal integrity* helps explain the many factors that determine one's accountability. It can be speculated that accountability is a personality trait, learned, or a combination of both. How a person deals with accountability is highly individual. Nurses take their professional accountability very seriously. A strong motivation for entering the profession is a desire to help others. This motivation is enhanced in the educational process whereby nurses' learn the professional code of behavior. Furthermore, values and cultural mores help shape a nurse's perception of and beliefs about accountability. Being accountable is part of an individual nurse's identity as a professional.

A nurse who is accountable does what a reasonable and prudent nurse would do who functions under nursing's code of ethics and appropriate standards. Being accountable can be very satisfying, especially when one has good experiences in nursing practice. On the other hand, accountability can engender many emotions and feelings. Thwarted accountability leads to frustration. Perceived failure to meet what one is accountable for can result in feelings of guilt and remorse. When someone or something blocks the actions one is accountable for, the result may be anger, fear, or anxiety. The emotional side of accountability is thus linked with personal integrity.

*Public good* is a strongly linked to the nursing profession's accountability to the public. The fact that a registered nurse has a license to practice nursing under the authority of a state statute establishes nursing's accountability to the public. The accountability of the licensed nurse is defined in statutes, rules, and regulations. Even though some states have more explicit nursing practice acts than others, all have mechanisms for interpretation of the law and the rules and regulations governing nursing practice. The statutes, rules, and regulations are periodically reviewed and changed or refined, especially when their relevance to current practice is challenged.

Nurses are accountable for ensuring that the nurse practice acts continue to be appropriate for current practice and that they deal effectively with contemporary issues so that public safety and welfare are protected. Most nurses, however, see their license as the "base" for practice rather than the "definition" of the practice. Accountability of the nursing profession goes beyond a statute of basic accountability. The nursing profession must make sure that practice acts embrace the public's ever-changing requirements for improving health. Nurses honored in Nursing's Hall of Fame, many of whom led major social reforms, are role models for leaders of the profession (Gerteis and others, 1993). Another application of public good is to consider the public as a whole when making policy decisions about health care. In this instance the public good takes precedence over a few individuals' welfare.

*Service of and by the profession* embodies the science of nursing, its knowledge base and its competencies. A nurse is accountable to other nurses to keep the profession viable. The public perception of nursing is based on each person's personal experience with individual nurses. Each nurse's accountability in the aggregate adds up to the reputation of the nursing profession. The whole profession is affected by the actions of each individual nurse. Each nurse is accountable for ensuring that his or her practice meets professional standards.

Nurses as a body also are accountable to keep their science current and to continuously update and revise nursing standards. Keeping up to date in nursing knowledge and competencies is each nurse's professional responsibility. Each nurse also has an accountability to the profession. The notion of the service of and by the profession incorporates commitment and loyalty to the profession. Nurses, as do professionals in other disciplines, are often accused of having a "vested interest" in matters affecting nursing practice and nurses. And well they should, because the profession is essentially a "virtual" body made up of all of its members. Each nurse has a stewardship role toward keeping nursing an effective profession.

As with any activity that affects the public, public trust is difficult to achieve and easy to lose. The nursing profession is no exception. Prominent among the many ways to keep nursing effective are endeavors in research, quality improvement methods, public policy developments, and supporting and contributing to nursing's positive image.

*Leadership* encompasses competencies for "taking the high road" in patient care, as well as in matters affecting nursing practice. It is common practice today to use the term *leadership* interchangeably with management. But management theories explain that not all managers are leaders and that not all leaders are managers.

Accountability for leadership means going the extra mile in every aspect of practice. For example, a nurse assumes a leadership role when taking care of patients, applying nursing knowledge to assessment of the patient's situation and to working with the patient and family to plan care and to implement the interventions that will improve health. The accountable nurse follows through, acquires new information when needed, and thinks of alternatives when the plans do not work well.

Nurses working together on a public policy issue or a project that advances and improves health for a group or a community is another example of leadership. Leadership is an accountable activity that keeps the profession viable. Leadership means that nurses are not comfortable with the status quo and always seek to improve their science to provide better care for individual patients, groups, and communities. Leadership means that nurses always seek to improve care and the care environment by improving their relationships with other health professionals and with those in the organizations or teams in which they work.

## ACCOUNTABILITY IN THE FUTURE

The four domains of accountability—personal integrity, public good, service to and by the profession, and leadership—are fundamental. They are threaded through nursing's past, and they will not change in the future. The context of nursing care, education, and regulation, however, will change. Today's major challenges will be resolved, and a new status quo will become the norm. Even as present-day issues and problems, such as cultural diversity, are resolved, new issues and problems will emerge through social and economic pressures for change. Nursing is accountable to ensure that patient care is the focus of deliberations and actions, even in the midst and confusion of change. This focus will also be reflected in the emerging nursing educational system, regulatory system, and nursing practice.

The purpose for nursing education and regulation will not change, even though the processes of becoming educated and of regulating the profession may. The nursing profession will continue to be assessed and evaluated according to the demonstrated practice of its individual members and on how well nursing meets its accountability to the public. One of the most profound changes will be the way nurses enter the profession. Licensure, as we now know it, will give way to a demonstration of competencies that are updated continuously and that will be applicable to the practice in its current context.

### Health Care Environment

The environment and context of patient care will affect nursing's accountability in the future. Therefore it is useful to consider what health care will look like in the future. Nurses have been and will continue to be central in the health care system, which ensures that they will help shape the new system that, conversely, will help shape the nursing profession.

Futurists predict that health care will be vastly different from the health care system we know today. Two strong factors, new technology and public policy on health and health care, have ignited change. Many think that this change, along with the new alternative financing and new businesses, is a transition to an entirely new way of financing and delivering a new value-driven health care system. We are experiencing only the beginning of transformation of the health care system. To be in synchrony with the worldwide changes of health care reform, the nursing profession must begin its own transformation.

Concepts of nursing's accountability developed in this chapter are framed with the assumption that the purpose of nursing has remained constant over time. Although nursing's purpose will continue to be a constant for the profession and for health care, the work of nursing will change dramatically as patient care and the health care delivery system changes. The challenge for nursing is to keep its eye on the constants while adapting and forging nursing's transformed work.

### Purpose of Nursing

The purpose of nursing is expressed in the way nurses perform their work. Nursing's accountability is value laden and is reflected in what nurses do and in what they believe their role to be in society. Nursing itself has created and sustained public expectations for nursing care. Nurses are known for valuing quality care. Accountability is ingrained in the nursing profession and embedded in its logic, its science, and its spirit. The result is that people view nurses favorably. They trust nurses and depend on them to be advocates for their care. To keep this public trust intact, nurses must attend to how their work reflects their values in a transformed health care system. Although nursing has a long history of positive trust and confidence, this trust must be constantly nurtured. It will not be easy to keep the public trust in an environment of change. Nurses must keep their purpose in the forefront in their science and in their actions.

Nursing has a solid foundation for the future. In its long history of service, nursing has developed a reputation envied by many. Over the past century nursing has developed from its early roots in healing, nurturing, and caring to a profession. The science of nursing has matured with considerable effort and skill to its current knowledge base and practice. Nursing science has matured in tandem with social and scientific discoveries and in concert with the environment. In different ways and in different times, nurses have contributed to social and cultural changes, working to improve health and life. Nursing also has been affected by these changes, as evidenced in the rich history of nursing's contribution to society.

## Preparing for the Future

Chronicles of how nurses have functioned in disasters, wars, poverty, and social injustices are a legacy for the future. The way nursing adapted to the institutionalization of health care, in which hospitals became the central place for care, is another chapter of growth and discovery. Nurses have become so integral with hospitals that nursing is often thought of as synonymous with hospital care, although in nursing's earlier history, care was provided almost exclusively in patients' home. In hospitals nursing is the only profession that stays with the patient over 24 hours, the most accessible and caring factor in recovery from illness, disease, and trauma (Finer, 1961). Now, nurses have entered another phase in their rich history. As hospitals become a smaller component of health care, nurses are again becoming more mobile, moving into the community to organize and provide patient care in very different ways.

In all of these changes, noted not only by the development of nursing science but also by different modes of dress, furniture, equipment, and focus, the essence of nursing has been evident. Nurses have consistently helped others to become increasingly independent in taking care of their own health. Whether helping to bring cleanliness to housing; treating the injured; or helping someone learn to walk again or to learn proper nutrition, exercise, and rest; nurses have held to their purpose: to improve health. In every setting where they have practiced, nurses have stayed close to patients. The helping and caring relationships nurses learned to foster early on in their careers are highly valued by patients and their families.

Nursing has arrived at a new pivotal point in the history of the profession in which the context of their care is significantly changing. During the past several decades, nursing has been largely focused on hospital nursing practice. Two-thirds of working nurses have been practicing in hospitals, and they have learned to focus their relationships in the context of hospital care. Now that the health care system is changing, nursing must preserve its purpose in a new and different context.

## Changing Environment

Keeping the focus on the purpose of nursing in a turbulent change environment is difficult. Even the way change occurs is changing. Our current excellent ability to adapt will not be sufficient for the massive changes of the future. Previously change took place in increments, was well planned, and was executed and incorporated into practice over time. There was time to learn the new technology and to develop new patterns of patient care. These experiences help but do not fully prepare nurses for the rapid-fire changes of the future.

Change inevitably disrupts current practice while it creates new expectations. Aspects of work that nurses count on, such as the assumed commitment to job security and support in maintaining the traditional role, no longer exist in hospitals or in business and industry in general.

Many professions, such as banking and engineering, have undergone radical transformations. Nursing is well positioned now to go through its own transformation.

Nursing is also fortunate to be moving into this change with a good track record. In the last century nursing has been a central part of the development of a massive health care industry. Nurses have moved and grown with the change. For example, there is great variety in the jobs that nurses hold today in all types of patient care arenas, from the central caring roles to the peripheral businesses. Nursing has a presence in patient care; in community care; and as a leader in organizations, policy, and education.

Health care transformation portends increasing specialization but from a broader base with increasing consolidation of like concepts and affinities. Health care technology, beyond our imagination, will allow patients to seek advice, consultation, and help for self-care from their homes. We can expect that new diseases will spring up overnight, challenging medical knowledge of cause and treatment. There will be new types of emotional crises that reflect the futuristic environment. As the health care system is less associated with buildings and structures, nursing will increasingly become more associated with flexible systems for continuity of care than with the settings in which care is provided. The health care system, designed to deal with new technology and new issues, will have new types of health care workers. These new workers will deal with high technology and with the care delivery from totally different perspectives. Nursing will have to work harder and faster to keep pace.

## Changing Work of Nursing

Nurses are particularly well equipped to deal with the future, always adapting to the health care needs of people. In the near future nurses will concentrate on the needs of the growing number of aging people who will require care quite different from the traditional nursing home concept of care. They will develop new interventions to deal with health care needs in a new environment. Nurses will help people adjust to a new interdependency with their environments. They will develop new research and insights on the human condition, health, and illness. They will continue to care for, heal, and nurture people in all stages and phases of life.

Nurses will develop an understanding of the environment and the new way that the business of health care is managed. The traditional process of separating the practice of health care from the economics of it will no longer apply. The cost and price of services will be currency for dealing and negotiating. Current developments are transitional toward a future in which humanistic aspects of patient care are revitalized, in the context of values in practice, and in which there is renewed emphasis on patient and professional decision making.

These changes will be made possible by the emerging science of nursing and by the new relationships that patients have with their own health care and with the physicians, nurses, and others who facilitate their health. Patients will perform self-diagnoses, treatment, and assessments of progress with support from health care providers. The nurse as knowledge worker will be a reality. In the past emphasis has been on doing—in fact, not many years ago a nurse felt guilty for sitting with a patient on a busy nursing care unit. Future work will be in designing patient care delivery and in planning how people can effectively assess their own health and mark progress toward improvements. The work of nursing will be to analyze the outcomes of care and to identify areas where new interventions can be designed or old ones can be improved or eliminated. The nurse of the future will have a battery of mature technologic devices at hand for use in patient care to help predict future health care needs and to develop ways to make sure that people continue to improve their health (Hesselbein and others, 1997).

In the future hospitals will continue to be special places that require specialized talents and skills of nurses. Some nurses will specialize in caring for people who suffer trauma, injury, and the effects of disease and illness. These nurses will have a myriad of new tools and techniques to provide care. Many nurses will be working directly with groups of patients assigned to their care for health management and chronic care management.

Community nursing centers are only the beginning of nursing's new developments, which emphasize health and will be facilitated by technology that will enable nurses to provide comprehensive services for the continuum of care in many sites. The team of physician, nurse, pharmacist, and other health care professionals will be the common work group, and this team will be working in an entirely different type of health care infrastructure. Just as part of nursing's culture ensures that nurses are close to people where they live and work, physicians and others will be increasingly mobile and equipped with the technology to interact with patients from afar.

A significant adjustment for nurses will be to give up their traditional practice of being accountable to the bureaucratic rules about how to behave in organizations. The layers of delegation in these organizations will be gone. Instead there will be a direct line between the patient and the assigned caregivers—the team that accepts accountability to provide care. What a relief to deal with a new system that focuses on what should be done for patients instead of sorting out who does what tasks in each part of multidisciplinary team care. Technology will allow monitoring of each profession's input, making it possible to focus more on the way the care is designed and implemented in alignment with the patient's situation and the environment.

This change from working in buildings in shifts with circumscribed units and functions to assignment to a continuum of care delivered in a variety of settings using various modes of intervention will have a major effect on nursing. An entire new infrastructure for the profession will inevitably be crafted to ensure adequate clinical support systems, peer review, and the important peer support in practice.

The relationship between education and practice will become blurred as professional nurses incorporate research, education, and policy aspects into their practice. Becoming a "whole" profession in one person is a sobering thought. It is comforting, however, to know that some aspects of the nursing practice infrastructure will not change, such as the emotion-laden interactions with people that nurses experience daily. What will not change is nurses' needs for support systems. Part of the clinical support systems will be available on line, but there will continue to be a need for professional dialogue to enhance understanding, to probe new areas of knowledge, and to discover new insights that improve the capability to provide nursing care.

Decision making will be the foremost professional requirement in the future work of nurses. Knowledge of scientific methods for research, surveys, and epidemiology will be core content, just as knowledge about society, groups, and the learning behaviors of people are essential to carry out care (Heibeler and others, 1998). Most importantly, learning from experiences will become a major way of developing the list of items to study. The health care team will use experiences to develop insights into opportunities for improvements and development.

## Business of Nursing

One of the areas of most interest in today's practice is aligning the business of health care with the practice. Nursing can make a unique contribution to this development because nursing does not have long-standing economic expectations. Nursing has only begun to develop a financial base for practice.

In the future, cost and price issues will be resolved in a most interesting way. Health care will be so technologically advanced and competencies of caregivers and patients will be so well understood that the complex structure of health care delivery will be transformed into a direct line of communication. What we know now as point of service is only the beginning of this profound change. In the future, health professionals will focus on the patient with new awareness of the accountability for quality care. A new type of reward system to recognize quality care will emerge from the bureaucratic cocoon to become an integral part of each person's practice.

Nurses have been and will be leaders in helping others understand the importance of focusing on patients. In fact, one of the reasons that nursing has sustained the public trust is that nurses are not entrepreneurs but are practical in the acquisition and use of resources for patient care. This knowledge will serve them well in the future because patients will have as much knowledge about the cost and price of their care as the caregivers, thus eliminating a source of conflict and discontent with intention and motivation (Parson and others, 1998). New incentives that relate clearly to decision making and outcomes of care will be devised to ensure cost effectiveness.

In the alignment of the business and practice components of health care, the nursing profession will predictably become more entrepreneurial, but price will be only one factor to consider in care decisions. As the transformation takes place, nursing's accountability lies in making sure that the change is carefully constructed to keep its value system intact. In this way nursing will keep the faith with its historic achievements and will ensure preservation and growth of its value system.

## CONCLUSION

A profession, such as nursing, is known by the way it deals with its accountability. Nursing has always guarded its accountability to safe patient care. In fact, nursing is known for its vigilance and advocacy for patients. The future will be shaped by the force of past accomplishments. Nurses will be thoughtful about their professional accountability, how accountability is learned and nurtured to focus clearly on the patient.

Positioning nursing to influence health care from the inside out is the accountability of individual nurses and the profession as a whole. This accountability begins with a strong sense of wanting to help others and a commitment to the next iteration of nursing. In the past, nurses were depicted as seeing nursing as an avocation. Nurses may have absorbed accountability as part of their being. Nursing then became a vocation. The next stage of development focused on management, with the development of roles and positions in the increasingly complex hospital structures. Nursing was expressed as duty. The aspiring nurse had to prove capability for accepting accountability. We are in the next stage of development, in which nursing's accountability comes from its knowledge and actions. The future will be built on this past, and the rich history of nursing's accountability will be passed on to future nurses who will create a new future.

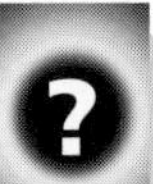

## *Discussion Exercises*

1. Discuss both the ethical and legal ramifications of accountability.
2. As health care and nursing change, nursing' accountability will change. Explain new areas of accountability for individual nurses, as well as changes in accountability for the profession.
3. Nurses are accountable for their own practice and, in some circumstances, for those of their colleagues. Describe an actual or hypothetical situation in which you were concerned about your accountability.

## References


Brown EL: *Nursing for the future,* New York, 1948, Russel Sage Foundation.

Finer H: *Administration and the nursing services,* New York, 1961, MacMillan.

Gerteis M and others: *Through the patient's eyes: understanding and promoting patient centered care,* San Francisco, 1993, Jossey Bass.

Henderson V, Nite G: *Principles and practice of nursing,* ed 6, New York, 1978, Macmillan.

Hesselbein F and others, editors: *The organization of the future,* San Francisco, 1997, Jossey-Bass.

Hiebeler R and others: *Best practices: building your business with customer-focused solutions,* New York, 1998, Arthur Andersen Simon & Schuster.

Parson ML and others: *Interdisciplinary case studies in health care redesign: strategies for improving patient care,* Gaithersburg, Md, 1998, Aspen.

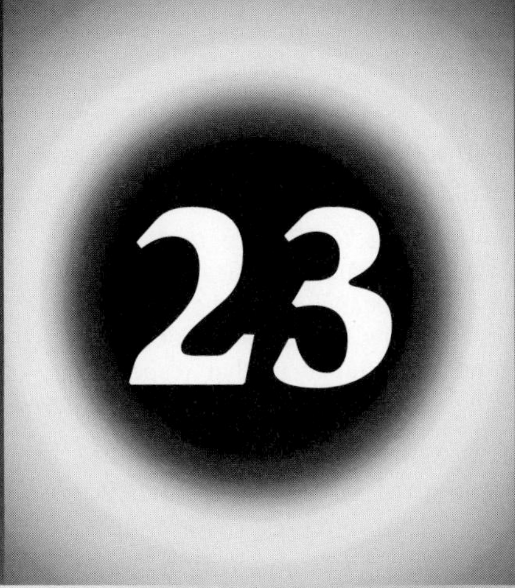

# Professional Licensure

**Jennifer Bosma**

*The people's good is the highest law.*

**Cicero**

## THE FOUNDATIONS OF NURSING REGULATION

Regulation is the government's intervention to accomplish an end that is beneficial to its citizens. In the tenth amendment to the U.S. Constitution, all powers not explicitly reserved to the federal government may be exercised by the states. For example, authority over interstate trade is reserved to the federal government in the Commerce clause of the Constitution (The practice of health care has been held to be interstate trade for the purposes of antitrust laws.) (U.S. Department of Commerce, 1997). Included in the powers remaining with the states is the "police power" to enact reasonable laws necessary to protect the health, safety, and welfare of their citizens.

State nursing practice acts establish regulatory/licensing boards as administrative agencies of the state and authorize them to exercise this power. Regulatory boards must maintain the balance between the state's responsibility to protect the health, safety, and welfare of its citizens and the rights and interests of practitioners in practicing their chosen profession.

### Public Protection

Why is there a need for the state to protect its citizens in health care? Other goods and services are driven by market forces. Generally, factors such as reputation, guarantees, and litigation work efficiently together to ensure that consumers get what they pay for.

There are three critical reasons explaining why market forces are insufficient to ensure the protection of the public in health care: information asymmetry, bundling of services under a managed care plan, and secondary harm.

Although consumer access to health information and advice is rapidly changing through the explosion of computer-based resources, consumers still generally have less ability to access and interpret information than do professionals. Bundling of services under a managed care plan reduces the consumer's selection of practitioners. If consumers select a provider not included in the network, they pay significant penalties for these services. Secondary harm occurs when an individual receives subpar care from an incompetent practitioner and, in turn, infects or harms others (Cox and Foster, 1990). Regulation compensates for these consumer dilemmas by ensuring that any licensed practitioner has met at least the minimum qualifications for practice. The consumer may rest assured that any practitioner with the state's imprimatur has met the standard and will be held accountable for his or her performance and behavior.

## Legislative Authority for Nursing Regulation

Under the authority conferred by the legislature under the state's nursing practice act, boards of nursing promulgate rules for the licensure of registered nurses (RNs), licensed practical nurses/vocational nurses (LPNs/VNs), and, in many states, advanced practice registered nurses (APRNs). The law and administrative rules usually include protection of the title, a scope of practice, legal standards of practice, and disciplinary grounds. State boards are required to specify the qualifications that any applicant for licensure must meet, such as a standardized educational program, demonstration of competence, and a record of behavior free from indications of potential harm to the public (e.g., felony conviction). Boards of nursing mandate that applicants provide validated sources of information about their education, competence, and prior behavior before the board decides whether to grant legal authority to practice, that is, issues a license. The authority of professional licensing boards in this regard is one to which the courts have consistently deferred beginning with the historic U.S. Supreme Court ruling in 1889 in *Dent v. State of West Virginia:*

> . . . No one has the right to practice medicine without having the necessary qualifications of learning and skill . . . Reliance must be placed upon the assurance given by his license, issued by an authority competent to judge in that respect, that he possesses requisite qualifications.

This authority carries with it strict constitutional responsibilities related to due process, property rights, and other rights of citizens. The fourteenth amendment to the U.S. Constitution has been found, in professional licensure case law, to require that state-imposed restrictions bear a rational relation to an individual's fitness or capacity to practice the profession (Massaro and O'Brien, 1983).

## Board of Nursing Accomplishments

Boards of nursing have led the way in a number of areas of regulatory improvement since nursing regulation began in the early 1900s. These serve as a foundation for projecting future scenarios.

### Disciplinary Actions

Disciplinary actions were rare in the early days of regulation. Beginning in the 1970s, boards promulgated legal standards of practice. Nursing practice acts were amended to require reporting of suspected violations by licensees. During the 1970s and 1980s the number of drug-related cases mushroomed, and boards developed effective and efficient ways to keep nurses impaired by substance abuse out of practice while allowing them opportunities for rehabilitation and return to productive and safe practice. While managing a larger caseload than any other health profession licensing board (as a result of the overall number of licensees), boards of nursing have refined their disciplinary procedures to reduce backlogs, prioritize cases according to the risk to the public, and effectively monitor all nurses with stipulations attached to their licenses. A number of boards also have collaborated to establish alternative-to-discipline programs for impaired nurses (e.g., diversion programs, so called because they divert a licensee to rehabilitation instead of sanction). In the 1990s boards have increasingly seen disciplinary cases related to impairments, such as sexual misconduct, as well as substandard quality-of-care cases. Boards are individually and collectively conducting research to determine the most effective ways of managing these extremely complex cases.

### Licensure Examinations

Initial licensure requirements have been honed to a well-defined set of expectations that are clearly related to the practice of the profession at the entry level. Licensure examinations are based on empirical job analyses that are performed on a national level every 3 years by the National Council of State Boards of Nursing. Test plans and passing standards are reevaluated on the same triennial basis to ensure that the content and pass/fail points for the examinations (NCLEX-RN and NCLEX-PN) are reflective of current competencies required for safe and effective practice.

A variety of accommodations have been made to meet the needs of candidates for licensure. Since the mid 1980s boards have made modifications for candidates with disabilities. A mechanism to screen foreign-educated nurses' qualifications in nursing and in the English language has been offered by the Commission on Graduates of Foreign Nursing Schools since the late 1970s and is recognized by most states. In 1994 boards of nursing were the first health care profession regulators to make the move to computerized adaptive testing, offered year-round in secure professional testing centers with high-speed turn around on results' reports, providing applicants with rapid licensure.

## A PROBABLE FUTURE FOR PROFESSIONAL LICENSURE

A probable future scenario assumes a "business-as-usual" future and presents what is likely to happen if nothing is done, which changes the course of events. Business as usual, in terms of the environment for professional licensure for nurses, implies phenomena such as the following:

The federal government will leave health care and professional regulation to the states but make occasional incursions through preemption or incentives tied to federal funding.

Public interest groups will demand evidence of the effectiveness of regulations to protect the consumer, and they will lobby for the right to change regulations that impede personal choice.

Tensions will mark relationships among health care practitioners, educators, administrators, and regulators.

The health care delivery system alternatively will ignore licensure laws and seek to be assigned the responsibility for corporate credentialing (e.g., institutional licensure) of professionals.

Advanced practice registered nurses will find it difficult to move from state to state as a result of differing scopes of practice, prescriptive authority, relationships to physicians, and educational requirements.

In the midst of these challenging circumstances, boards of nursing will use creativity and innovation to assure the public that nurses are qualified and practice safely:

RNs and LPNs/VNs will enjoy mobility from state to state because licensure requirements are similar and a common, computer-based examination is used nationwide.

Nurses who violate the laws governing practice will be fairly and efficiently disciplined, which is due to the processes boards have in place for investigation, formal and informal hearings, legal counsel, training for board members, and other necessary resources; boards of nursing are widely acknowledged for their diligence in carrying out discipline.

Other states will be able to discover prior disciplinary action before issuing a license by endorsement because an online database will be available to all boards across the nation.

Board-approved schools of nursing consistently will graduate students who pass the licensuring examinations at rates exceeding 90%.

Overlaid on these general conditions related to professional licensure will be regulatory issues concerning the legal roles and relationships of various types of practitioners performing nursing activities, including unlicensed assistive personnel (UAP) and other licensed practitioners performing overlapping activities. Extrapolating the forces shaping the present licensure system and the current regulatory issues, one can envision a probable future scenario.

## Advanced Practice Registered Nursing

The practice of advanced practice registered nurses (APRNs) will continue to be state bound because pressures from associations of related health professionals will perpetuate state-level differences in licensure requirements and practice parameters. APRNs will continue attempts to change state legislation, and the patchwork pattern will shift but will not become uniform across the nation. The resulting differential distribution of APRNs from state to state, combined with differing practices regarding reimbursement and laws relating to scope of practice and physician relationship, will exacerbate problems with consumer access to care in underserved areas.

Differences in regulatory approaches for various categories of APRNs also will persist. One approach will subscribe to the model used in medicine, whereby the license is issued for generalist practice and specialty credentialing is handled via private certification. Another approach will acknowledge the reality that physicians "got there first" and reserved to their exclusive scope of practice areas such as diagnosis and prescribing. As a result, explicit statutory authority will be the only way to ensure a solid legal foundation for advanced practice. In different states legislation will reflect these varying approaches not only in terminology but also in the way in which advanced practice nurses are educated, function, and are reimbursed for services.

Variation regarding qualifications also will persist from state to state and across the various types of advanced practice. Although nurse practitioners generally will be educated at the graduate level in their clinical specialty and take the corresponding certification examination to assess entry-level competence, examinations will not have emerged in all specialties for clinical nurse specialists and graduate programs will not have become the norm for midwifery. Requirements for prescriptive authority may have gained uniformity for nurse practitioners through curriculum and regulatory guidelines, which were the result of a successful public/private partnership between the U.S. Public Health Service Division of Nursing and the Agency for Health Care Policy and Research (U.S. Department of Health and Human Services) and the National Council of State Boards of Nursing and the National Organization of Nurse Practitioner Faculties. However, variation will continue to restrict which drugs may be prescribed in different states, and the prescriptive privileges for clinical nurse specialists will continue to be problematic.

## Unlicensed Assistive Personnel

On the other end of the practice spectrum, the regulation of unlicensed assistive personnel (UAPs) will reflect the ambivalence that has been evident historically, with some states having no legal recognition of this level of practitioner other than allowing for delegation to UAPs by licensed nurses, whereas others will regulate UAPs using approaches that span the spectrum from private certification, to registry, to licensure complete with scope of practice. Ambivalence between protecting the public by regulating UAP practice, preferably by a board of nursing, and concerns that regulating UAPs confers a legitimacy that leads to dangers such as independent practice and a confusing proliferation of levels of nursing personnel (all referred to by consumers as "nurses") will continue.

This ambivalence was reflected historically in two situations 10 years apart. In 1987 the Nursing Home Reform Act was passed as part of the Omnibus Budget Reconciliation Act (OBRA), establishing various regulatory requirements for nurse aides employed in long-term care facilities receiving federal funds. The legislation did not specify which state agency would be responsible for the regulation. A few boards of nursing actively sought to be assigned responsibility, whereas others were adamant in declining it out of philosophic opposition or practical resource considerations. Similarly, in 1997 the American Nurses Association simultaneously recommended that it would "continue to support federally regulated UAPs in home health and long-term care while opposing any new categories for regulation," and ANA also recommended support of a range of strategies for appropriate use of UAPs that will recognize states' individual circumstances in regulation of UAPs by providing guidelines to state nurses associations (SNAs) pursuing regulation and opposing attempts by other groups to regulate UAP.

Because in this probable scenario there has been no resolution of the underlying philosophic differences, states will continue to polarize in the regulations they adopt, with some refining the regulation of UAPs to distinguish levels or specialties and others refining their delegation paradigms. Neither approach will be successful in creating clarity, consistency, or rationality (related to consumer safety) in employers' utilization of UAPs or consumers' expectations of UAPs.

## Federal Incursion

The probable future for professional licensure includes federal incursions into state regulation. This will extrapolate the trend evident in the 1987 OBRA, as well as other health care regulatory arenas such as clinical laboratory services, mammography, and insurance coverage for maternity stays. The interference of differing state standards with interstate commerce, such as telehealth, will result in federal prescription of standards that must then be implemented by the states. As the "business" of health care delivery proceeds through its fundamental change, other needs will emerge, causing the industry to lobby Congress for overrides of state discretionary differences, such as those that hinder the ability to move practitioners around the country in special purpose teams, the ability to export health care services, and the ability to implement best practices or protocols consistently in all states served.

## Public Interest Groups

The effects of public interest group criticisms in this probable scenario will result in draining support and resources from regulatory boards. Areas in which nursing boards excel will be overlooked, although credit occasionally will be given for the continuing improvements that boards have made in competence assessment, especially recent additions of cutting-edge technology, to increase fidelity to actual clinical performance and decision making. Cooperative efforts among regulators of various health professionals will result in strides toward strategies for ensuring continuing competence. However, the complexity of defining and equitably measuring competence in specialized professions will make this progress slower than public interest groups would like.

Nursing boards will be able to cite successes in competency assessment and their exemplary record in discipline to avert drastic action by state legislatures, such as deauthorizing boards ("sunsetting"). However, generalization of some instances of regulatory board failures and a continuing lack of data on regulatory outcomes will undermine support for boards' requests for the resources and authority needed for continuing quality improvements.

## Practitioners, Educators, Administrators, and Regulators

Tensions will continue to mark interrelationships among practitioners, educators, administrators, and regulators as a result of unclear definitions of roles and responsibilities for ensuring competence and utilizing them to the full extent of their competence. Practitioners will live with daily consequences of the education that they perceive is a mismatch for the practice demands they face. Educators will decry the impossibility of fitting all that is expected into the curriculum, especially with the dearth of rich clinical experiences for their students. Administrators will bemoan the lack of competence of practitioners produced by the educational system and "blessed" by the regulatory system. Regulators will be blamed by practitioners, educators, and administrators for stifling creativity and posing barriers. Little progress will be made on more productive relationships as a result of lack of systematic analysis and consensus building about society's needs, the services to be provided by the health care delivery system to meet societal needs, the types of nursing roles required by that system, the education needed to prepare persons to fulfill those roles, and the regulation that facilitates those roles while ensuring that the public is protected against incompetent or unethical practice.

The health care system will continue to value licensure when it ensures quality services, controls risk, and minimizes liability. The health care system will devalue licensure when it limits options for staffing, imposes a burden to document competence, or demands expense to verify credentials periodically that provides no utility to the system. When regulation is perceived as overwhelming and burdensome, an irrational and dangerous situation will arise. In *The Death of Common Sense* (1995), Philip K. Howard notes that regulatory goals enjoy wide support but that it is the often formalistic implementation by government, with a web of requirements such that total compliance is impossible, that has fostered a 'culture of resistance' that destroys cooperation. In this probable scenario, as the direction of society becomes increasingly national, and even global, the continuation of a system in which state boundaries create a web of requirements such that total compliance is impossible will encourage flagrant neglect of compliance with the law.

This probable scenario is marked by unresolved issues within several areas, including legislation, federal/state interests, public interest, health care provider relationships, and the health care delivery system. The lack of resolution will cause the licensure system to grow increasingly out of sync with a fundamentally changed health care system attempting to meet the needs of a very different population base across states, the country, and even the globe. It prevents the leaps of change required to reengineer licensure for a new age in health care delivery. Even in the midst of these considerable challenges, boards of nursing will effectively carry out and incrementally improve the protection of the public. Systems for initial licensure, including examinations and license processing, and discipline will continue to be at the cutting edge of psychometric, technologic, and regulatory best practices.

## A PREFERABLE FUTURE FOR PROFESSIONAL LICENSURE

This scenario presents a future envisioned to be optimal in some way, but it will require mobilization of efforts to occur. This preferred scenario will be characterized by the following:

The federal government will acknowledge that professional licensure is efficiently, effectively, and responsively handled by the states, combining the best of local enforcement with a national perspective.

Public interest groups will cite professional licensure as an arena where public/private partnerships have served to advance the public good.

The health care delivery system will know and comply with laws and regulations pertaining to the practitioners it contracts with and employs, and the data exchanged between system administrators and regulators will provide mutual benefits.

This positive environment is based on the following significant accomplishments by boards of nursing.

Licenses for LPNs/VNs, RNs, and APRNs are mutually recognized by the states, offering mobility for all nurses and improved access for consumers. Scope of practice and initial and continuing licensure requirements have become nearly identical because mutual recognition has increased the public and professional support for harmonization.

Nurses are held accountable by boards for their competence, not only when they enter practice but also on a continuing basis, resulting in high public regard for the profession.

Interstate disciplinary processes are carried out with the effectiveness and efficiency long associated with nursing boards' in-state proceedings. Recently, a comprehensive information system has given the public and health care employers online access to relevant data to assist them in ensuring quality of the providers they select.

Boards have begun to address the realities of globalization by exchanging licensure and disciplinary information with nursing regulatory bodies internationally and by implementing potential methods of harmonization on a demonstration basis.

Advanced practice nursing, the use of assistive personnel, practicing nurses, educators, administrators, regulators, the health care system, and others will all benefit in this preferred scenario.

## Advanced Practice Registered Nursing

Pressure will be brought to bear by multistate health care systems to influence the passage of regulation to harmonize practice parameters, such as relationships between nurses and physicians regarding prescriptive privileges. One key ingredient in the success of the legislation was the standardization of educational requirements for APRNs at the graduate level and inclusion of credible content and uniformity in curricula nationwide. A second key to success was agreement reached by professional and regulatory bodies about a consistent approach to regulation and competency assessment of APRNs: the profession acknowledged the need for statutory authorization while regulators worked collaboratively with professional certification bodies to ensure that their certification programs were demonstrably appropriate and therefore best used for regulatory purposes. Advanced practice roles will continue to evolve, and a "core curriculum/core competency" solution will be developed by certifying bodies in conjunction with regulatory bodies. This will ensure that educational and examination criteria are available and sufficient to support regulatory decisions even when formal certification examinations or credentialing do not exist for evolving roles.

## Unlicensed Assistive Personnel

The ambivalence of previous decades over the regulation of UAPs will be largely resolved through a nongovernmental solution. Private groups will develop voluntary mechanisms by which health care institutions commonly ascertain the competence of UAPs for their particular roles and assignments. Motivation for institutions to adopt this voluntary mechanism for ensuring the quality of UAP services include competing on the basis of quality, fulfilling various institutional accreditation standards, and ensuring adherence to institutional risk management policies.

Regulators, in collaboration with practitioners and educators, will design workable and enforceable guidelines for delegation and supervision of care provided by UAPs, with the degree of autonomy of the relationship between UAP and the consumer dependent on the condition and competence of the consumer to supervise the services rendered. Enforcing observance of the guidelines will require creative approaches to establish jurisdiction and effective sanctions over UAPs practicing below standards, but this will be made possible through strong consumer group support for extending the jurisdiction of regulatory boards to all those who provide any aspect of nursing care to consumers. Nursing boards will be able to effectively limit the work of UAPs who violate standards for competent and ethical care.

Consumer groups will be instrumental in discouraging employers from adding new types of health care workers who lack defined standards and have ambiguous accountability. As a part of this "driver's seat" influence over health care quality, consumer groups will be instrumental in educating the public to demand professionals who are qualified and competent, as well as cost effective, to provide the services and achieve the health outcomes they need.

### Practitioners, Educators, Administrators, and Regulators

Clarification will occur through empirical study that identifies the unique contributions of each nursing role and its required competencies, coupled with policy analysis of the number and nature of roles required for the health care delivery system to fulfill the needs of consumers. Clear, consensual documents will be created and updated periodically by a consortium of practitioners, educators, administrators, and regulators. These documents will describe the needs of the health care consumer and the delivery system for nursing services, the roles required to meet those needs, and the competencies for which the educational system accepts accountability to develop in their graduates.

Regulators will be acknowledged as supporting creative and well-founded changes in practice, as well as focusing regulation on producing continuous improvement in health outcomes for consumers. When a practitioner must demonstrate initial or continued competence, regulators will have collectively succeeded in creating and improving the assessment tools required to effectively ensure safe practice to consumers. Regulators will have worked with employers to exchange data to evaluate the continuing competence of individual practitioners without duplicating data collection efforts. In return, employers will have access to a central information system, which they can use to ensure quality of nursing care and to market their services.

### Other Groups

The federal government and public interest groups will have observed the progress toward rational and effective regulation of state-based professional licensure. As a consequence, they will have become supportive of the states continuing to bear primary responsibility for ensuring competent nursing practice. Although professional licensure is unlikely to be the most richly endowed among government services, state legislatures will have shown a greater inclination to provide funding and to grant appropriate authority now that effective partnerships are in place.

### Health Care System

The health care system will have become strongly supportive of nursing personnel in consensus roles. Regulation will be regarded as reasonable and an ally in ensuring quality care rather than as an obstacle to be circumvented.

## CONCLUSION

The preferable scenario differs from the probable scenario primarily in that key issues (e.g., federal/state controversies, advanced practice regulation, UAP regulation, health care providers' roles) will have been resolved. Mobilization of efforts will be required to bring about this preferred scenario. Consensus on optimal solutions and who will best implement them will take strong leadership, willingness to lay aside some aspects of organizational agendas, and, most of all, perseverance to devote resources and priorities to achieving outcomes that are in the best interests of the health and welfare of the public. The results will be worth the effort.

#### Acknowledgment

The author gratefully acknowledges the assistance of Vickie Sheets, Sharon Weisenbeck, and Patricia Calico with this chapter.

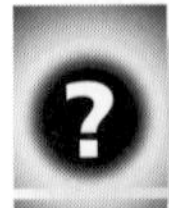

### *Discussion Exercises*

1. An optimistic perspective on a preferable future for regulation in nursing is offered in the chapter. What predictions do you think are likely to occur? Unlikely? Why?

2. Regulation of health care professionals is designed to protect the public from unsafe practices and to ensure the minimal competencies of practitioners. What methods, other than licensure, would you suggest to accomplish these goals?
3. National licensure and institutional licensure have been suggested as alternatives to state licensure. What are the pros and cons of each?

## References

American Nurses Association: House of delegates, Washington, DC, June, 1997.

Cox C, Foster S: *The costs and benefits of occupational regulation,* Washington, DC, 1990, Bureau of Economics, Federal Trade Commission.

*Dent v State of West Virginia:* 129 U.S. 114 [32 Led 623, 9 Sct 231], 1889.

Howard P: *The death of common sense,* New York, 1995, Random House.

Massaro T, O'Brien T: Constitutional limitations on state-imposed continuing competency requirements for licensed professionals, *William Mary Law Rev* 25(2):253, 1983.

U.S. Department of Commerce: Telemedicine report to congress, 1997.

# 24 Educational Accreditation

**Sherril B. Gelmon**
**Janis P. Bellack**
**Akiko M. Berkman**

*It is a capital mistake to theorize before one has data.*

**Sherlock Holmes**

Accreditation is a public hallmark of quality. It reflects that a program or institution has engaged in a rigorous process of internal and external review and is recognized as meeting specified standards of educational excellence. Thoughtful reviews of the higher education accreditation process and accreditation in health professions education may be found elsewhere (Filerman, 1984; Millard, 1984; Dickey, 1985; Gelmon, 1995). Here, the focus is on accreditation in nursing, taking into account the forces in higher education and specialized accreditation that have shaped the continuing evolution of nursing accreditation. As nursing education programs try to respond to these rapid and dramatic changes, the criteria and processes for accreditation of nursing education programs must change in ways that encourage innovation and flexibility but preserve and enhance program quality.

## SPECIALIZED ACCREDITATION

Several key assumptions underlie contemporary discussions of accreditation in higher education in the United States (Young and others, 1983). Accreditation initially developed as a voluntary, nongovernmental process. Such a system of guided self-evaluation and self-improvement is central to voluntary self-regulation of educational programs. The primary value of accreditation can be found not in its outcomes but rather in its process of self-evaluation and peer review (Gelmon, 1997a).

Today, specialized, or programmatic, accreditation plays a valuable role in our society by assuring the public that the accredited program guarantees that students have met certain standards and are prepared for entry or advancement within a particular profession (Association of Specialized and Professional Accreditors [ASPA], 1993). The accreditation process in higher education in the United States includes a common set of components: self-study; preparation of documentation; on-site peer evaluation; presentation of findings in report format; decision making regarding accreditation status; and ongoing periodic review, updates, and reporting.

## Evolving Process of Accreditation

As a point-in-time review, accreditation as we know it today is increasingly out of step with the rapid pace of educational change, which has been hastened by the speed of societal change. Most educational programs are accredited on 5- to 10-year cycles. This means that programmatic changes that occur between accreditation site visits may go unreviewed for years by the agency whose stamp of approval ensures that the program meets certain quality standards.

Furthermore, revising accreditation standards to keep pace with external changes is typically a lengthy and arduous process. By the time newly revised standards take effect, changes in higher education and health care may have rendered them obsolete or at least out of step with the current environment. Although it is important to maintain consistency and stability in accreditation standards and procedures over a certain period to ensure equitable application across institutions or programs, rigid adherence to published standards very well may be out of touch with current educational and professional practices, with accreditation inhibiting change and innovation in curriculum and program delivery as an undesirable and unintended consequence (Kirkwood, 1973; Bender, 1983; Shugars and others, 1991).

Fortunately, accreditation has great potential to evolve from its "old" way to a new process that is more responsive to the challenges facing higher education (Gelmon, 1997b). The forces driving change in higher education have created tensions for accreditation, which are delineated in Figure 24-1. These tensions illustrate how accreditation can evolve in concert with changes in higher education and health care and be receptive to and even encouraging of innovation. For example, greater emphasis can be placed on consultation and guidance through the use of peer experts.

Accreditation can change from its traditional focus on content and compliance to a future focus on processes and improvement and encourage an evolution from a highly prescribed, structured format that simply perpetuates usual practice to one that emphasizes the competencies of new graduate health professionals and their capacity for lifelong learning. To do this, accreditation can promote learning in "real-work" clinical experiences in a variety of settings, as well as in the traditional classroom. These learning experiences in turn can foster a high degree of personal development, with an emphasis on the acquisition of skills and knowledge that will have relevance for future professional practice and community citizenship.

## Current Reality of Specialized Accreditation

Rising costs associated with accreditation have become major issues for college and university administrators, as well as for the accreditation agencies. The accreditation process consumes considerable human, physical, and financial resources. Many question whether accreditation adds value to higher education and the public, and, if it does, whether the margin of value is worth the high cost of the investment (Mayhew and others, 1990; Dill and others, 1996). Although historically administrators viewed the investment in accreditation as beneficial to their institutions, the benefits today are not as clear (Prager, 1993). Given the many demands on institutional resources, administrators may be less inclined in the future to invest in specialized accreditation of individual programs. The challenges that accreditation faces now not only have prompted the creation of a new national

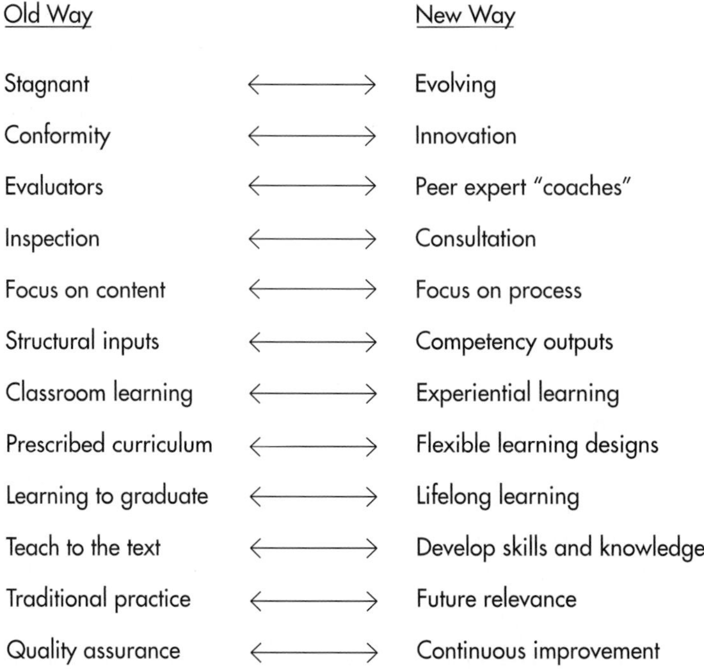


**Figure 24-1** Tensions in accreditation.

coordinating body for postsecondary accreditation but also have fueled a drive to seek ways to improve the accreditation process.

Specialized accreditation in the health professions today reflects the environmental and political forces of the past few decades. The Pew Health Professions Commission has called repeatedly for reform of accreditation in its reviews of health professions education and work force regulation (Shugars and others, 1991; O'Neil, 1993; Pew Health Professions Commission, 1995). In 1996 the Commission created a Task Force on Accreditation of Health Professions Education and charged this interdisciplinary group with engaging the broad community of accreditors, professional associations, and higher education organizations in a series of forums on accreditation and also with developing policy recommendations to improve health professions accreditation (Center for the Health Professions, 1996). The task force expects to report its recommendations for widespread dissemination in the near future.

## Benefits, Criticisms, and Barriers

Ideally, specialized accreditation of health professions education programs is a reliable indicator of program quality and a process by which certain benefits accrue to the programs themselves, their respective professional bodies, their "customers" (students, graduates, employers), and ultimately the public. There are many reasons that specialized accreditation emerged as a measure of program quality and why its supporters continue to advocate its importance (Center for the Health Professions, 1996). Specifically, specialized accreditation in the health professions includes the following:

Provides a hallmark of program excellence and achievement beyond minimum standards

- Formalizes the shared values of a profession and integrates them with those in health care and higher education
- Provides public policy makers with a strong tool to ensure that the public's interest and investment are protected
- Ensures that programs are responsive to changing public needs and demands
- Facilitates professional marketability and mobility through a broadly recognized and valued credentialing process
- Provides an opportunity for peer review and collaboration for program improvement
- Provides leverage for programs to preserve and strengthen institutional support and ensure equitable access to institutional resources
- Encompasses a broad range of measures of program quality, including structures, processes, and outcomes

Despite its strengths, accreditation has been criticized increasingly on a number of fronts and by a variety of stakeholders (Center for the Health Professions, 1996). Some of the more common criticisms include the following:

- The focus has been on single point inspection and compliance rather than continuous program improvement.
- Current policies and practices are often more regulatory and punitive than voluntary and consultative.
- Specialized accreditation is costly, burdensome, and duplicative of other institutional/program reviews; time and resources spent might be better directed to teaching, learning, research, and service.
- Proliferation of multiple accrediting bodies has resulted in fragmentation and segmentation of specialized accreditation.
- The current system of specialized accreditation prevents crossdisciplinary or interdisciplinary standard setting and program review.
- Specialized accreditation tends to protect and elevate professional self-interests above those of the public.
- Specialized accreditation is highly prescriptive in some disciplines, thus discouraging experimentation, flexibility, innovation, and the ability to be responsive to local/state needs and specific institutional missions.
- There is a high degree of variation among the criteria and processes of specialized accreditation and minimal evidence that these criteria and processes are valid and reliable.
- There is little solid evidence to support that accreditation does what it purports to do, that is, ensure program quality.
- Current accreditation processes provide minimal opportunity for involvement/input by certain key stakeholders, for example, practicing health professionals, employers, consumers, policy makers, and payers.

The need and demand for change in the current system and processes of specialized accreditation are being driven by a variety of forces, both within and external to the programs and institutions (Center for the Health Professions, 1996). These include the following:

- Constrained resources and a desire to improve efficiency and cost effectiveness
- External demands for accountability, especially from state legislatures, funding agencies, and consumers
- The growing focus on outcomes assessment, outcomes management, and continuous improvement in all sectors, for example, industry, health system, and education
- The rise of managed care and integrated delivery systems, which demand rapid deployment, workforce flexibility (cross-training), and cost control
- The rapid proliferation and use of technology (information technology, communication technology, distance education)
- Growing interest in expanding opportunities for collaboration among the various accrediting agencies—to improve the processes, reduce duplication, and achieve cost savings while ensuring program quality

Unfortunately, many barriers exist in the current environment that inhibit change and protect the status quo (Center for the Health Professions, 1996). Some of the barriers are endemic to the change process, whereas others are specific to specialized accreditation. The most commonly cited barriers include the following:

- Established traditions in health professions education and general resistance to change
- Decentralization and overspecialization of the health professions, with each accrediting agency and profession wishing to preserve its autonomy and "turf"
- Self-interests of the professions and their respective accrediting bodies and the desire to maintain established hierarchies
- Well-entrenched structures and processes within the current system of specialized accreditation
- Wide variation in accreditation practices among the different health professions and their accrediting agencies
- Wide variation among health professions educational programs (e.g., length of program, requirements, professional vs. technical), thus requiring different measures of program quality
- Accreditation as "big business"
- Rigid, prescriptive criteria and policies of the current approval bodies, especially the U.S. Department of Education
- A generally litigious society

This is the reality we find ourselves in today. How did we get here?

## HISTORY OF EDUCATIONAL ACCREDITATION

### Early Years

The nature and evolution of accreditation in higher education in the United States dates back to 1862 when Congress passed the Land Grant Act. This act granted federal land to the states to facilitate the establishment of state universities. As these "land grant" and other universities and colleges flourished, Congress and the public began to question the quality of education being delivered. Accreditation emerged as a response to meet expressed concerns.

The commonly accepted purpose of accreditation is to promote and ensure the highest quality in education. However, the process for ensuring program quality through accreditation has changed over time. In the late 1800s and early 1900s the federal government and the institutions struggled to make higher education more accountable to the public. One of the principal weaknesses of the higher education system in the United States was its lack of centralized control (Blauch, 1959). The absence of a "ministry of education," similar to that found in many other countries, was viewed as a limitation in the system (U.S. DHEW, 1977). Thus voluntary accreditation emerged as a way to achieve greater control in ensuring the delivery of high-quality education by colleges and universities while avoiding government regulation, historically feared in the United States. Thus accreditation bodies developed initially in response to a recognized need for nongovernmental peer reviews and, second, to address specific regional and professional standards for ensuring quality.

Early on, accreditation was four pronged (Blauch, 1959). First, agencies were charged with responsibility for accreditation criteria and standards for higher education programs. Second, inspection of institutions was provided by competent authorities to determine if the institution met these standards. Third, a list of institutions that met the public standards was published regularly. Finally, periodic reviews were instituted to make certain that these institutions continued to meet the established standards.

The earliest accreditation organizations in the professions appeared around the turn of the century (Blauch, 1959). Dates of establishment include osteopathy in 1897, law in 1900, medicine in 1904, and nursing in 1916, although most did not begin publishing lists of accredited programs until several years later. A significant point of leverage for reform of higher education was the publication in 1910 of the Flexner Report, prepared by the American Medical Association (AMA) in conjunction with the Carnegie Foundation (Kells, 1994). This report prompted the adoption and enforcement of specific standards for medical education, resulting in the closure of a large number of inferior medical schools and generating a ripple effect across other professions and academic institutions. By providing a template for educational standards and program review, the Flexner report served as a catalyst for reevaluating what was meant by "quality" professional education.

Regional accreditation of colleges and universities grew out of membership associations that had been established to improve the relationship between secondary and higher education and to strengthen college admission standards. Although six regional associations were established between 1885 and 1924, it was the North Central Association of Colleges and Secondary Schools that took the lead in accreditation, adopting its first standards for colleges in 1909, publishing its first list of accredited colleges in 1916, and incorporating standards for junior colleges and teachers colleges by 1918 (Blauch, 1959). With increasing professionalization and specialization of the workforce and proliferation of academic programs to educate these new professionals, multiple accrediting agencies were established over the years to create program-specific standards and ensure the quality of specialized programs.

## Recent Past

Over the past 70 years accreditation has shifted from a fairly rigid to a more flexible approach. Accrediting agencies have taken the initiative in adapting their processes to encourage institutional and program individuality rather than mandating that all academic units look alike. There also has been a shift from strictly external review to a review process that relies heavily on internal self-evaluation and self-regulation. These changes reflect changing societal expectations and demands (Young and others, 1983).

The federal government has become increasingly involved in accreditation. Specific activities include federal legislation that linked eligibility for federal funds (such as those authorized by the 1952 Serviceman's Readjustment Act) to accreditation, other "gatekeeping" mechanisms that connected student loan or special educational program funds to accreditation, and state legislation that tied eligibility for professional licensure and practice to graduation from an accredited program. State involvement in judging the quality of educational programs began in New York as early as 1784, with an emphasis on teacher education and liberal arts, although most state agencies did not begin accrediting or approving educational programs until early in the twentieth century (Blauch, 1959).

The proliferation of accrediting agencies and associations during the first half of the twentieth century prompted calls for coordination of accreditation, and in 1949 the National Commission on Accreditation (NCA) was established to coordinate accrediting bodies and control the expansion of specialized accreditation (Blauch, 1959). The NCA was an institution-based organization that did not include the accreditors on its governing board. It established a series of operating principles, most of which are still in effect as fundamental components of the decentralized pattern of oversight and review of higher education in this country. The specifications of these principles follow.

The six regional associations would be responsible for formal accreditation of colleges and universities in their respective region.

The regional associations would deal only with national professional accrediting agencies recognized by the NCA, and colleges and universities would deal only with officially recognized professional agencies.

Professional accreditation agencies would meet certain requirements established by the NCA and would coordinate their activities with the regional associations.

No more than one agency would be recognized in a particular field of study, thus limiting the number of accrediting agencies and the potential for duplication of effort or competition.

The policies and procedures of all recognized accrediting agencies would reflect qualitative indicators, as well as quantitative measures.

In 1964 the Federation of Regional Accrediting Commissions in Higher Education (FRACHE) was established as a forum for the regional associations to share concerns about institutional accreditation (Bemis, 1991). FRACHE worked closely with NCA, but over time the number of specialized accreditors continued to increase, prompting rising concern about effective coordination among regional and specialized accrediting agencies. Although a Council of Specialized Accrediting Agencies existed within the NCA, it became increasingly apparent that there was a compelling need to improve coordination among multiple accrediting agencies. The push for more effective coordination by a nongovernmental organization eventually resulted in the creation in 1975 of the Council on Postsecondary Accreditation (COPA).

Initially, COPA concentrated its attention on recognition of specialized and professional agencies but in 1980 assumed recognition of the regional associations as well (Bemis, 1991). One of COPA's main purposes was to monitor accreditation bodies to ensure that they met certain standards. COPA also provided a network for collaboration and information sharing among the various accrediting groups.

## Problems Emerge

In the early 1990s the U.S. Congress expressed concerns about the significant increase in default rates in federal student loan programs, suggesting that default rates were linked to poor academic quality and reflected the failure of accreditation agencies to adequately monitor these programs. Students who do not graduate or who graduate but are unemployable often default on their loans. Despite the fact that the overwhelming majority of high default rates occurred in financially unstable trade and proprietary institutions, Congress passed a new Higher Education Act (HEA) in 1992 that mandated greater governmental oversight of the accreditation process and increased the gatekeeping responsibilities of the accrediting agencies.

The 1992 HEA expanded the gatekeeping and regulatory functions of the Department of Education (DOE), converting the DOE from an agency concerned only with monitoring loan default rates and controlling access to federal training funds to an overseer and regulator of the entire accreditation process. Thus the 1992 HEA shifted the culture and philosophy of accreditation from one of peer review and professional judgment to one of government regulation and prescriptive monitoring (Tanner, 1996). It is evident that these changes to accreditation have added regulatory functions to specialized accreditation, thus moving it beyond a solely voluntary, peer-review process.

Concurrent with these developments, the long-established system of accreditation in higher education began to unravel, and in 1993 the board of COPA voted to dissolve the organization. The following year a special committee of former members of COPA established a new entity, the Commission on Recognition of Postsecondary Accreditation (CORPA), to serve as a temporary mechanism for recognizing regional, specialized, and proprietary accrediting organizations until a new oversight entity could be established.

During this time many of the specialized and professional accreditors worried that their professional and organizational needs would not be met once COPA dissolved, and the next year an organization was established to address the unique needs of specialized and professional accrediting agencies. This new organization, the Association of Specialized and Professional Accreditors (ASPA) became an important catalyst for developing common practices for specialized and professional accreditation and for information sharing within this community. Today, ASPA continues to be an effective resource through its clear mission and goal of meeting the needs of the specialized accrediting community.

In 1994 the National Policy Board on Higher Education Institutional Accreditation (NPB) was formed by leaders of the regional accrediting associations and national higher education organizations to constitute a national coordinating body to succeed COPA. The NPB included representation from the nine regional accrediting commissions and seven organizations of higher education whose members are college and university presidents (National Policy Board, 1994). The NPB assumed responsibility for creating an organization that would take COPA's place in overseeing regional and specialized accreditation and developed a proposal for a new oversight organization, which met with widespread opposition. The regional accreditors viewed the NPB's proposal as intrusive and undermining their responsibilities for setting regional standards for accreditation, whereas college and university leaders expressed concern that the NPB's standards would interfere with institutional autonomy and prerogative (Dill and others, 1996). The proposal failed to garner sufficient support, and the NPB quickly dissolved.

### Council for Higher Education Accreditation Established

Following the NPB's dissolution a work group of college and university presidents formed to explore other ways to achieve coordination and recognition of accrediting agencies. In 1995 this group proposed the creation of a Council for Higher Education Accreditation (CHEA), which was overwhelmingly endorsed by the nation's college and university presidents. The principal difference from its predecessors, COPA and CORPA, is that CHEA is "owned" by the institutions, whereas COPA and CORPA represented and were supported by the accrediting agencies (Braskamp, 1996). It is interesting to note the similarity in structure and governance of CHEA to that of the National Commission on Accreditation (NCA), created some 40 years earlier.

CHEA became operational in 1996 and has several functions (CHEA, 1996). First, it provides a recognition function for the regional associations, as well as specialized and professional accreditors. Second, it acts as a lobbyist for the community of accreditors. Finally, it has responsibility for ongoing evaluation of the accreditation process and for recommending improvements. CHEA assumed the functions of CORPA in late 1996, and CORPA was dissolved.

Within this historic context, accreditation of nursing education programs evolved and was influenced by the many forces driving change in postsecondary accreditation in general. We turn now to consider accreditation in nursing education against the backdrop of this larger context and the evolving changes within the profession of nursing itself.

## NURSING ACCREDITATION AT THE END OF THE TWENTIETH CENTURY

Currently, specialized accreditation of nursing education programs is conducted by several organizations. The National League for Nursing (NLN) has been the principal specialized accrediting agency for practical, diploma, associate, and baccalaureate and higher degree nursing education programs since 1952. In addition, the American College of Nurse Midwives (ACNM) independently accredits nurse midwifery programs, and the American Association of Nurse Anesthetists (AANA) independently accredits nurse anesthesia programs. Accreditation of continuing education programs in nursing is conducted by the American Nurses Association (ANA). NLN and AANA were recognized by the former COPA and are currently members of ASPA. The ACNM did not choose to be recognized by COPA or to join ASPA. In 1996, after several years of considering the issue, the American Association of Colleges of Nursing (AACN) decided to formally pursue the possibility of accrediting baccalaureate and graduate degree programs in nursing, potentially adding another player to the accreditation process in nursing.

It is important to understand that until 1992 the regional accrediting commissions served as the institutional accreditors and "gatekeepers" of federal funds, including student loans and program training funds, for the vast majority of practical, associate, baccalaureate, and higher degree nursing education programs. However, the NLN served a dual role as both specialized and institutional accreditor for all diploma programs and for those practical nursing education programs not located in regionally accredited institutions of higher education. The NLN's recognition as an accrediting agency by the U.S. Department of Education (DOE) ensured access to federal funds for these programs.

In the early 1990s the NLN accreditation criteria were radically changed to encourage "innovation and responsiveness to local [program] needs while achieving a national standard in the critical outcomes of nursing education" (Tanner, 1996). Although viewed by some as compromising the older, more specific accreditation standards, the NLN was one of the first specialized accrediting agencies to address the barriers that rigid accreditation criteria imposed on professional programs trying to respond to rapid changes in the environment. The changes were made to allow programs more flexibility and to place greater emphasis on outcomes (what students had learned, what competencies they had acquired) than on structures or processes (admissions criteria, teaching methods, allocation of credit hours). Tanner (1996) argues that the 1992 Higher Education Act promulgated a throwback to old "input criteria" and "checklists and counting" rather than a forward move to educational outcomes, which are more difficult to measure.

In 1995 the NLN came under "severe and critical scrutiny" by the DOE for what the DOE said was NLN's failure to comply with many of the DOE's new criteria (NLN, 1996). NLN was first scheduled to be reviewed under the new DOE regulations in May 1995; NLN requested a 6-month delay in its review under the new DOE criteria and was granted a deferral on its application until November 1995, when it was reviewed. In a letter dated February 1996 the NLN was notified by U.S. Secretary of Education Richard Riley that it was not in full compliance with 35 of the 77 mandated criteria. The DOE deferred the NLN petition for renewal of continued recognition to give the NLN time to demonstrate that "it was putting forth serious effort and acting in good faith to come into compliance" and requested that a progress report be submitted in March 1996. The NLN submitted its progress report as requested. An analysis by the DOE staff, reported in June 1996, noted that NLN was not in compliance with 11 of the 77 criteria, five of which were related to the DOE's new regulatory standards for accrediting agencies. The NLN presented specific timetables for achieving compliance within the next 6 months.

Despite NLN's plan the staff recommended to the DOE's National Advisory Committee on Institutional Quality and Integrity (NACIQI) that NLN's recognition as an accrediting agency be withdrawn. At its June 1996 meeting the NACIQI voted to recommend withdrawal of NLN's recognition; NLN subsequently filed an appeal. A September 1996 status report from the NLN revealed that the association was able to demonstrate its compliance with 71 of the 77 criteria. The NLN noted that the remaining six criteria were "all in progress" and as of January 1997 the NLN would be in compliance with all but one, which could not be met "until the three year study of [the reliability and validity] of NLN Criteria is completed" (NLN, 1996). This study was initiated to meet one of the DOE's required criteria.

In December 1996 Secretary Riley upheld NLN's appeal and continued its recognition for 6 months with a request for a progress report to be submitted in March 1997. In January 1997 a new NLN Accrediting Commission (NLNAC) began operations. The NLNAC was formed in response to a DOE requirement that the accrediting body of any professional association must function as a "separate and independent" entity. In March 1997 NLNAC submitted the requested progress report, and in June the NACIQI voted to recommend to Secretary Riley that the NLNAC be granted preliminary approval as a recognized accrediting agency for all nursing education programs. A follow-up report must be submitted by the NLNAC to the DOE in 12 to 18 months, which is standard procedure when the DOE recognizes a new accrediting agency, which the NLNAC is considered to be.

In response to members' concerns about accreditation, the board of directors of the American Association of Colleges of Nursing (AACN), whose 500+ members are deans or directors of baccalaureate and graduate nursing education programs, began investigating the possibility of developing its own mechanism for accrediting baccalaureate and graduate degree programs. In 1996 AACN appointed a task force on nursing accreditation "to explore the fiscal, professional, regulatory, and statutory aspects of specialized accreditation, and . . . what role, if any, AACN should play in the accreditation of baccalaureate and graduate nursing programs" (AACN, 1996). The AACN noted that its principal reason for creating the task force was "the proliferation and lack of coordination of specialized accreditation within nursing . . . and the rapidly expanding number of nurse practitioner education programs" (AACN, 1996). The task force subsequently proposed that the AACN lead the development of a new alliance model to bring the various accrediting groups in nursing together and also called for the establishment of a new entity whose sole purpose would be the accreditation of baccalaureate and graduate nursing programs. The AACN affirmed its intent to pursue this new accreditation function regardless of the result of the DOE review of the NLN, and in October 1996 AACN members approved the task force's proposal by a 4:1 margin.

In January 1997 AACN appointed a steering committee to plan the new alliance and accrediting entity. The steering committee subsequently proposed the creation of two organizational entities: the Commission on Collegiate Nursing Education (CCNE) and an accreditation alliance of nursing organizations involved in accreditation and credentialing. AACN envisions that the alliance will evolve into a "wholly separate and unified accreditation entity" that will "bring uniformity and a more streamlined and coordinated approach to accrediting baccalaureate and graduate nursing programs . . . by putting into place common standards, common data sets, and a common process" (AACN, 1997a; AACN, 1997b). A draft of CCNE's accreditation standards was disseminated in June 1997, and final approval and adoption by the AACN membership occurred in late 1997.

Meanwhile, NLN chartered its new NLN Accrediting Commission (NLNAC) as a "separate and independent" entity; approved bylaws; hired an executive director; and appointed a 15-member panel of commissioners representing nursing education, nursing service, and the public. Accreditation criteria for all program types were modified to include DOE mandated standards; evaluation of member programs continues under the revised criteria, guidelines, and procedures. Improved mechanisms for internal consistency and quality control of the accreditation process were put into place in 1997, additional staff were employed, and efforts were made to ensure more rapid dissemination of information related to changes in the process to interested parties, including the more than 1400 NLNAC-accredited programs (NLNAC, 1997). NLN, through NLNAC, affirmed "its resolve to refocus on accreditation as the central service of the organization" and restore its stature "as the nursing profession's foremost accreditor for all educational programs at all levels of nursing" (Ryan, 1997). NLNAC's ability to accredit programs at all levels of nursing education may be particularly attractive to those schools and institutions that have multiple levels of nursing education, for example, associate and baccalaureate, practical nursing and associate, and those few schools that offer associate through doctoral degrees in nursing.

Critics of AACN have expressed concern that AACN's decision to pursue a role in accreditation divides nursing and thus weakens its potential to influence accreditation regulations at the national level. Both NLN and AACN have been criticized by members of the nursing education community for their failure to come together on this issue and work collaboratively to strengthen nursing accreditation for AACN's and NLN's member institutions. The AMA and the Association of American Medical Colleges (AAMC) have successfully created such a shared model of accreditation of undergraduate medical education programs through their separate and independent Liaison Committee on Medical Education (LCME). Similar alliances exist in accreditation of health management, public health, counseling, teacher education, and other professional programs.

AACN has been criticized for being an elitist member organization of nursing deans and directors with no opportunity for membership by the larger nursing education community and for seeking to separate nursing accreditation by program level, with the potential for aggravating long-standing tensions among nurse educators across the continuum of nursing education. NLN has been criticized for neglecting its own internal problems, which are perceived by many as having created NLN's difficulties with the DOE in the first place. NLN's fiscal and organizational problems, coupled with its long-standing resistance to addressing the issue of differentiated practice and credentialing, undermined its credibility and the trust of its members (both agency and individual) in the mid 1990s. Although NLNAC affirmed its intent to accredit all levels of nursing education programs in 1996, NLNAC may have lost ground when AACN was moving forward aggressively with a well-organized, highly visible strategic plan to enter the accreditation business. Where does this leave nursing accreditation as the twenty-first century approaches?

## NURSING ACCREDITATION IN THE TWENTY-FIRST CENTURY

The previously discussed review, along with interviews with a number of key leaders in nursing education and nursing accreditation, led us to generate both probable and preferable futures of accreditation in nursing. The key leaders we interviewed affirmed the same advantages and the same concerns and criticisms of accreditation that are summarized earlier in this chapter. The issues identified include:

Redundancy and duplication of accreditation processes

Lack of effective integration and coordination of accreditation processes

More than one accrediting agency, which allows for choice and competition but may cause confusion

Uncertainty about value added by accreditation

Failure of accreditation to distinguish true quality

High costs associated with accreditation—fiscal, human, technical, time, operating

Inflexibility of accreditation standards, compromising the ability to be responsive to rapid changes in the environment

Lack of opportunities for input by important stakeholders, particularly students; practicing nurses; policymakers; employers; and consumer advocates

Our projected probable future is based on current evidence and input from a variety of sources. Alternatively, we pose a preferable future—our vision of what accreditation in nursing can be—that we believe has greater potential for preserving the value of accreditation, strengthening the accreditation process, overcoming perceived barriers in the process, and creating a shared model of responsibility and public accountability for high-quality nursing education into the future.

### Probable Future

Given the changes in higher education and health care and what has transpired in the last few years with regard to accreditation of nursing programs, we project that the probable future will involve two separate entities—NLNAC and CCNE—that will serve as recognized agencies for general accreditation of nursing programs. The former will continue to accredit all levels of nursing education, whereas CCNE will accredit baccalaureate and higher degree programs only. Therefore duplicate accreditation services will be available to these latter programs, increasing the total dollars invested by the nursing education community in accreditation despite the fact that the total number of nursing education programs will not increase. On the other hand, competition for customers may compel both CCNE and NLNAC to hold costs down and achieve internal efficiencies that they may not be motivated to achieve otherwise.

With both NLNAC and CCNE involved in accrediting baccalaureate and higher degree programs, schools with these programs have a choice of which agency to belong to and seek accreditation from. Also, those nursing schools with multiple levels of nursing education will be forced to either stay with NLNAC, which has core criteria that cut across all program levels, or choose NLNAC to accredit their programs offered at below the baccalaureate level and CCNE to accredit those at the baccalaureate and graduate levels. Some schools, initially at least, will probably choose to be accredited by both NLNAC and CCNE, taking a "wait and see" approach as the school tests the processes, costs, and value of each accrediting agency. Thus resources will be invested in duplicate accreditation that could be spent more effectively and profitably elsewhere, especially in this era of constrained finances in nursing education.

We also project that the probable scenario of two nursing education accrediting agencies may tempt programs to choose between the two on the basis of cost (least expensive) and the extent and scope of reporting required by the criteria and guidelines. Specific criteria may influence the decision and could potentially weaken nursing's progress in advancing itself within higher education. This scenario, over time, could lead to a weakening of accreditation standards, as CCNE and NLNAC compete for the business of a limited pool of nursing schools. Faced with the need to survive, NLNAC and CCNE might resort to "dumbing down" standards and requirements to hold onto customers. This would not be a conscious or intentional aim but would occur under the rubric of "streamlining" and "improving" the standards in response to customer needs. Still, the effect would be the same.

Furthermore, with both AACN and NLN offering accrediting services, there is a possibility that regulators such as the individual state boards of nursing or the policy-making National Council of State Boards of Nursing (NCSBN) may step in and claim both regulatory and accreditation functions for nursing education and practice. Given recent calls by the Task Force on Healthcare Workforce Regulation of the Pew Health Professions Commission (Finocchio and others, 1995) to simplify and streamline interstate and interprofessional regulation of the health care workforce, it is not far fetched to imagine this occurring. The NCSBN has already investigated the possibility of a second licensure level for RNs at the advanced practice level but has not taken action yet.

Finally, it is probable that some cooperation and collaboration between AACN and the advanced nursing practice accreditors (ACNM and AANA) will be established, including one or more of the following: shared site visits, similar reporting cycles, common reporting formats, and even agreed-on core criteria, with separate subspecialty criteria. However, there are many financial, professional, and political barriers to such an arrangement, and currently too many incentives exist for maintaining the status quo. These include the desire of the subspecialty organizations to maintain their autonomy and authority in accrediting their respective educational programs, the fiscal stability and professional prestige of the accrediting arms of the AANA and the ACNM, and the location of many nurse anesthesia and some nurse midwifery programs in other than AACN-member schools of nursing (many are housed in schools of medicine or allied health). Furthermore, it is not clear which organization would ultimately have authority for this "wholly separate and unified" entity; presumably it would be AACN. However, will AANA and ACNM willingly accept a subordinate role in the accreditation of advanced practice nursing programs?

Is there an alternative that would be acceptable to all entities involved in specialized accreditation of nursing education programs? We offer our preferable scenario, which encompasses the various nursing accreditors but calls for an integrated approach to specialized accreditation in the health professions, using an interprofessional model.

## Preferable Future

At a time when concerns abound about the duplication, fragmentation, and excessive cost of accreditation, two entities for accrediting nursing education programs seem both unnecessary and counterproductive. Not only does it create a competitive situation in which baccalaureate and higher degree nursing programs will be forced to choose one or the other, but also the justification for having two accrediting bodies is not sufficiently compelling and may further confuse an already confused public.

Protecting the public from harm is not a function of accreditation; that is what regulation and professional licensure are intended to do. Instead, accreditation is aimed at assuring the public, and specifically prospective students of a program and the employers of the graduates, that the program meets certain quality standards agreed on by the professional community. Accreditation also should promote innovation, responsiveness to changing needs, ongoing self-assessment, continuous improvement, and periodic objective assessment by external peers.

The preferable future for nursing accreditation is an alliance model in which all specialized accrediting agencies in nursing join together and share the responsibilities and rewards associated with the business of accreditation. Given current realities and the likelihood that institutional leaders' concerns about duplication, fragmentation, and costliness will continue and may even escalate, it is time for the agencies engaged in accreditation—both existing and emerging—to put aside their respective organizational agendas and come together for the benefit of all of nursing education (general, specialized, subspecialized, basic, advanced, continuing).

In this preferable scenario the general accrediting agencies for undergraduate and graduate nursing education, specifically NLN and AACN, will share responsibility for accreditation similar to the model in place in medical education accreditation. This will involve the joint establishment and support of a single accrediting commission, with clearly defined links to the two parent organizations. Furthermore, ACNM, AANA, and ANA will link their respective criteria and activities with the single accrediting commission to serve those nursing education programs with subspecialty offerings in nurse midwifery and nurse anesthesia, as well as those with continuing education programs. Peer review panels with the necessary specialized expertise in program type and focus will be appointed by the commission on the recommendation of the respective associations to ensure expert review.

This preferred alliance model will streamline the entire accreditation process for nursing education programs, making it more cost effective and reducing the number of separate self-studies, site visits, and accreditation fees that now consume so many resources and so much time. These resources could be better spent by faculty and administrators in achieving their professional aims. However, it is unlikely that this preferable model will emerge. Given the tensions between voluntary and regulated accreditation; the existing barriers to collaboration among the various nursing accreditors; and the strong professional, economic, and political incentives for preserving the status quo; it is not likely that our proposed preferable model will come to pass.

## Outcome of Preferable Future

Regardless of the actual structure that emerges in the future—an alliance model or continuation of multiple accreditors of nursing education programs—in the preferable future accreditation will become a continuous internally driven and externally monitored process of evaluation and improvement. As has been suggested elsewhere (Gelmon, 1996), such an approach will involve adopting a model of improvement, using the following questions to frame the accreditation process.

Tell us what you want to be. (What is your aim? What are you trying to produce?)
Tell us how you are going to do it.

Tell us how you are going to measure and evaluate your success.

Tell us how you are going to use the results of this evaluation to improve what you are doing, and if necessary, make changes in what you do.

This continuous improvement approach will shift the focus of accreditation from one of single-point inspection and compliance to one of seamless data gathering, self-assessment, decision making, and improvement, in which up-to-date and reliable information may be accessed by the accreditors as needed so that they can ensure ongoing program quality.

We also envision a preferable future of "virtual accreditation," in which the entire process of data gathering, assessment, and program improvement is continuous and facilitated by the use of state-of-the-art technology. Accredited programs will maintain fully digitized Web sites that accreditors and others (e.g., prospective and enrolled students, state agencies, employers) can "visit" to review the information that assures them that the program meets established standards of quality.

## CONCLUSION

The history of accreditation in higher education has been fraught with controversy and conflict, as has the recent history of accreditation in nursing education. We cannot predict the future; we can only speculate on what is preferable, what is probable, and what may be viewed as inevitable. Nursing education clearly faces a number of challenges with respect to accreditation. It is our desire that these issues be addressed and resolved in the near future so that nursing as a profession may concentrate its energies on continuing to improve the professional preparation of new entrants into the field of nursing to meet the needs of our evolving health and social services system.

For continuing updates on nursing accreditation, visit the following Web sites:

AACN/CCNE: *http://www.aacn.org*

NLN/NLNAC: *http://www.nln.org/nlnac.htm*

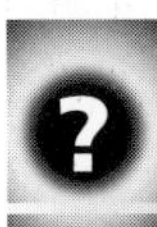

### *Discussion Exercises*

1. To what do you attribute the historic difficulties in accrediting higher education in the U.S.?
2. Compare and contrast accreditation of higher education with accreditation of nursing education.
3. Do you agree with the authors' idea of "virtual accreditation"? Discuss ways it could work.

## References

American Association of Colleges of Nursing (AACN): Fact sheet: an alliance for accreditation of nursing higher education, *http://www.aacn.org,* 1996.

American Association of Colleges of Nursing (AACN): AACN moves to establish alliance to accredit nursing higher education, *http://www.aacn.org,* January 13, 1997a.

American Association of Colleges of Nursing (AACN): Accreditation news notes, *http://www.aacn.org,* February, 1997b.

Association of Specialized and Professional Accreditors (ASPA): *The role and value of specialized accreditation: a policy statement,* Arlington, Va, 1993, The Association.

Bemis JF: *Northwest Association of Schools and Colleges 75 year history 1917-1991,* Boise, Idaho, 1991, Northwest Association of Schools and Colleges.

Bender LW: Accreditation: misuses and misconceptions. In Young KE and others: *Understanding accreditation,* San Francisco, 1983, Jossey-Bass.

Blauch LE: *Accreditation in higher education,* Washington, DC, 1959, U.S. Government Printing Office.

Braskamp L: Personal communication, 1996.

Center for the Health Professions: *Backgrounder: the task force on accreditation of health professions education,* San Francisco, 1996, University of California.

Council for Higher Education Accreditation (CHEA): *CHEA news,* Washington, DC, 1996, The Council.

Dickey FG: Accreditation in the allied health professions. In Hamburg J, editor: *Review of allied health education: 5,* Lexington, Ky, 1985, University Press of Kentucky.

Dill DD and others: Accreditation and academic quality assurance: can we get there from here? *Change* 28:17, 1996.

Filerman GL: The influence of policy objectives on professional education and accreditation: the case of hospital accreditation, *J Health Adm Educ 2*:409, 1984.

Finocchio LJ and others: *Reforming health care workforce regulation: policy considerations for the 21st Century,* San Francisco, 1995, Pew Health Professions Commission.

Gelmon SB: *Accreditation as a stimulus for continuous improvement in health management education: a case study of ACEHSA,* fellowship thesis, American College of Healthcare Executives, 1995.

Gelmon SB: Can educational accreditation drive interdisciplinary learning in the health professions? *Joint Commission J Qual Improvement* 22:213, 1996.

Gelmon SB: Accreditation, core curriculum and allied health education: barriers and opportunities, *J Allied Health Educ,* 26(3):119, 1997b.

Gelmon SB: Facilitating academic-community partnerships through educational accreditation: overcoming a tradition of barriers and obstacles, Rockville, Md, 1997a, Bureau of Health Professions, U.S. Public Health Service.

Kells HR: Self-study process: a guide for postsecondary and similar service-oriented institutions and programs, Phoenix, 1994, American Council on Education/Oryx Press.

Kirkwood R: The myths of a accreditation, *Educ Rec* 54:211, 1973.

Mayhew LB and others: *The quest for quality,* San Francisco, 1990, Jossey-Bass.

Millard RM: The structure of specialized accreditation in the United States, *J Educ Library Info Sci* 25:87, 1984.

National League for Nursing Accrediting Commission (NLNAC): NLN accreditation, *http://www.nln.org/nlnac,* June, 1997.

National Policy Board: Proposal for a new national non-governmental recognition authority, Washington, DC, 1994, The Board.

O'Neil EH: *Health professions education for the future: schools in service to the nation,* San Francisco, 1993, Pew Health Professions Commission.

Pew Health Professions Commission: *Critical challenges: revitalizing the health professions for the twenty-first century,* San Francisco, 1995, UCSF Center for the Health Professions.

Prager C: *Accreditation of the two year college,* San Francisco, 1993, Jossey-Bass.

Ryan SA: President's message: we still have much to do, *NH&C: Perspectives on Community,* 18:94, 1997.

Shugars DA and others: *Healthy America: practitioners for 2005,* Durham, NC, 1991, Pew Health Professions Commission.

Tanner CA: Accreditation under siege, *J Nurs Educ* 35(6):243, 1996, editorial.

Task Force on the Accreditation of Health Professions Education: Results of environmental scanning exercise, working paper, San Francisco, 1996, University of California.

U.S. Department of Health, Education, and Welfare (DHEW): *Invitational conference on the federal government's relationship to the nationally accrediting agencies,* Arlington, Va, 1977, The Department.

Young KE and others: *Understanding accreditation,* San Francisco, 1983, Jossey-Bass.

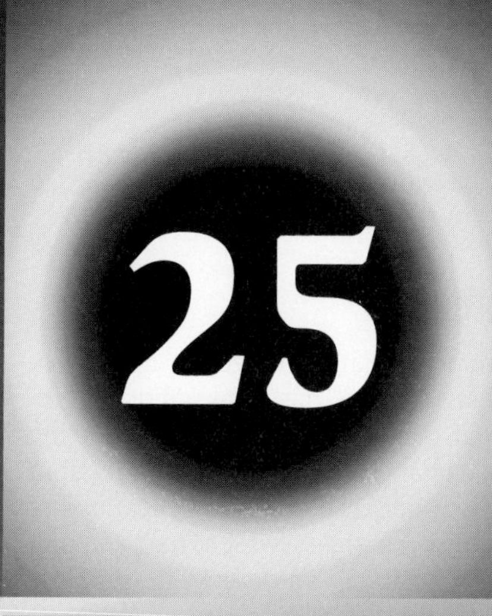

# 25 Ethical Issues

**MaryCarroll Sullivan**
**Myra J. Christopher**

*Never doubt that a small group of committed citizens can change the world; indeed it is the only thing that ever has.*

**Margaret Mead**

As one millennium comes to a close and another is about to begin, it is appropriate to consider the present situation and future prospects for nursing. Few professions have undergone the radical transformation that nursing has in such a relatively short time. It is only during the latter half of the twentieth century that nursing became a profession. How that status came about and what has occurred in the succeeding decades provides an interesting historiography of nursing and nursing ethics. This transformation, however, is likely to be only a preview of the dramatic changes nursing is likely to undergo in the first half of the twenty-first century as a result of continued health care reform efforts, a cultural shift regarding end-of-life care, and the emergence of "genomic" medicine.

This chapter provides a historic overview of ethics in nursing. Perhaps, more importantly, this chapter speculates about the changes nursing is likely to undergo in the future, and questions are raised regarding the ethical implications of these changes.

## NURSING AS A PROFESSION

In view of the sociologic definition of profession, it is difficult to understand why nursing was accorded professional status only recently. A profession is ". . . an occupation that regulates itself through systematic, required training and collegial discipline; that has a base in technical, specialized knowledge; and that has a service, rather than profit, orientation enshrined in its code of ethics" (Starr, 1982.) Arguably nursing met these criteria long before it was popularly accorded the status of profession and certainly long before it gained collegial appreciation as such from other professional groups. What is important, however, is the more popular, albeit somewhat pejorative, understanding of the term *professional.*

If polled, many people would probably characterize a profession as a discipline, which is self-regulating and operates with a certain degree of independence, at least in terms of setting its own agenda. Seen in this conceptual framework, nursing has been recognized as a profession since the middle of the twentieth century. In recent years and despite its newly attained professional status, nursing has come under tremendous assault. Although it still can be arguably described as self-regulating, it probably no longer is able to claim that it always sets its own agenda. The ability of nursing to be self-regulating and to set its agenda may be even further impaired in the near future as a result of the deprofessionalization of both medicine and nursing because of the transition from a fee-for-service health care delivery model to a managed care model. In ethical terms, such a situation would be a tremendous setback for the professional status of nursing and could be a serious threat to nursing's capacity to express moral agency.

## Moral Agency: Responsibility and Accountability

Two characteristics must be present for moral agency to occur. The first is *responsibility.* The moral agent must be able to make choices about how one is going to act. Additionally, the moral agent must be able to assume the blame or the credit for the consequences of one's action.

The second characteristic of moral agency is *accountability* (see Chapter 22). The agent must be able to rationalize, explain, or defend the choices taken that resulted in said consequences. The combination of these characteristics creates professional autonomy.

Nursing is being influenced by a number of factors today; some of these influences will have still greater effect as we move into the next century. It is important to assess the impact of these influences to determine their effect on the ethics of nursing. Most importantly, we must ask: Do they limit or constrict professional autonomy?

## Legal Changes

One of the more dramatic changes in nursing of the past several decades has come about in response to legal changes with regard to nursing practice. These changes are discussed in detail in the following chapter. The ethical implications of just one of these changes, which has a direct bearing on professional autonomy in nursing, must be considered.

A significant change in the legal status of nursing is one that is somewhat a backhanded compliment: *Nurses are now named as defendants in their own right in malpractice suits.* In previous decades most nurses were not named as parties but rather their potentially liable actions were collapsed into suits against physicians or hospitals. The assumption in these legal strategies was that nurses were either acting under the orders and therefore the licenses of physicians or that nurses fell into the category of "servants" to the hospital corporation. In either case the implicit or explicit assumption was that nurses did not bear the responsibility of their actions. That thinking, which in a sense protected nurses from litigation, had to logically extend into the presumption that nurses were thus incapable of acting as moral agents; they were unable to claim responsibility for the consequences of their actions. Additionally, there were the pragmatic concerns on the part of plaintiffs' attorneys that juries, like most of the public, liked nurses, and that a nurse did not provide enough of a deep financial pocket to make the suit practical.

In recent years that has all changed. Nurses are named as defendants. They are held responsible for their actions and must account for them. Although the practical ramifications of that change in legal regard is one that is not particularly pleasant for nurses, it nevertheless implies moral agency on their part, which seems to emphasize a broad view of nursing's professional autonomy.

## FROM FEE-FOR-SERVICE TO MANAGED CARE TO . . . ?

The latter part of the twentieth century saw a fundamental shift in the way in which health care was delivered. The traditional fee-for-service model in which medicine had been practiced and health care had been delivered saw a sea change. The discrepancy between costs and charges, at times because of the inability to distinguish between the two, gave way to allegations of a system and providers within it who had little sense of accountability or responsibility. Using the definitional understanding of ethical behavior previously cited, one must conclude that there was much that was unethical, if not illegal, in the delivery of health care. Charges were made that the system was inherently and increasingly unjust. A change was deemed necessary, and in response a shift away from the traditional delivery method occurred.

In the early 1990s it appeared that the transition from fee-for-service would be toward some sort of national health care model. For a variety of reasons citizens of this country turned their backs on such proposals and chose instead market-driven health care reform. At the heart of this shift was the financial or economic model that provides reimbursement for health care goods and services and offers incentives to contain costs. As health care in the United States moved from a fee-for-service model to a managed care model, every player in the health care system was affected and we experienced firsthand what many have referred to as the "corporatization of medicine." Nursing has felt the impact of this economic shift and experienced it in some ways that are quite paradoxical.

### Impact of Managed Care on Nursing

The impact of the managed care movement has had a dramatic effect on the way in which nurses practice their profession and an equally dramatic effect on the setting in which they practice. In each of these areas the ethical ramifications are noteworthy.

Before the era of managed care, most nurses were oblivious to the costs of the health care they delivered. Equipment and supplies were there to be used, patients were there to be treated, facilities were there to be utilized. The introduction of the financial or economic aspect to health care into the design of a care plan or the discussion of a significant health care decision was seen as crass or just wrong.

A decade into market-driven reform, the average nurse practices with a constant awareness of the effects of cost-containment efforts linked to these reform initiatives. For many in nursing the negative repercussions of losing sight of the bottom line have been part of their experience. In its winter 1996 to 1997 'Communique,' the American Nurses Association Center for Ethics and Human Rights reported the results of a national survey exploring nurses' perception about the impact of cost containment on patient welfare and nursing. Of those responding, 69% reported that they confront ethical issues daily to weekly and that 49% of those issues were related to "cost-containment issues that jeopardize patient welfare."

As a result of cost containment, nurses have seen their numbers decrease to what many feel are dangerously low levels as hospital staffs downsize by means of attrition or outright firing to reduce the largest entry on any business' ledger: staff salaries. Staff nurses whose patient load is dangerously large are left in a position of having to constantly triage, often unable to do more than the absolute necessities. In addition, new categories of paraprofessionals have been introduced, and often nurses are expected to train and oversee their work. The combination has resulted in a dramatic decrease in morale among nurses.

There seems to be an underlying frustration at the heart of this phenomenon, which is less articulated and less articulative. This frustration has its roots in the deprofessionalization of nursing and the moral burnout associated with health care reform. Interestingly, at the same time that staff nurse positions are being cut, nurses are being placed in roles with tremendous decision-making responsibility and moral authority.

Many CEOs in managed care plans have nursing backgrounds, and as a result, many health plans now allow enrolled members to make appointments with clinical nurse specialists and forego visiting a physician at all. In integrated systems nurses may independently staff and run outreach clinics in rural communities that then feed patients into tertiary care centers. One of the most interesting examples of nursing's increased responsibility and accountability may be the emergence of the nurse care manager in both integrated systems and managed care plans. These nurses assume responsibility for planning and coordinating care for high-risk patients, ushering them in and out of the system as they deem necessary and appropriate. Responsibility and accountability are heightened for nurses in these roles from both a legal and ethical perspective.

## Impact of Managed Care on Ethical Decision Making

It is often nurses who, because of their two-dimensional role of patient caregiver and patient advocate, have the perspective needed to step back from the situation and ask the question that shifts decision making from a strictly clinical or scientific basis to an ethical one: "Just because we can do *X*, should we do it?" This shift from the physically possible (can) to the morally ideal (should) is the work of ethics, and it is a task for which nurses are particularly well suited because of their relationships with patients and families. The amount of concentrated time that nurses spend with patients and their families allows them a better opportunity to elicit the values and goals that have informed the lives of the people in their care than many physicians have. This aspect of the nurse/patient relationship is particularly true of nurses who work in an acute care setting, but it is increasingly true of nurses in outpatient environments also, many of whom become the primary care provider for people whose main access to health care is in home health or clinic settings.

There are two fundamental questions in ethics: *What is my duty?* and *To whom is that duty owed?* When those questions are posed in the context of a critical look at nursing in the era of managed care, they must be answered on multiple levels and from more than one perspective.

### Individual

The first response to these questions is from the individual nurse's self-perception. The answers for the staff nurse or the nurse in independent practice should be: "My duty is to provide the best care (or competent care) that I am able to give, and my duty is first to the patients I serve and then to the organization within which I offer that service." For the nurse executive or the nurse manager, the answers should be: "My duty is to see that my patients/members receive competent care, and my duty is first to the patients/members and then to the plan within which I offer my service."

### Profession

From a professional perspective, however, the response may be somewhat different. This response should recognize the responsibility of colleagues for each other. There ought to be a cohesiveness that promotes a sense of professionalism rather than undermines it. There needs to be a sense of duty to protect the agenda and practice parameters of the profession characteristic of other, older professions, such as medicine and law. This self-protection need not reflect a defensive posture, but it may well serve to defend the professional gains made by nursing in the past decades as the profession comes under attack by outside influences. The reality is that nursing's agenda is set by external powers not generated by nurses in response to nurses.

### Society

At an even broader societal level, the voice of nursing has been conspicuously absent from debates and discussions about development of large integrated systems, national health policy, and from the bioethics movement. Nursing is challenged to find its place at the table without leaving behind its patient care focus.

In the future these problems and their related ethical issues will change, but they will not go away. Many believe that managed care is a necessary step in evolving from a fee-for-service model to a national delivery system. Some argue that we will evolve to five or six health care delivery corporations, probably all for profit. Others believe that the American public will quickly become disenchanted with the "corporatization" of medicine, but most are not prepared to speculate about what an alternative model might be.

At the same time the health care delivery system is being restructured and nursing is facing numerous professional challenges, many are questioning what care is being provided (or not provided), particularly for seriously ill and dying patients.

## CARE OF SERIOUSLY ILL AND DYING PATIENTS

There is probably not a more comprehensive topic to address in health care at this time than the care of the seriously ill and dying. The ethical implications are vast because the way in which we approach this care defines us as a society and as individual practitioners. The serious and appropriate approach requires a multidisciplinary perspective, broad in its scope and far-reaching in its consequences.

One study, the Study to Understand Prognoses and Preferences for Outcomes and Risks of Treatment (SUPPORT), revealed to the health care community that we have failed miserably in our attempt to successfully balance the remarkable benefits and advances in technologic progress with the need to have a thoughtful and value-based rationale for employing those technologies in the face of impending death (SUPPORT, 1995). According to the results of the study, the vast majority of Americans die after having been in pain, alone, patients in the intensive care unit, in comas, or on ventilators within 72 hours of their death. Approximately one third of the families of the almost 10,000 patients included in the survey were financially destroyed by their terminal hospital stay. "Do-not-resuscitate" orders were not written in most of these cases, until 2 or 3 days before death. Even when advance directives existed for patients, those directives were not adhered to in the majority of cases. Neither were hospice referrals made in a timely fashion.

This study was done in two phases with patient populations of approximately 5000 in each phase. When the first phase produced the results reported above, the investigators decided to designate nurses at each of the study sites to guarantee and facilitate discussions during which patient preferences were elicited, documented, and communicated to the entire care team. The implicit understanding in this intervention of placing the nurse in the roles of facilitator, mediator, and patient advocate spoke volumes about the perception of nurses by the study's designers and principal investigators. This perception that nurses could influence decisions about care was never challenged.

Despite the existence of these nurses in the study's second phase, the results of the second phase were unchanged from those of the first, and a clarion call was sounded for all health care professionals. As is true with many research studies, critical suggestions or changes may be offered regarding the methodologies or the framework of this study. What remains unchanged, however, is the instinctive reaction to the results of the study. Most providers in health care found the outcomes announced in SUPPORT to be congruent with their own anecdotal experiences and empiric observations. With the general findings of SUPPORT to serve as a foundation, there are urgent issues that need to be included on the agenda for nursing ethics in the new millennium.

With reference to the fundamental questions, *What is my duty*? and *To whom is that duty owed*? the results of SUPPORT demand that nurses have a duty to improve the care of the seriously ill and dying.

Because the scope of that response could be overwhelming, there are several possible ways to approach the task. One helpful and manageable way is to follow a clinical theme schemata. This thematic "map" is the basis for a multiyear, multifaceted project being initiated by the Midwest Bioethics Center in Kansas City. The goal of this project is to define specific strategies to improve the care of the seriously ill and dying in their community. Called *PATHWAYS*, this project offers an agenda to meet this somewhat daunting, but nevertheless compelling, challenge for health care providers in the twenty-first century. There are five main topics that comprise the theme-based response to this challenge: *palliative care, advance directives, "do-not-resuscitate" orders, treatment abatement guidelines,* and *psychospiritual care.* Each carries explicit ramifications for nurses.

## Palliative Care

*Palliative care* is a term heard with increasing frequency in clinical settings. Unfortunately, each reference to it seems to presume a common understanding that our experience tells us does not exist. For example, many people equate the term "palliative care" with "palliation," which refers to the end product of comfort measures. There is an unfortunate tendency to narrowly construe the concept of palliative care to pain relief measures. Although pain control or management is undoubtedly a significant component in a well-constructed palliative care plan, the scope of palliative care far exceeds that narrow construction.

This distinction is not just a matter of semantics. The way in which one defines and understands palliative care will profoundly affect the way in which one cares for the seriously ill and dying. The impact of one's definition of palliative care will be felt throughout the spectrum of patient care, not just with terminally ill patients. For this reason it is essential to perceive palliative care in the most sweeping and comprehensive way possible.

In addition to pain management techniques and procedures, palliative care encompasses a broad range of concerns. Certainly there are many clinical needs to be addressed. In addition to pain control, managing other symptoms that have an adverse effect on the quality of patient's lives must be a priority. Beyond pain and physical symptoms there are myriad other sources of patients' suffering, and these areas comprise the rest of the palliative care agenda. Social, emotional, and psychologic needs, as well as legal and financial matters, must be recognized and resources provided. Spiritual support must be made available.

Palliative care is a holistic approach that is as much an attitude or mindset as it is a paradigm for action. The role of the nurse is crucial. When the time comes that patients recognize that they are terminally ill, sometimes that status has to be enunciated by the care providers, and at other times patients know before any announcement is made. There is a duty on the part of caregivers to communicate by word and deed that the moment has not come to give up, cease treatment, or stop being aggressive. Rather, the time has come to shift modalities and redirect aggressive energy and effort to palliation rather than cure. This attitude will be communicated successfully to patients only when the caregivers they trust embody the attitude themselves.

Nurses must learn about palliative care in all of its complexity so that they can spontaneously make or request physician referral for palliative care services and so that they can convincingly communicate the positive, energetic, and aggressive treatment modality that palliative care is to their patients. Furthermore, nurse educators must revise their curriculum and develop plans for educating and supporting practicing nurses to better understand palliative care and to explore the ethical issues linked to the transition from aggressive acute care to aggressive palliative care.

## Advance Directives

Advance directives are documents in which people stipulate the parameters of their health care in anticipation of the time when they are not able to articulate their wishes because of incapacity.

These documents take various forms and are known by various names, depending on the jurisdiction within which they are completed. Some examples of advance directives are *living wills, health care proxies,* and *durable power of attorney for health care.*

## Living Will

The living will is a testamentary document. The document serves as the voice of its author when that person is unable to speak. The most obvious drawback to this type of advance directive is the static nature of the document. Once written, it is meant to provide a kind of definitive guide for caregivers and family members as to the wishes of the incapacitated patient. The problem is that the document is inflexible and open to (mis)interpretation. The intent behind its creation was to have the patient prospectively address and respond to all possible questions that may surface at the time when these answers are needed. Clearly, those are unrealistic expectations to have of any piece of paper, and experience with the living will has served to underscore its deficiencies.

## Health Care Proxies and Durable Power of Attorney

Health care proxies and durable power of attorney (DOA) for health care are categorically different from the living will. In these two cases the person completing the directive designates someone else as a surrogate who will speak for him or her when he or she is incapacitated. The health care proxy or DOA document does not serve as the voice of the patient but provides a substitute decision maker. The ethical obligation of both designator and surrogate is to collaborate in substantive anticipatory discussion so that the surrogate can voice opinions and decisions that are consistent with the values and goals of the person for whom he or she is speaking.

The most important aspect to these documents is the opportunity their very existence provides for having discussions about the end-of-life issues that will surround that time in all of our lives. We need to focus less strictly on the particular piece of paper and consider more carefully the intention behind the document. To fully appreciate what that intention might be, it is absolutely essential that the designator, family members, and the surrogate have frequent and in-depth dialogues about the quality of life that is acceptable, the interventions that are warranted, and the values and goals that would inform decisions that cannot be anticipated in advance.

## The Nursing Role

The nursing role with regard to advanced directives is multifaceted. In the development of the nurse-patient relationship, the nurse is frequently the health care provider with whom the patient has the most frequent and the most unintimidating encounters. A logical inquiry to include in the history-taking interview is to ask if the patient has an advanced directive. Whether the answer is yes or no, the opportunity for conversation about advance care planning is presented. These conversations may be documented so that there is a record of both the conversation and its content, and so the documentation can provide valuable evidence as to the evolution of a patient's thoughts and feelings about end-of-life issues.

Implementing these directives is also within the realm of nursing responsibility, although this is frequently more easily said than done. Most of those resisting the directive are genuinely concerned that the wishes stated therein are outdated or not based on informed consent to or refusal of treatment simply because significant time has elapsed between the formulation of the directive and the events that make it relevant. Sometimes that resistance is based on a feeling that clinical judgment is being subjugated to a static piece of paper. In either case the skills of advocacy and sometimes conflict mediation are necessary elements of the nursing skill set to assist families and health care professionals to make reasoned and ethical care decisions.

## Assisted Suicide

Some have argued that a logical extension to allowing people to make advance directives regarding end-of-life care is allowing people to request assistance in dying. Although the U.S. Supreme Court decided that there is no constitutional right to physician-assisted suicide *(Washington v. Glucksberg, Vacco v. Quill)*, their decision did leave the door open for states to consider whether terminally ill patients have a right to seek and receive assistance in dying.

This is not exclusively a physician issue. Asch (1996) reported that a survey of 850 nurses who practiced in intensive care units revealed that 141 of them said that a patient or a family member had asked them to participate in euthanasia or assisted suicide. One in five or 129 of the nurses said they had carried out these practices at least once, and 35 said they had hastened a patient's death by pretending to carry out treatment that had been ordered. Much criticism was raised about Asch's research. Nevertheless, nursing as a profession must be prepared to take a significant role in the public dialogue and debate about assisted suicide.

## Do-Not-Resuscitate Orders

As was revealed in SUPPORT, do-not-resuscitate (DNR) orders continue to be problematic in clinical situations. The problems are related to the writing of the orders, especially the point in the hospitalization at which they are written and using an advance directive rejecting resuscitation. Many clinicians try to justify the delay in discussing DNR orders or the failure to implement an advance directive on the basis of the irreversible nature of the decision not to resuscitate in the face of cardiopulmonary failure. That argument for justification just does not work. There is no acceptable excuse for delaying discussion about resuscitation orders. As indicated previously, end-of-life issues ought to be incorporated into the conversational agenda of patient/clinician encounters from the earliest meeting.

Because of the rapport that exists between most nurses and their patients, as well as with patients' families, the nurse may be the ideal person to raise the issue of DNR orders. In many institutional policies and attitudes, that discussion is one designated specifically to the physician. Traditionally, the nurse has felt that the topic is one that should be first broached by the physician, with follow-up discussion frequently left for the nurse to clarify issues or respond to questions asked by patients or their families. Certainly no one would argue that nursing responsibility extends to making certain that the issue gets raised either with the patient or with the attending physician. The difficult part, and one that is of crucial importance, is that the issue is introduced and resolved in a timely fashion. Because nurses tend to spend more time with patients, they may be able to raise the subject at regular intervals, over time, in a way that does not create apprehension and yet ensures comprehensive discussion and resolution.

Many believe that the whole DNR discussion is "upside down," that it was wrong to make cardiopulmonary resuscitation a standing order for all those who die in our hospitals and nursing homes, and that we should reverse the current policy and be required to write resuscitation orders. Outcomes-driven health care decision making will surely fuel this debate as we critically examine the consequences of our current policies. Nurses must play a critical role in deciding about this important health matter and in helping institutions consider existing policies.

## Treatment Abatement Guidelines

The context of the nurse/patient relationship has always been one of accessibility and intimacy. It will become more so as the managed care system continues to ration the time that patients have with their physicians. Patients have always turned to their nurses for information to supplement what they have heard or understood from their physicians about diagnosis, prognosis, and therapeutic options. It is logical to extrapolate from these traditional roles in nursing as communicator and interpreter that nurses will play an extensive role in discussions about medical futility and treatment abatement.

Once again, the nursing role has several components. In addition to responding to patient inquiries about statements made by physicians or questions about the whys and wherefores of the clinical course being pursued, nurses have an obligation to advocate for their patients. Ethical decision making always begins with accurate information. Nursing has a critical role to play in conducting research and reporting results of outcomes studies to help patients and providers better understand when treatment may be truly futile.

### Patient Advocacy

Patient advocacy sometimes takes the form of adopting a kind of "devil's advocate" role in questioning the rationale behind therapies being offered or undertaken. This obligation becomes particularly urgent when those therapies yield little or no benefit or when the benefit gained is disproportionate to the burdensomeness of the therapy. Burdens to be considered include pain and suffering, as well as financial, psychologic, or emotional hardship. They must be gauged against the gains offered by the proposed therapies. The burden of treatment and its intended and realistic outcome must be consistent with the values and goals of the patient. Once again, the values history is an essential part of the nursing assessment. An articulated values system becomes the standard against which qualitative decisions regarding life-sustaining treatment will be gauged.

### Medical Futility

The patient's values are used increasingly in situations in which the question of medical futility arises. Medical futility is difficult to recognize and even more difficult to accede to when to do so may mean acknowledging that there is nothing more that clinical intervention can offer. In addition to the values history obtained in previous encounters or at admission, the nurse is the sole member of the care team who is likely to have had extended conversations with patients. Although this time is being shortened as economic constraints affect staffing ratios, nurses have more exposure to patients and families than any of the other clinical disciplines. It becomes imperative that nurses learn to incorporate the kind of inquiries that will flesh out of the nuances of the values history into their conversations with patients and families. When the time comes that the family or care team needs to help the patient with capacity think through decisions about treatment abatement or, even more difficult, to make substituted judgments for patients without capacity, evidence as to their wishes will be crucially important to substantiate decision making that is truly reflective of or in the patients' best interests.

## Psychospiritual Care

This topic is one that is frequently neglected in the construction of a nursing care plan. Formerly, the admission form included a question about a patient's religious status. That question gradually disappeared from most admission sheets. Despite the rise of the "holistic health" movement in the late 1970s to address all significant aspects of patients' needs, attention to the religious life of patients was eliminated from the realm of clinical concern. Whether this was due to an antireligious bias or a response to somewhat arbitrary privacy boundaries is difficult to tell. Deleting religion from the roster of clinical information makes it difficult to solicit or listen to the spiritual needs of the patient. Unless a serious psychopathology presented or was claimed by the patient, the psychologic or emotional needs of patients have been equally ignored. Many argue that the basis for these deficiencies is the discomfort most clinicians feel about these subjects. Regardless of the reasons for the deficiencies, these subjects deal with essential characteristics that make us human.

The nursing duty in each of these areas is at once simple and very difficult. Nurses, because of their relationship with patients, are generally the staff members to whom patients feel most comfortable confiding fear, anger, frustration, and other emotions. We must extend that comfort zone to allow patients to voice their other, even more private, needs or concerns. At times, that will require outright interrogation about whether patients would like to take advantage of pastoral care or other spiritual resources. The same explicit offer may be necessary or appropriate for psychologic or emotional counseling.

For some patients overt reference to these services may be offensive. In these situations, as with many others, extra sensitivity is required. That consideration adds only to the duty to carefully address concerns in the psychospiritual realm; it does not diminish that duty.

This discussion of palliative care is punctuated with words like *duty* and *obligation*; this is not by accident. Palliative care, with its multiple dimensions, must be seen as a moral imperative. As we look into the future, with a population living longer in an environment of ever-advancing biotechnology, we see a model of nursing practice that accommodates the broadening scope of nursing practice requirements. The fact that these will be requirements and not suggestions or recommendations is what argues for acceptance in viewing the palliative care model as an imperative or obligatory method of care. More importantly, it is the model that acknowledges the full humanity of all patients, in each of its dimensions, and attempts to respond to the full range of their needs. For this reason, nurses have an ethical duty to learn and initiate the palliative care model to be able to offer it to their patients.

While we are refocusing and refining our current model of health care, a third era of medicine is racing toward us, one that is more ethically complex than anything we have yet faced, the coming of what some have called "genomic medicine." A book on the future of nursing would be incomplete without some discussion about the Human Genome Mapping Project and its implications for society and nursing (see Chapter 10).

## ETHICAL IMPLICATIONS OF GENETIC ADVANCEMENTS

The Human Genome Mapping Project (HGMP) is an international research project begun in 1990 with the intention of mapping the entire human genome. The U.S. government initially committed $3 billion to this project, the largest of its kind and one that will unquestionably and permanently alter, if not replace entirely, our current medical model.

We have already had glimpses into the future that will be associated with the emerging knowledge and the technology associated with it. In early 1997 the world was shocked by the news that a British scientist had reported cloning an adult ewe named Dolly. Virtually every week reports of lesser import are made about new genetic markers being identified or new gene therapies being tested. Because of the dramatic advances made in computer science in the 1990s, progress has come at a much more rapid pace than had first been imagined. Not uncommonly, it appears that science races ahead and ethics runs behind.

Fortunately, James Watson, one of the scientists awarded the Nobel prize for the discovery of the double helix and the original director of HGMP, convinced Congress to earmark 1% of the HGMP budget for ethical research and study, and the "working group on the ethical and legal and social issues related to mapping and sequencing the human genome" was formed. This group has identified nine topics they deem to be of "particular importance":

1. Fairness in the use of genetic information with regard to insurance
2. The impact of knowledge of genetic variation on the individual
3. Privacy and confidentiality of genetic information
4. The impact of the HGMP on genetic counseling with regard to prenatal screening, presymptomatic testing, carrier status testing, testing for polygenic disorders, and population screening versus testing
5. Reproductive decisions influenced by genetic information
6. Issues raised by the introduction of genetics into mainstream medical practice
7. Uses and misuses of genetics in the past, relevant to the current situation

8. Questions raised by the commercialization of genetic products
9. Conceptual and philosophic implications of the initiative

Nurses are already dealing with some of these issues, but the moral dilemmas associated with this new medical model are probably limited only by our imagination.

Nowhere else at this point in the biotechnologic evolution is there such a dramatic example of the need to constantly refer back to the foundational questions of ethics: "Just because I *can* do something, *ought* I to do it?" "What is my duty in this situation?" and "To whom is that duty owed?"

Because of the still experimental nature of much of the applied science of genetics, the potentially conflicting and competing claims that derive from the tension between the need to diagnose or treat the genetic matter of a specific patient and the significance of *any* outcome for the good of increasing human knowledge, whether that outcome benefits the specific patient at hand, will present some of the moral ambiguity for nurses involved in counseling patients or for those just engaging in conversations with patients about newly available testing or therapy. Although in the past those nurses were a small number of professionals working directly in genetics or genetics counseling settings, increasingly more nurses will need to ask themselves about their roles in advising, critically questioning, and advocating for their patients as genetics becomes incorporated into many specialty practice areas.

## CONCLUSION

In examining even cursorily the ethical implications of several areas for nurses, many questions are raised for which there are no clear answers. What has become clear, however, is that nurses in the twenty-first century must becom[e com]fortable with and, more importantly, good at asking the tough, critical questions. They must adopt the philosophic position that has been paraphrased by many different cultures in the past and that seems more urgent and necessary now than ever: the value and validity of a searched-for truth is found in the rigor and the quality of the search, by the questions asked along the way, and by the testing of the routes taken.

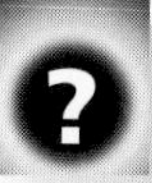

## *Discussion Exercises*

1. What is the ethical issue in nursing that concerns you the most? Describe the ethical dilemma and explain divergent positions.
2. In addition to the programs designed to address ethical care of patients described in the chapter, do you know of similar programs? If not, describe a program you would like to see designed.
3. What was your preparation to care for seriously ill and dying patients? What would you have liked to have learned?

## References

American Nurses Association Center for Ethics and Human Rights: *Communique*, Winter, 1996-1997.

Asch DA: Role of critical care nurses in euthanasia and assisted suicide, *New England J Med* 334(21):1374, 1996.

Starr P: *The social origins of professional sovereignty: the social transformation of American medicine,* New York, 1982, Basic Books.

The SUPPORT Principal Investigators: A controlled trial to improve care for seriously ill hospitalized patients: the study to understand prognoses and preferences for outcomes and treatments (SUPPORT), *JAMA* 274(2):191, 1995.

*Vacco v. Quill* 117 SCR 2293.

*Washington v. Glucksberg* 117 SCR 2258, 117 SCR 2302.

# 26 Nursing and the Law

**Diane K. Kjervik**

*I like the dreams of the future better than the history of the past.*

**Thomas Jefferson**

Because of its basis in precedent, the legal system reacts to more than initiates changes and thus can be influenced more readily than other professional systems. Nursing therefore is in a position to create its future legally. Either preferable or probable scenarios will occur depending on the amount of attention nursing gives to its legal future. The law's involvement with nursing sweeps broadly from definitions of what nursing is to what nurses do (standards of practice), outcomes to be achieved, and contexts of care. This chapter reviews the areas of law most likely to be affected by nursing action or inaction: torts, agency, contracts, labor law, and civil rights. Also because the best nursing law rests firmly upon ethical principles, ethical components of the evolution of nursing law are addressed.

## THE LAW

### Torts

Tort law examines the breach of a legal duty that results in injury to someone (Gifis, 1995). Although both intentional and unintentional acts are included in torts, the unintentional acts (professional negligence or malpractice) are of greatest concern in nursing. As nursing changes its standards of practice (which the law refers to as *standards of care*), the law will use these standards as well. The challenge nurses face is making sure that their standard is the one adopted by courts of law . . . not physician-defined nursing standards. In some states physicians are allowed to testify on the standard of care for nursing, but the preferable course is for nurses to do so (Aiken, 1994). Nurses must be willing to testify as expert witnesses for both defense and plaintiff so that they are not seen as biased in the eyes of the court and the jury. Because of the discomfort of facing a cross-examination, nurses may not wish to serve as expert witnesses but should consider assuming these roles on occasion.

The law requires that proximate cause be shown in a malpractice case, for example, that the breach of the standard led to patient injury. As nursing intervention research becomes more sophisticated, we will know more about what action causes what outcome. Ironically, not only will our clients know more about what they can expect of us, thereby improving the trust in nurse-patient relationships, but also data on expected outcomes will enable nurses to better defend themselves if they are sued for malpractice.

Just as individual nurses can be held liable for malpractice, so too can the corporations in which they work be held liable for the safety and well-being of their clients (Carroll, 1996). The standards of corporate negligence are currently inconsistent, but as they evolve, nurses in risk management positions and nursing administrators particularly will feel the effects. The opportunity before them, however, is to influence the direction of the evolution.

## Agency Law

When a nurse is sued, the nurse's employer is often also liable under agency law. Using the principle of respondent superior, the employer is liable for acts of the employee. Whether the nurse is acting within the scope of employment is a key legal consideration, so it behooves nurses to know what is expected by the employer as articulated in hospital policies, JCAHO requirements, and in-service education. Ideally, the nurse participates on practice committees to develop job expectations.

Credentialling and licensure requirements influence what employers expect of nurses, and nursing must continue its active involvement with these functions. Professional nursing organizations for staff nurses and advanced practice nurses (APNs) currently publish standards of practice, offer certification examinations, and provide continuing education to enhance workforce competency. As cross-training for various functional subspecialty continues, nursing certification will respond accordingly. For instance, the American Nurses Credentialling Center now offers a functional certification for case managers as an "adjunctive certification module" (American Nurses Association, 1997). In addition, telenursing will more frequently enable nurses to interact with clients in distant sites. Telenursing raises numerous licensure law issues that are currently being debated, such as multistate licensure (Gobis, 1996). Preferably, nurses would hold a multistate license that would provide mobility and flexibility for nurses (see Chapter 22). More standards of practice are national rather than local; thus the national or multistate license is a wise policy choice.

## Contracts

Employment contracts are the most common contracts in which nurses are involved. Most are "at will," giving the nurse and the employer the right to end the contract when either wishes to do so without penalty. Exceptions are made for terminations based on discriminatory reasons. In the future nurses are likely to sell their services to hospital or managed care organizations (MCOs) as a group to provide specific services (e.g., staff intensive care units). These contracts will contain definite terms, such as dates of initiation and termination, credentialling requirements, malpractice coverage, and hourly or capitated rate for services. Faculty in schools of nursing already practice under such arrangements, and as research, teaching, and practice roles are integrated, contracts for these combined roles will become more common.

## Labor Law

The effectiveness of unions in the future is hard to predict, but over the past 15 years, their strength has waned. Nurses in a number of states are represented by their ANA state affiliate or another union and work contractually under a collective bargaining contract, which is mediated by the National Labor Relations Board (NLRB). In a recent decision the NLRB nurses in Montana appealed a decision by the hospital not to bargain with their union because according to the hospital, the nurses were all supervisors. The NLRB rejected the hospital's decision (American Nurses Association, 1997). In the future proactive nursing groups will anticipate the reduction of union representation and will begin to establish their own corporations that sell services to hospitals, MCOs, and other health care entities (see Chapter 20).

The need for nurses to speak with a strong, if not unified, voice will be more important than ever in the new century. For years nurses have been associated with the medical establishment and have either benefited or struggled with the result of that union. There can be no doubt, however, that the changes in the medical profession as a result of cost-containment efforts will affect nursing.

Although many primary care APNs will find jobs where physicians used to be, baccalaureate prepared nurses will move into the community for practice sites. Unions may help some of these nurses, but many will be left to the support they can get from one another and in coalition with politically sophisticated organizations that legally will challenge managed care at every step. An example of this is the "gag rules" that prohibited managed care workers from recommending other providers to the MCOs' clients. Such gag rules have been challenged successfully on legal and ethical grounds and will continue to be in the future (Martin and Bjerknes, 1996).

Whether nurses continue union representation or choose to disaffiliate with the union, the law will be involved with their choice of "voice." The collective bargaining process is a creature of statute, as is corporate law. Petitioning the government for statutory change is a mechanism to change the law. Many professional nursing organizations lobby for preferable changes and will continue to do so more often in coalition with other education and service organizations.

### Civil Rights

Protection of vulnerable persons such as those with handicaps is granted under the law. Nurses will probably continue to align themselves with the consumers of their services and act as advocates on their behalf. This will benefit nursing and consumers, both of whom are challenged by the managed care environment. Gag rules that prevent health care providers from disclosing information about alternatives and the systematic removal of the more expensive treatments by legislation, courts and executive branch rulings are examples (Bursztajn and others: 1997). Speaking freely within the nurse-patient relationship is critical to both establishing trust and effective problem solving.

Nursing is committed to diversity of its workforce and respect for its patients and their families. Policies that promote diversity, such as affirmative action, are being challenged legally, and many nurses have the opportunity to speak on behalf of diversity in this forum. The preferable course is for nurses to examine their legal and policy options that promote or impede diversity and take corresponding action. Community health nurses are particularly concerned and involved with public policy development, such as clean water and air policy that improves the health of communities. Policy that is evenhanded in its intent and application so that poor, disabled, or otherwise vulnerable people receive full benefit of the environmental policy should be promulgated.

## LAW AND ETHICS

Whatever course nursing law takes, its ideal development will be guided by ethical frameworks and opinions. Just as the law reacts to societal problems and maintains stability by honoring precedent, ethics is proactive, anticipating and contemplating societal problems. With regard to genetic cloning, for instance, ethicists responded immediately to the news about the newly cloned sheep in Scotland with predictions about ethical dilemmas that might arise. The law, on the other hand, sits back waiting to pronounce judgment on the acceptability of the practice until it is approached by concerned consumers or health care providers. As the legislative branch makes law and responds more quickly than the other branches of government to the need for change, members of state legislatures and Congress are approached to act and do so sometimes quickly and other times very slowly, if at all. Petitioning Congress or state legislatures is also less financially burdensome than seeking a judicial remedy. The executive branch that "executes law" does not create new law but carries out law passed by the legislative branch. When faced with policy choices within its discretion, however, the executive branch will establish ethics panels to guide its deliberation; for example, the National Institutes of Health has set up ethics panels to guide decisions about informed consent and the use of fetal tissue for research.

## INFLUENCING POLICY

Nursing is poised to influence societal policy because of its increasing strength and visibility and consumer confidence in its advocacy, commitment to caring, and technical skills. Partnerships between nursing service, education, and research sectors will be enhanced by adding ethical and legal insights and practice to its repertoire. Nursing law, ethics, and policy scholarship will assist nursing to choose partnerships and practices that are consistent with its caring mission. Care of patients who have abortions, patients with human immunodeficiency virus (HIV), and those seeking assisted suicide are several noteworthy examples.

Nursing law scholars have addressed pressing questions such as whether nursing's relationship to consumers is that of advocate, fiduciary, or both (Sanchez-Sweatman, 1997), involuntary detention of patients with tuberculosis (TB) (Abbott, 1997), privacy of health information in the computer age (Koennecke, 1997), advance directives (Fade, 1995), and assisted suicide (Kjervik, 1997). These analyses can guide the choices that nursing makes about what to lobby for and what research, education, or service projects to fund.

To a great extent the issues identified by nursing law scholars revolve around the tension between self-determination and safety to the public. Although infection by multidrug-resistant TB or HIV, assisted suicide, or removal of life-extending treatment are experienced individually, friends, relatives, and others are affected (or infected) by these experiences. The law has been and will continue to be the mediator of policy choices that affect life and death.

As the world's population and demands on resources increase, the law guided by ethical considerations will carve resolution between competing demands. Whether nurses will be advocates, fiduciaries or entrepreneurs or play other roles in this resolution will be greatly affected by the law. Privacy of the individual will become more of a treasure as it erodes, and nurses will need to decide what role they will play in its protection.

For nurses to understand their role in lawmaking so that they can employ legal tools to achieve their goals, nursing schools must have legally and ethically sophisticated curricula. Weiler (1997) expresses concern that current accreditation criteria do not require legal aspects of practice to be included in nursing curricula, yet students need information about legal standards of care, scope of practice, documentation, and numerous other aspects. Weiler points out: "Nursing must make a commitment to teaching legal aspects of nursing practice before that integration[of law into curriculum] can occur consistently on a national level." The opportunity facing nursing is whether to choose the road of legal sophistication and activism or the path of reactivity. Nursing has learned enough about power to use it. The power of law in achieving nursing goals is obvious and necessary to success.

## NURSING LAW AND THE FUTURE

In the twenty-first century, nursing law will evolve to a point of intellectual, as well as practical, significance. Nursing leaders worth their salt will incorporate ethics, law, and policy analyses into their discourse. Centers addressing nursing ethics, law, and policy, such as the one at the University of Texas at Galveston, will flourish if nursing leaders seize the opportunity to grow with the law rather than in spite of it. Although the law is reactive, it does act, and, when it does, nursing's agenda should be at the table guiding and informing legal decisions.

Nursing law has become more sophisticated since the foundation in 1982 of its first national organization, the American Association of Nurse Attorneys. Since that time a national organization for legal nurse consultants has appeared, and the *Journal of Nursing Law* began publication in 1993. Although some nurses who become attorneys leave their nursing identities behind, most nurse attorneys are boundary spanners who navigate the borders between nursing, medicine, law, ethics, and policy. Most are practicing attorneys who represent either injured patients as plaintiffs or hospital and health care professionals as defendants in malpractice cases. Some represent the health care industry as corporate counsel or work in executive branch agencies such as licensure boards or workers compensation boards. A small percentage are employed full time in academia, but many teach individual courses or classes on nursing law. Scholarship that incorporates both ethics and law is just beginning to emerge (Aiken, 1994; Hall, 1996), and the future agenda will include more boundary-spanning scholarship.

## CONCLUSION

Nurse attorneys serve, teach, and educate others and so are natural allies in the missions of schools of nursing. Legal expertise in contracts, credentialling, and risk management strategies will be valuable and necessary. Similarly, nurse attorneys will assist health care service agencies and policy makers. Nursing law has come of age and invites nursing to draw on its legal talents to reach nursing goals.

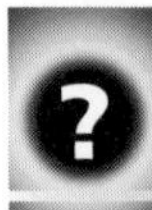

## *Discussion Exercises*

1. What laws regarding health care would you change?
2. Nursing has become more active in health policy endeavors in recent years. Select a health care issue of interest to you (e.g., legislation regarding managed care, restrictions on nurse practitioners' practice) and design a plan to influence public policy. Delineate each step and identify potential collaborators, as well as potential opponents.
3. Select a potentially controversial issue in health care and explain how it might be resolved legally.

## References


Abbott KM: Involuntary detention of TB patients: an age-old problem in a modern context, *J Nurs Law* 4(1):7, 1997.

Aiken TD: *Legal, ethical, and political issues in nursing,* Philadelphia, 1994, FA Davis.

American Nurses Association: Employers can't label staff nurses "supervisors" to avoid negotiation, *Am Nurs,* 1997.

Bursztajn HJ and others: Medical negligence and informed consent in the managed care era, *Health Lawyer* 9(5):14, 1997.

Carroll MM: Nursing malpractice and corporate negligence: how is the standard of care determined? *J Nurs Law* 3(3):53, 1996.

Fade AE: Advance directives: an overview of changing right-to-die laws, *J Nurs Law* 2(3):27, 1995.

Gifis SH: *Law dictionary,* ed 4, Woodbury, NY, 1995, Barron's Educational Series.

Gobis LJ: Telenursing: nursing by telephone across state lines, *J Nurs Law* 3(3):7, 1996.

Hall JK: *Nursing ethics and law,* Philadelphia, 1996, WB Saunders.

Kjervik DK: Assisted suicide: the challenge to the nursing profession, *J Law Med Ethics* 24(3):237, 1997.

Koennecke EW: The nurse's legal responsibility for protecting the privacy of health information in the computer age: senate bill 1360, *J Nurs Law* 4(1):53, 1997.

Martin JA, Bjerknes LK: The legal and ethical implications of gag clauses in physician contracts, *Am J Law Med* 22(4):433, 1996.

Sanchez-Sweatman LR: The nurse and patient: is it a fiduciary-advocate relationship? *J Nurs Law* 4(1):35, 1997.

Weiler K: Legal implications for professional practice. In McCloskey JC, Grace HK, editors: *Current issues in nursing,* ed 5, St. Louis, 1997, Mosby.

# V

# Nursing's Scientific Future

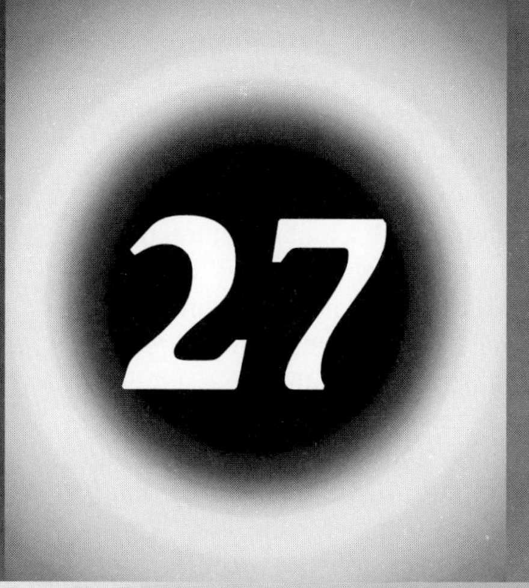

# 27 The Future of Nursing Research

**Patricia A. Grady**

*Limited expectations yield only limited results.*

**Susan Laurson Willig**

Nursing research is emerging as a major force in generating a body of scientific knowledge that adds a vital and necessary perspective to the conduct of the nation's health research effort. While the search for cures continues, research on prevention and improved care is critical. Nursing research is well positioned to address this need because its long traditions in patient care have built a strong foundation for generating research hypotheses aimed at addressing health problems in the individual. With its focus on human health and behavior, nursing research subsumes a complex set of questions that require multiple approaches that span basic laboratory studies and clinical research, as well as investigations into prevention of disease and promotion of healthy life choices.

In conducting research particular emphasis is placed on addressing questions in populations with special health problems and needs, such as older people, women and minorities, residents of rural areas, and the economically disadvantaged. Through research we may discover how cultural and ethnic identity affect behavior and differences in risk patterns. Research also can elucidate the intertwined influences of socioeconomic status, geographic location, and other factors on health-related attitudes, decisions, and behaviors.

## A DECADE OF NURSING RESEARCH AT THE NATIONAL INSTITUTES OF HEALTH

During the last decade nursing research has explored the biologic and behavioral aspects of critical health problems. Clinical research has grown as new technologies have become available and as the capability to move science from bench to bedside has been amplified. The AIDS crisis, breast cancer, brain and spinal cord injury, and brain disorders are among the leading foci of this effort.

The future of nursing research is strongly rooted in its many research accomplishments to date. In a review of the state of the science at the National Institute of Nursing Research's (NINR) tenth anniversary meeting in September 1996, nurse researchers celebrated the field's accomplishments and acknowledged that there are many intriguing leads for future study. The research presented a decade of federal support for nursing research, spanning nursing research theories, behavioral and basic physiologic fields, the interplay of economics and health care delivery, and the importance of managing treatment side effects. Other presentations described research targeting specific needs for nursing knowledge. These include translating basic science into clinical care, approaches to managing behavior in the presence of cognitive impairment, the importance of developing culturally relevant educational programs in preventing HIV infection and intervening in low-birth-weight (LBW) risk, development of transitional care from hospital to home to achieve health and savings in health care costs, basic research on disorientation, inquiries into the effect of pain on immune responses, and investigations into biologic predictors of chemotherapy-induced nausea.

Each of these topics, as presented at NINR's tenth anniversary meeting, is described and serves as an example of the development of research areas of study. Suggestions for future research needs are made.

## Translating Basic Science Into Clinical Care

Dr. Sue K. Donaldson of Johns Hopkins University described a model of nursing research that focuses on the laws and processes that affect the well-being and optimum functioning of human beings, whether sick or well (Donaldson, 1996). She noted that nursing research seeks to build a knowledge base that will support clinical care by enhancing overall independent functioning. Consequently, the focus of nursing research can involve preclinical, clinical, and health services research. Nursing research is integrative research, combining basic science with a biobehavioral perspective to produce interventions that can be tested in clinical trials and demonstration projects.

Dr. Donaldson cited two examples of nursing research that demonstrate this integrative model. The first was a collaboration between a pathophysiologist who had conducted basic research on myocardial infarction and sudden cardiac arrest and a nurse researcher who had conducted extensive patient-oriented studies on biofeedback (Cowan and others, 1990). Working together, these researchers have developed a cognitive behavioral intervention that allows patients to reduce the variability of their heartbeat and thereby reduce the risk of a second heart attack.

The second example involved a study of chronic urinary incontinence, which affects 10 million people in the United States, including 50% of nursing home residents (Sampselle and others, 1997). Many patients, as well as many health care professionals, believe it to be an unavoidable and untreatable consequence of aging and cognitive impairment. As early as the 1950s, research has shown that exercising the pelvic floor muscles is very effective in reducing incontinence. Several groups of nurse researchers have worked to improve the effectiveness of these exercises through biofeedback (Burns and others, 1985; Burns and others, 1993) and to develop new diagnostic tools; others have conducted basic research on the types of muscle fibers involved and the most effective way to exercise them (Ferguson and others, 1990). The resulting interventions have been tested successfully in large, randomized clinical trials and are now the subject of additional studies.

## Cognitive Impairment: Managing Behavior

Dr. Kathleen Buckwalter of the University of Iowa outlined the work of nurse researchers in developing interventions for behavioral problems caused by chronic irreversible dementias such as Alzheimer's disease (Buckwalter, 1996). In addition to primary or cognitive symptoms, these conditions also produce a number of secondary symptoms, including changes in personality, emotion, and behavior, that are troubling to caregivers and consume significant amounts of time and resources. These secondary symptoms, which include wandering and repetitious or inappropriate behaviors, as well as depression and delusions, have received less attention from health care professionals and researchers than cognitive symptoms such as memory loss and inability to think abstractly.

Researchers have used a conceptual model that stresses the interaction between the person and the environment. According to this model the progressive degeneration of the cerebral cortex diminishes the individual's ability to process stimuli, resulting in a lower stress threshold and a higher potential for anxiety and dysfunctional behavior (Hall and Buckwalter, 1987). Consequently, researchers have sought to identify potential stressors—fatigue, caffeine, competing stimuli, and unexpected changes in routine—and control them at a level that is comfortable for the patient. Particular emphasis is placed on interventions for home caregivers and for staff and family caregivers in institutional settings.

Dr. Buckwalter and her colleagues have recently completed a clinical study that follows 246 caregiver couples for 6 months, using several educational and support interventions and collecting data through behavioral logs and periodic visits. Data from this trial are still being analyzed, but the study has already led to other projects involving rural populations, pharmaceutical effects, and differences in male and female caregiver's educational needs. The next stage of this also will focus on the transition from home to institutional care.

## Cultural Relevance for HIV/AIDS Prevention

Dr. Loretta S. Jemmott (1996) of the University of Pennsylvania described the efforts of her multidisciplinary team to translate theory into practice by designing culturally sensitive interventions to reduce behaviors that put adolescents at risk for sexually transmitted HIV infection. HIV infection has had a disproportionate impact on the African-American community, which makes up 12% of the U.S. population but has 28% of the AIDS cases—52% of female cases, 30% of adolescent cases, and 52% of pediatric cases.

Using focus groups and questionnaires, researchers discovered that attitudes, expectations, and self-confidence rather than knowledge alone were the factors that determined whether male adolescents used condoms or engaged in risky behaviors. Consequently, the investigators designed community-based interventions that would not only increase knowledge but also change attitudes about condom use and build self-confidence through the use of films, games, exercises, and role-playing. A prominent feature of these interventions was pride in race and community and was expressed in the message, "Respect yourself, protect yourself—you're worth it."

After 3 months' participation in the study, the experimental group reported having sex less often, having fewer partners, and using condoms more frequently than the control group. These results were duplicated in a second trial with female adolescents, with the finding that attitudes rather than information were the determinants of condom use. These results are now being translated into large-scale interventions in cooperation with the Urban League of Metropolitan Trenton, with funding from several institutes of the National Institutes of Health and the New Jersey Department of Health.

## Culturally Appropriate Intervention in Low-Birth-Weight Prevention

Dr. Dyanne Affonso (1996) of Emory University described another study to design and test a community-based, culturally appropriate intervention to prevent low birth weight. The study population was taken from an ethnically diverse community on the island of Hawaii, in which several minority groups—Hawaiian, Filipino, and Japanese—had unusually high rates of LBW babies. Pregnant women tended to drop out of standard prenatal programs because the programs seemed unrelated to their lives. Focus groups revealed that these women wanted alternatives and preferences rather than prescribed care; they wanted an interactive system that educated them about what was happening inside their bodies during pregnancy.

To recruit subjects researchers used a "neighborhood women's health watch." To ensure the cultural competency of their intervention, they worked with traditional healers to understand the belief systems of the various communities. The study included an incentive system that provided not only information and care but also nutritional vouchers from local businesses. It sought to make prenatal care a community affair rather than just an obstetric event.

The intervention has had several positive outcomes. Women in the experimental group made more prenatal visits, had longer gestational periods, and gave birth to infants with somewhat higher average birth weights. The women also scored higher on subjective measures of long-term quality of life. Costs were no higher than $1260 per woman for prenatal and postpartum care. Cost effectiveness will be addressed in future studies, but these costs may be low compared with the costs of treating higher numbers of LBW babies.

## Improvements in Transitional Home Care

Dr. Dorothy Brooten (1996) of Case Western Reserve University presented a program of research that included several NINR-funded studies of the use of advanced practice nurses in the transition from the hospital to home. In 1980 when the system of prospective payment was introduced, researchers became concerned with the health outcomes of early discharge of high-risk, vulnerable patients. Initial research focused on very-low-birth-weight infants (under 1500 grams), a group with high morbidity and mortality in the first year accompanied by very high health care costs.

Researchers developed and tested a "transitional home care" model consisting of comprehensive discharge planning, evaluation of patient readiness and environmental adequacy, and home visits and telephone contacts by nurse specialists. Randomized clinical trials demonstrated that this model could reduce the mean hospital stay by 11 days, reduce hospital charges by 27%, and reduce physician charges by 22%, with no significant difference in health outcomes for the infants.

When these findings were published in 1986 (Brooten, and others, 1986), NINR provided funding to apply this model to three groups: women with emergency cesarean deliveries, pregnant women with diabetes and hypertension, and women with abdominal hysterectomies. In each case the intervention significantly reduced both the length of hospital stay and hospital charges, while maintaining or improving health outcomes and greatly improving patients' satisfaction with their care. Most recently, researchers have applied the model to the care of women who are at high risk of having very-low-birth-weight infants because of diabetes, hypertension, or preterm labor. In this latter case home visits were substituted for half of the physician care. Preliminary results indicate that the experimental group had longer gestation periods, infants with higher birth weights, and shorter hospitalizations both before and after delivery.

Other groups have modified this model for controlled trials with elderly cardiac and surgical patients, both with and without home visits. The results suggest that home visits by nurse specialists are important for maintaining health outcomes over the long term. Analysis across these studies will provide insights about how the model works in various patient groups. However, it is already clear that important factors in the model's success are the continuity of care provided by the home visits and the experience and expertise of the nurse specialists.

## Disorientation: Using Cues to Assist in Wayfinding

Dr. Barbara Therrien (1996) of the University of Michigan described efforts to develop an animal model to guide the development of clinical interventions for disorientation in humans, such as patients with Alzheimer's disease. Most people find their way to a goal using either place navigation, which allows people to develop mental "maps" of their surroundings, or cue navigation, which is based on visual guideposts and landmarks. Place navigation is governed by the hippocampus—the largest memory structure in the brain—which is vulnerable to ischemia and is a prime target of disease, including Alzheimer's disease. Cue navigation, which depends on other brain structures, is a less-efficient and more limiting form of wayfinding, but it can be very useful in unfamiliar or confusing environments or when the hippocampus has been damaged.

Researchers found that by using an animal model, whose hippocampus is physiologically similar to that of humans, they could produce a model of impaired place navigation that mirrors clinical disorientation. In subsequent experiments researchers found that introducing a single visual cue improved the wayfinding performance of those with unilateral lesions. Animals with bilateral lesions showed improvement when the cue was enhanced with a pulsating sound or a flashing light. When a distraction was introduced, these improvements were somewhat dampened, particularly in females.

Having found that lesioned females became more severely disorientated, more easily distracted, and more resistant to therapy, researchers began to study the effects of the estrus cycle on wayfinding and disorientation. They found that females with damaged brains learned faster during proestrus, when estrogen levels are highest. This result suggests that estrogen may have a positive influence on learning through cue navigation. These and other findings will provide valuable guidance in the development of clinical therapies for human patients, including postmenopausal women.

## Pain and Its Immunologic Implications

Dr. Gayle Page (1996) of Ohio State University described a series of animal experiments that have demonstrated implications of pain management for sustaining the immune response. Dr. Page focused on the interaction of natural killer (NK) cells and the MADB106 tumor, a syngeneic mammary adenocarcinoma that metastasizes to the lungs when injected intravenously (Page and others, 1993; Page and others, 1994). Initial experiments demonstrated that the tumors were highly sensitive to NK control but only during the first 24 hours after injection, suggesting that this model might be adequate for studying the relationships among surgery, pain, immune competence, and metastatic development.

In preliminary studies male animals who underwent abdominal laparotomy under anesthesia developed 2.5 times as many metastases in their lungs as did the control group who received anesthesia but did not undergo surgery. This result was consistent with numerous studies showing that surgery increases host susceptibility to metastasis. When the animals were given a slow-release dose of morphine preoperatively, however, there was no increase in the number of metastases. Researchers concluded that these outcomes were due to the negative impact of pain on NK cell activity and the positive impact of pain management on immune response.

When these experiments were repeated in females, there were three times as many metastases in proestrus animals, who have higher levels of circulating estrogen. This result was consistent with the literature on the effect of the estrus and menstrual cycle on NK cell activity in animals and humans. This work has implications for timing and pain management in surgery for breast cancer and possibly for all types of surgery in which immunosuppression is an additional concern. The investigators believe that this research provides a foundation for adopting the position that the alleviation of pain is not simply a matter of mercy. It should be viewed as a physiologic necessity.

## Biologic Predictors of Chemotherapy-Induced Nausea

Dr. Gary Morrow (1996) of the University of Rochester reviewed the findings of several years of study on nausea in patients with cancer.

About 60% of patients receiving chemotherapy experience side effects in the first 24 hours after their first treatment; others experience nausea 1 or more days following treatment (Morrow, 1995). Women experience nausea after chemotherapy more often than men and young patients more often than older patients. However, there is no reliable predictor of precisely which patients will get sick. Most patients who have experienced nausea will continue to do so during subsequent treatment cycles. In fact about 25% get sick just thinking about the next treatment. As a result of these responses, cancer patients may drop out of chemotherapy or have their doses reduced. Any deviation from optimal dosage compromises ultimate survival, so the ability to manage side effects has major consequences for the success of chemotherapy.

A growing body of evidence suggests that side effects are at least partially avoidable. Nausea involves the autonomic nervous system, and researchers have used spectral analysis of heart rate and respiration to measure variability in autonomic reactivity. The results indicate that autonomic reactivity increases in response to chemotherapy and with it the likelihood of nausea. However, patients with low parasympathetic reactivity before treatment are less likely to experience nausea, whereas those with high reactivity are more likely to experience nausea.

These findings have important implications for managing nausea. Given the rising cost of sophisticated antiemetics, these side effects pose a significant economic issue, as well as concerns about quality of life and survival. Further research is needed to translate the work of these investigators into patient-oriented clinical practices.

## STRENGTHENING THE NURSING RESEARCH BASE FOR THE FUTURE

As it enters the twenty-first century, the nation continues to benefit from the revolution in scientific innovation. Every day, advances in science and technology are providing more in depth information and newer and better tools that will allow researchers not only to answer today's questions but also to pose and answer questions not yet formed. Ten years from now nursing research must ask itself whether it has done "the research that matters," that is, the research that considers the full range of issues that affect the health of people in the United States, as well as the way those problems are addressed by a health care delivery system that even now is facing restructuring and serious challenges to continued quality of care. Areas in which nursing research will play a defining role include cognitive impairment, pain, genetics, and innovative therapies, as well as risk assessment, behavior modification, and disease prevention.

### Multidisciplinary Integration to Promote Robust Science

It is important to integrate basic, applied, and health services research using a broad range of qualitative and quantitative approaches. Nursing research has played a major role in promoting collaboration with other disciplines and professional groups to bring the perspectives of diverse disciplines to bear on issues of human health and patient care.

In all cases a sound theoretic grounding is essential. The outcomes of care extend beyond the individual to include the family and even the physical setting. In the future, as organizational factors play a larger role, researchers will be asked to move beyond the outcomes of morbidity and mortality and place greater emphasis on functional status, caregiver burden, satisfaction with care, quality of life, and, of course, costs of care and cost effectiveness.

Increasingly, the scientific challenge for nursing research will be to determine which interventions are most effective, and within what settings, and how these interventions must accommodate different populations. Of particular importance in this context is the effect that gender and ethnic differences can have. As a result researchers must track interventions across the entire trajectory of illness. This approach will require sophisticated understanding of both prevention and treatment, including the social and cultural context of health, as well as efforts to enhance the capacities of communities to become directly involved in promoting the health of its members.

Collaborations with many other disciplines in areas of mutual interest are important to maintaining the vigor of the field. Areas especially well suited for this approach are long-term care for at-risk older people, genetic testing and counseling, behavioral aspects of infectious diseases, the special needs of women with physical disabilities, and environmental influences on risk factors related to chronic illness.

## Chronic Conditions: Portent of the Future

During the next two decades the baby boom generation will enter the time of life when chronic illness becomes a fact of life. Furthermore, as many more people enter extreme old age, the need for caregiving will overwhelm traditional systems. In a study published in 1996 in the *Journal of the American Medical Association*, investigators at the University of California, San Francisco, estimated that by the year 2030, 148 million people in the United States will have chronic conditions that will incur direct health care costs of $798 billion (in 1990 dollars) (Hoffman and others, 1996). These projections contrast with the 90 million people in the United States who were living with chronic conditions in 1987 with direct health care costs of $272 billion. Those figures do not include institutionalized persons or the indirect costs of care. Even at the present time the need to care for individuals with chronic conditions is a high demand on our system of care. As the California team observes in the article, by 1995 100 million individuals had two or more chronic conditions. Today nearly every family in this country is now affected by the chronic health conditions of one or more of its members.

This predicted demographic shift in the age of our population, along with an accompanying rise in chronic illness and disability, provides an important opportunity for nursing. Nursing research will need to continue to pursue research along four growing areas of investigation: managing symptoms, avoiding complications of illness and disability, managing and controlling pain, and supporting family caregivers.

## Research Needs in Mixed Behavioral and Physiologic Conditions

Another model for future directions in nursing research can be seen in the research needed to understand conditions that appear to mix both behavioral and physiologic functions, for example, irritable bowel syndrome and fibromyalgia. These disorders involve extensive health care expenses in prescriptions, physician visits, lost time from productive activities, and hospitalizations each year. Currently, these poorly understood conditions are diagnosed very indirectly through a resource-intensive process of eliminating other causes.

Existing research suggests interesting links between physical and psychologic functions that need investigation through enhanced collaboration among researchers in multiple fields such as neuroendocrinology and psychology. As a next step research is needed to design screening programs to distinguish between behavioral and physiologic causes. The results of this research also will have important implications for developing future cost-effective therapies.

## Continuing Research Focus on Cardiovascular Health

Another fruitful area for research is in cardiovascular health. Although the incidence of the disease is decreasing, it is still the number one killer of more than 950,000 people in the United States each year and accounts for at least $2 billion in Medicare expenditures (Graves, 1994). Those who live with the disease may undergo invasive therapeutic procedures, such as angioplasty or bypass operations. Extensive lifestyle changes are usually required to preserve health.

The roots of cardiovascular disease (and many adult-onset conditions) are often buried in childhood. The visibility of the disease increases with age, but the disease process begins long before symptoms are apparent. Behavioral interventions early in life are key to achieving a healthy adulthood. Nurse investigators have designed and tested interventions to reduce cardiovascular risk factors. These programs need extensive, rigorous evaluation and adaptation in a variety of community settings to achieve their potential.

## Research Opportunities in Neuroscience

Two out of three people in the United States seek treatment in any given year for problems involving the brain or nervous system at tremendous costs to themselves and the health care system (Dana Alliance for Brain Initiatives, 1996). The nation must continue to support research dealing with symptoms typically associated with stroke, epilepsy, Parkinson's disease, and spinal cord injury, for example. Symptoms include problems with mobility, pain, sleep, and depression. In addition, research is needed on issues related to successful family caregiving, from both patient and caregiver perspectives. Collaborative studies addressing these issues will be important to the nation's health in the next century as the number of caregivers per patient is reduced with the aging of the population.

Managing traumatic brain injury also involves nurse researchers. On a national scale the combined acute care and rehabilitation costs of central nervous system trauma, including traumatic brain and spinal cord injury, are $10 billion per year (National Institutes of Health, 1995). Adding indirect costs, such as lost productivity, brings the total cost of these injuries to the nation to $35 billion a year (National Institutes of Health, 1995). Much of the disability that results from traumatic brain injury is caused not by the initial injury but by the cascade of biochemical events triggered by the injury. If untreated, brain tissue and cells are deprived of sufficient oxygen, resulting in metabolic by-products that contribute to the progressive deterioration of the brain. Additional research is needed to develop interventions that prevent such secondary disability. Prevention, treatment, and rehabilitative needs associated with traumatic brain injury in children and young adults is a critical area about which we have limited information.

## Research Needs in Long-Term Transplant Survival

As a result of previous investments in health research, 12,000 people in the United States benefit from an organ transplant each year (Teraski and Cecka, 1992). Many of these patients, the majority of whom have received kidney transplants, have survived into their 50's and 60's and are following long-term drug regimens, including immunosuppressive therapies. These regimens are not without side effects, such as osteoporosis, cancer, neurologic impairment, cardiac dysfunction, and atherosclerosis. In seeking answers about symptom management or prevention of these complications, nursing research must foster partnerships with other health disciplines to ensure a holistic approach to achieving a good quality of life for long-term transplantation survivors.

## Research Addressing End-of-Life Issues

Complex issues associated with the end of life have been receiving considerable national attention. Studies of bioethic, biologic, and behavioral issues directly related to the end of life are a pressing need. Research on these issues can be conducted through multiple methodologies including qualitative and quantitative behavioral and physiologic methods. Research is needed to understand the social, psychologic, and physical circumstances that surround the end of life and will need to address four critical issues: (1) managing the transition to palliative care; (2) understanding and managing pain and other symptoms, such as nausea and depression, at the end of life; (3) measuring results, such as relief of symptoms; and (4) documenting costs for patients and family caregiving during end-stage illness (see Chapter 25).

## Research Issues in Environmental Health Science

Environmental conditions that may contribute to chronic illness are another concern for nursing research. Such conditions can threaten the health of everyone, but for those who live or work near hazardous substances or potentially toxic influences, they can lead to disability and death. Environmental influences also can create the conditions that spread infectious disease. Worldwide global warming could have unknown consequences. For example, there is preliminary evidence that small rises in temperatures where it is typically low can substantially increase the transmission of malaria (Martens and others, 1995). The threat may be particularly great for vulnerable communities with poor health services but low prevalence of malaria.

In the United States more immediate environmental dangers include exposure to chemicals, radiation and noise at work, barriers to using personal protective wear, pesticide exposure among farm workers, the possible effects of dioxin exposure on endometriosis, the effects of pesticide exposure on neurologic function, and the toxic effects of waste sites. NINR is concentrating on disadvantaged and underserved populations who may have an increased risk of exposure to toxic substances and other hazards yet have the least amount of information about the consequences of that exposure. Efforts to intervene at the community level to overcome existing environmental health problems and prevent new hazards from occurring are proving to be more effective when community members are involved.

## The Need to Understand and Manage Pain

Since it was founded a decade ago, the NINR has dedicated many of its resources to research on managing the symptoms of chronic conditions. None of these symptoms is more common than pain, which afflicts the acutely ill and can seriously compromise the quality of life indefinitely for those with chronic conditions and for their families. Pain prompts nearly 40 million visits to health care providers each year and costs the nation more than $100 billion annually in health care expenditures and lost productivity (National Advisory on Neurological Disorders and Stroke Council, 1992). Furthermore, pain can prolong hospital stays and impede recovery.

Among the most interesting recent discoveries made by NINR-funded scientists is research demonstrating differences in men and women in finding pain relief. Two kappa-opioids, nalbuphine and butorphanol (commonly known as Nubain and Stadol), have been found to produce significantly greater pain relief in women than in men, even though the women reported higher amounts of pain initially. Past studies suggesting that kappa-opioids were less effective than mu-opioids in the management of pain may have relied too heavily on male patients to be able to detect evidence that kappa-opioids may be a better analgesic choice for treating women's pain. Women undergoing surgery, who have suffered nerve damage, cancer, and other disease conditions, may benefit immediately from these findings. Unlike the powerful morphine-like opioids, prescribed for moderate-to-severe pain, kappa-opioid compounds are generally free of the associated side effects (Gear and others, 1996).

These findings raise further questions about effective management of pain and about the design of comprehensive studies. For example, we need to understand better the role of hormones on the perception of pain. How does estrogen or testosterone mediate pain? Do women have more kappa receptors on certain nerve cells than men, thus enabling kappa-opioids to block pain better? Another question to investigate is whether there are age and gender differences in the way the brain regulates pain relief. New policies on the inclusion of women and children, as well as continued emphasis on inclusion of all populations in health research, will be important because pain continues to be an important area of research with many yet unanswered questions about better pain management for everyone.

## Nursing Research Opportunities in Genetics

The generation of scientific knowledge about human functioning is occurring quickly and will accelerate even more rapidly as mapping of the human genome is completed. We already have some previews of things to come. We can identify individuals who are at high risk for sickle cell disease, cystic fibrosis, Huntington's disease, and some cancers. At the same time, scientists continue to work to understand the importance of the interrelationship of genes, the environment, and personal lifestyle choices on the disease process and how that process can be altered.

What is considered the "promise" of science also is raising some public concern. Although an array of information about progress in genetics research is appearing in the media, there is doubt about the accuracy and predictive ability of current genetic tests. People will be faced with decisions about whether to undergo testing for genetic diseases, followed by more decisions about what to do and whom to tell when the results are positive. Some screening outcomes may require people to make inconvenient or unpleasant changes in lifestyle in an effort to allay the effects of a genetic disposition to disease. Other people may be confronted with the prospect of developing a disease that disables and kills but has no treatment. Difficult questions are already being raised by the possibility of transmitting a genetic condition to offspring. A host of other issues will arise as genetic therapies become available. In every case the common denominator is understanding options and making choices.

Health professionals must have the knowledge and skill to help people with this process. Because of its unique patient-oriented perspective, nursing research has an especially important role to play and will need to address issues related to symptoms associated with conditions in which genetics play a key role; cognitive decision making and learning styles, family education and counseling, and risk behavior and risk reduction.

Because advances in our understanding of human genetics have implications for many scientific disciplines and most health care providers, these research efforts are best suited to an interdisciplinary framework. To promote this approach, in 1996 NINR convened a group of clinical and basic scientists from multiple disciplines to identify unique nursing research and training opportunities in genetics. The immediate results were twofold: NINR is now offering postdoctoral and senior fellowships that link training in nursing research and genetics. NINR is also encouraging currently funded investigators to add genetic components to their ongoing projects.

# CONCLUSION

Nursing research is at the frontiers of science, building the foundation of knowledge that supports improvements in human health and well-being. The contributions of nursing researchers affect diverse fields. The nursing research enterprise has supported innovative research on behavioral factors in health and disease, on the management of cognitive impairment and pain, and on outcomes measures and the relevance of cultural factors in biomedical research. The results of this research have applications in a wide range of fields, including cardiovascular health, HIV prevention, prenatal care, and extended care for elderly patients.

The breadth and depth of these accomplishments confirm the importance of nursing research. The future vitality of nursing research will continue to be ensured by the many questions that still remain to be answered and the innovative ideas of nursing researchers. The last 10 years have advanced the field. The next decade will be a time of even greater innovation and accomplishment.

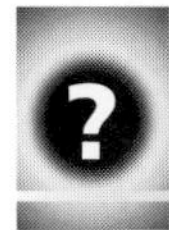

## *Discussion Exercises*

1. Nursing research has come of age at the end of the twentieth century. What are some of the political, social, and economic forces that enabled this progress?
2. Name the three most important areas you believe nursing research must address immediately.
3. In spite of plentiful nursing research that demonstrates effective interventions, far too little research becomes integrated into nursing practice. Why? What strategies should the profession use to encourage utilization of nursing research in practice?

## References


Affonso D: Improving pregnancy outcomes. Advancing health through science: the human dimension, Tenth Anniversary Research Symposium conducted by the National Institute of Nursing Research, Bethesda, Md, September, 1996.

Affonso D and others: Neighborhood women's health watch: partners in community care, *Adv Practice Nurs Q* 1(3):1, 1995.

Brooten D: Transitional home care: health and economic improvements. Advancing health through science: the human dimension, Tenth Anniversary Research Symposium conducted by the National Institute of Nursing Research, Bethesda, Md, September, 1996.

Brooten D and others: A randomized clinical trial of early discharge and home follow-up of very low birthweight infants, *New England J Med,* 315:934, 1986.

Buckwalter K: Cognitive impairment: managing behavior. Advancing health through science: the human dimension, Tenth Anniversary Research Symposium conducted by the National Institute of Nursing Research, Bethesda, Md, September, 1996.

Burns PA and others: Kegel's exercises with biofeedback therapy for treatment of stress incontinence, *Nurs Pract* 10(2):28, 1985.

Burns PA and others: A comparison of effectiveness of biofeedback and pelvic muscle exercise treatment of stress incontinence in older community-dwelling women, *J Gerontol* 48(4):M167, 1993.

Cowan MJ and others: Power spectral analysis of heart rate variability after biofeedback training, *J Obstet Gynecol Neonatal Nurs* 26(4):375, 1990.

Dana Alliance for Brain Initiatives: Delivering results: a progress report on brain research, Dana Alliance Pub, p 2, New York, 1996, Dana Alliance Press.

Donaldson SK: Translating basic science into clinical care. Advancing health through science: the human dimension, Tenth Anniversary Research Symposium conducted by the National Institute of Nursing Research, Bethesda, Md, September, 1996.

Ferguson KL and others: Stress urinary incontinence: effect of pelvic muscle exercise, *Obstet Gynecol* 75(4):671, 1990.

Gear RW and others: Kappa-opioids produce significantly greater analgesia in women than in men, *Nat Med* 2(11):1248, 1996.

Graves EJ: National hospital discharge survey: annual summary, 1992, *Vital Health Stat* 119:1, 1994.

Hall GR, Buckwalter KC: Progressively lowered stress threshold: a conceptual model for care of adults with Alzheimer's disease, *Arch Psychiatr Nurs* 1(6):399, 1987.

Hoffman C and others: Persons with chronic conditions: their prevalence and costs, *JAMA* 276(18):1473, 1996.

Jemmott LS: Cultural relevance: HIV/AIDS prevention. Advancing health through science: the human dimension, Tenth Anniversary Research Symposium conducted by the National Institute of Nursing Research, Bethesda, Md, September, 1996.

Martens WJ and others: Potential impact of global climate change on malaria risk, *Environ Health Perspect* 103:458, 1995.

Morrow G: Psychological aspects of anticipatory nausea and vomiting. In Chapman S, editor: Managing nausea and vomiting in the medical practice, Stonington, Me, 1995, Caduceus Medical Publishers.

Morrow G: Biologic predictors of chemotherapy-induced nausea. Advancing health through science: the human dimension, Tenth Anniversary Research Symposium conducted by the National Institute of Nursing Research, Bethesda, Md, September, 1996.

National Institutes of Health: Disease-specific estimates of direct and indirect costs of illness and NIH support, {Appendix: injury—trauma (central nervous system)}, Bethesda, Md, 1995, U.S. Department of Health & Human Services.

National Advisory on Neurological Disorders and Stroke Council: Progress and promise 1992: status report on the NINDS implementation plan for the decade of the brain, NINDS Pub, p 2, Bethesda, Md, 1992, U.S. Department of Health & Human Services.

Page GG: Pain and its immunological implications. Advancing health through science: the human dimension, Tenth Anniversary Research Symposium conducted by the National Institute of Nursing Research, Bethesda, Md, September, 1996.

Page GG and others: Morphine attenuates surgery-induced enhancement of metastatic colonization in rats, *Pain* 54:21, 1993.

Page GG and others: The role of LGL/NK cells in surgery-induced promotion of metastasis and its attenuation by morphine, *Brain Behav Immunity* 8:241, 1994.

Sampselle CM and others: Continence for women: evidence-based practice, *J Obstet Gynecol Neonatal Nurs* 26(4):375, 1997.

Teraski PI, Cecka JM: The UNOS scientific renal transplant registry. In Teraski PI, Cecka JM, editors: *Clinical transplants* Los Angeles, 1992, Regent of the University of California.

Therrien B: Disorientation: using cues to assist in wayfinding. Advancing health through science: the human dimension, Tenth Anniversary Research Symposium conducted by the National Institute of Nursing Research, Bethesda, Md, September, 1996.

# 28 The Growth of Collaborative and Interdisciplinary Research

**Sue K. Donaldson**

*Work hard. Take chances! Be very, very bold!*

**Lillian Hellman**

The origins of nursing research and doctoral programs in nursing are interdisciplinary and collaborative. However, growth in this realm has been stunted by researchers and leaders in nursing, perhaps as a result of insecurities and professional identity crises. Nursing has fostered forms of communication and knowledge that are accessible only to those within the discipline. Poor interdisciplinary communication has limited the impact of the perspective of nursing and nursing knowledge on the greater whole of health-related research. The price that nursing will pay for continuing on its current course includes obscurity and limited impact of nursing knowledge, further stunting of the development of nursing research and the discipline and truncation of support of nursing research. Obscurity and insignificance of nursing knowledge will seriously undermine the relevance of nursing professional practice in the managed care environment.

Nursing can change its course and use collaborative and interdisciplinary opportunities and strategies to develop an exciting knowledge base that is valued as a source of solutions to health care problems and a source of futuristic directions for health promotion. The changes needed to expand the scope of nursing research and the impact of nursing knowledge are neither costly in terms of money nor difficult in terms of barriers presented by researchers from other fields. The most difficult challenges to growth in collaborative and interdisciplinary research arise from beliefs and preferences of nurse researchers and leaders and the limited interdisciplinary experience of doctoral students and younger researchers in nursing. Nursing must create rewards and challenges within nursing to effect the changes needed for survival and growth as a discipline and profession.

## BRIEF HISTORY: TRIMMING OF OUR INTERDISCIPLINARY ROOTS

The relative insularity of nursing knowledge and nurse researchers is shocking in view of the fact that their roots are multidisciplinary and interdisciplinary and the result of collaborative efforts. The dramatic growth in the number of nurse researchers and doctoral programs in nursing in the 1970s was due to education and mentoring of nurses in other disciplines and, most significantly, the basic sciences. The major formal program for increasing the number of doctorally prepared nurses was the federally funded Nurse Scientist Training Program. A significant cadré of nurses were educated in doctoral programs in the basic sciences, both social and biologic, as a part of the U.S. Public Health Service Nurse Scientist Training Program, which was operative from 1962 to the late 1970s.

A subsequent national program that promoted interdisciplinary research collaborations between nurse researchers and researchers in other fields was the Robert Wood Johnson (RWJ) Clinical Nurse Scholars Program. The RWJ Clinical Nurse Scholars Program was particularly effective because it socialized nurse researchers who were committed to the clinical practice of nursing into the mainstream culture of science and clinical research. Both the Nurse Scientist Training Program and the RWJ Clinical Nurse Scholars Program provided research training in environments where professional and disciplinary boundaries were ignored and priority was placed on focusing all available expertise to address gaps in knowledge and answer significant questions.

Schools and colleges of nursing expanded their faculties with the former nurse scientist trainees and engaged them in the planning and implementation of the doctoral programs in nursing. The nursing faculty with PhDs from other disciplines created a critical faculty mass for mentorship of predoctoral students and assured institutions of higher education that the doctoral programs in nursing would conform to the standards of their more established PhD-granting divisions. Some faculties of nursing actively sought an interdisciplinary collaborative model for research and doctoral education in nursing, whereas others did so only to comply with institutional requirements.

During the 1970s and early 1980s the majority of nurses active as researchers were the products of non-nursing doctoral programs, and this is undoubtedly a major reason for the early interdisciplinary collaborative flavor of the emerging doctoral programs in nursing. Some of the doctoral programs retain this characteristic, such as the joint PhD in nursing and psychology at the University of Wisconsin, Madison, and the required graduate minor in another established discipline at the University of Minnesota.

Despite these early influences and programmatic requirements intended to shape an interdisciplinary collaborative model for doctoral programs in nursing and nursing research, the majority of current graduates from doctoral programs in nursing have not had significant involvement in interdisciplinary collaborative research. They have not and do not plan to share critical thinking and planning with researchers from non-nursing fields.

Unfortunately for nursing the postdoctoral training model has neither been a dominant one nor has this experience been required for faculty positions, even in institutions offering doctoral education in nursing. Postdoctoral training has been a mechanism for expanding the new PhD's collaborative and interdisciplinary experience. Some schools of nursing have made a commitment to interdisciplinary postdoctoral training using their own resources, such as the postdoctoral program in basic sciences at Rush University, Chicago, during the early 1980s, or using corporate funding and partnership, such as the continuing Johnson and Johnson, Inc. postdoctoral fellowship in wound healing at Johns Hopkins University School of Nursing, Baltimore. The National Institute of Nursing Research (NINR) also is currently supporting nursing postdoctoral fellows in the Human Genome Mapping Project and at the National Institute of Aging, National Institutes of Health (NIH).

However, the number of nurse researchers with postdoctoral training experience remains small. Rather, the trend seems to be for nurses to plunge into faculty and other research careers directly from doctoral programs. These new graduates use faculty time and resources to grow into the role of researcher. Schools and colleges of nursing have used their research monies to fund faculty engaged in postdoctoral training rather than to fund the generation of preliminary data for extramural research proposal submission. Beginning faculty researchers confuse their need for postdoctoral research mentorship with career mentorship and are frustrated when they are not given the latter rather than the former. Only reluctantly do these beginning faculty researchers seek or establish interdisciplinary collaborations. These practices in nursing, which tend to foster the premature placement of doctorally prepared nurses in faculty research roles, disadvantage nurse researchers and limit the growth of nursing knowledge.

Some schools and colleges of nursing encourage and reward interdisciplinary collaboration and collaborative ventures for faculty and students. They are characterized by the following:

1. Faculties comprised of nurse and non-nurse members
2. Research products and publications authored by researchers from several disciplines
3. Joint appointments of nursing faculty in other research divisions
4. Non-nurse researchers as joint appointees in nursing or as faculty of the doctoral program in nursing
5. Interdisciplinary research and doctoral degree programs
6. Publication and presentation of research findings at non-nursing meetings
7. Service on editorial boards or as editor for non-nursing research journals and on research review committees outside of nursing
8. Leadership in national/international research organizations beyond nursing, such as within NIH or the American Heart Association

Although interdisciplinary joint appointments and primary appointments are not a guarantee for collaborative research, they do create a structure that facilitates interdisciplinary crossfertilization. The dearth of these interdisciplinary appointments in nursing, despite the significant number of nurses with doctoral degrees from non-nursing research disciplines, suggests an unnecessary insularity on the part of nursing. It also suggests that nursing research, that which builds the discipline of nursing, is not viewed as highly significant to societal health or as a valued counterpart to perspectives of other research disciplines.

This is perhaps the result of nursing investing its research and philosophic resources into the identification of a unique perspective and syntax at the expense of development of the substantive structure of the discipline (Donaldson and Crowley, 1978). Except for sociologists, non-nurse researchers are unlikely to want to conduct enquiry or develop theories that define or validate nursing. Kasper (1995) asserts that nursing has developed inadequately as a discipline because nurse researchers have produced processes and not substantive structure or knowledge. These manifestations of the inward focus of the discipline of nursing has created barriers to interdisciplinary collaborations in research, where the focus is on developing knowledge as an outcome.

The most puzzling of academic practices in schools and colleges of nursing is that of requiring that students in doctoral programs in nursing be nurses. This is an understandable requirement for doctoral programs leading to the DNSc, or equivalent degree, whereby development of a clinical role including clinical nursing research may be included. However, there is no valid argument for this requirement in the nonprofessional doctoral programs. If medicine and other professional schools had followed this pattern, the nurse scientist program would have been imperiled and the number of basic biologic scientists (i.e., non MDs) would be very small. There are definable realms in the discipline of nursing that do not require that the researcher be a nurse. The National Institutes of Health recognizes this and has awarded research grants to non-nurse principal investigators through the National Center for Nursing Research and its successor organization, the National Institute of Nursing Research. The research grant awards from the NINR to non-nurse principal investigators affirms that the principal investigator (PI) does not have to be a nurse to conduct research of importance to nursing; furthermore, these grant awards engage talented researchers from other disciplines in the work of building the knowledge of the discipline of nursing.

Nurse researchers rarely have non-nurse co-principal investigators (Co-PIs); they use non-nurse researchers more as consultants and as advisors. Similarly, it is rare to have a non-nurse researcher serve as the primary mentor for a doctoral student in nursing, even when the non-nurse researcher may be the best match for the expertise and resources required for the student's dissertation project. Nurse researchers and doctoral students in nursing usually limit their significant research experiences to interactions within nursing. Nurse researchers also present and publish primarily for each other, and an unintended consequence is that nursing has developed a scientific language and jargon that is not easily deciphered by the outside world.

In summary, at this point nursing has only a small cadré of researchers with PhDs or postdoctoral training in basic sciences and other non-nursing research disciplines and is engaged in relatively little interdisciplinary collaborative research. Furthermore, nursing has insulated its research enterprise and discipline by minimizing the number of non-nurse principal investigators, faculty researcher appointees, PhD students, and postdoctoral fellows. The interdisciplinary collaborative research efforts for activities central to the discipline of nursing usually consist of non-nurse researchers serving as consultants, advisory committee members, or readers rather than Co-PIs and primary mentors. The majority of students earning a PhD in nursing have not taken core research courses in another discipline and do not train as postdoctoral fellows in nursing or any other research discipline before taking a research position. Thus, the potential for interdisciplinary collaborative research is present in nursing, but it is not being actualized or fostered in the future generation of nurse researchers. The current status of nursing is one whereby interdisciplinary collaborative roots have been trimmed at the expense of stunting the growth and maturation of the discipline and of nurse researchers.

## PROBABLE FUTURE: EXPENSIVE COCOON

If nursing continues in the present mode, there will be a heavy price to pay. The insularity of nurse researchers and doctoral programs in nursing guarantees three things: (1) obscurity and limited utilization of nursing knowledge, (2) underdevelopment of disciplinary knowledge and research, and (3) truncation of support for nursing research.

### Obscurity

The first guarantee of obscurity will result from nursing knowledge and research being invisible to others. There are relatively few nurses among the totality of researchers, and this ratio of nurse to non-nurse researchers is unlikely to change much over the next 10 years. Thus, the current practice of designing, presenting, and publishing nursing research primarily for a nursing audience is unlikely to change the thinking and perspective of the general scientific community. If nursing research and knowledge do not involve and influence researchers and practitioners beyond nursing, then nursing research will not have a major impact on human health. In fact other disciplines will "rediscover" nursing knowledge and, in ignorance, claim it as theirs. Changes in the health care system have heralded the era of the health team, comprised of a variety of professional and nonprofessional providers (e.g., medicine, public health, physical therapy). If nursing research–based knowledge is only visible and understandable to nurses, it is unlikely to be used as the basis for care delivery by the team.

### Disciplinary Underdevelopment

Disciplinary underdevelopment, the second guarantee of nursing's current path of relative avoidance of interdisciplinary collaboration, is equally serious. Nursing does not have a body of researchers or a research infrastructure of sufficient size, diversity, and maturity to study all of the relevant realms of human health. The nursing perspective offers the hope of unique and creative solutions to health problems and promotion, but it will not have an impact unless nursing is able to sell its perspective to non-nurse researchers and to seduce them into incorporating it into their thinking and research designs.

Funding for research is also becoming more targeted and directed toward specific areas of concern rather than the ideas of individual investigators. Thus, in the future research will be conducted in interdisciplinary teams rather than by investigators working within the boundaries of a given discipline. Nurse researchers will not be able to function in these teams unless they become more interdisciplinary. Equally important, research funding will be directed to these interdisciplinary research teams. Nursing research will starve, as well as be ignored, if it continues to be conducted in isolation, fulfilling the third guaranteed outcome of nursing if it continues on its current course.

## PREFERABLE FUTURE: NURSING INTERDISCIPLINARY LEADERSHIP

In the preferred future nursing has a leadership role in the planning, management, and delivery of health care because of the extensive and relevant research knowledge base of the discipline. Nurses ground their careers, clinical services, and roles on interdisciplinary models and knowledge that emanates from research of the discipline. Nurses, because of their interdisciplinary breadth and collaboration, are the preferred team leaders in outcomes research and care delivery. The new health care system reflects the nursing perspective of partnering with patients and making their experience in the health care system a positive one that increases their autonomy and satisfaction. Because of effective teamwork and health promotion, health care costs drop and accessibility to clients improves along with client health status measures as functional abilities and quality of life.

Researchers in nursing are nurses and a mixture of all other related disciplines who focus on health-related questions and problems from the perspective of nursing. Results of nursing research are presented at all relevant national/international scientific meetings and in a wide variety of interdisciplinary journals; nursing research is frequently cited in the media and presents a challenge to other researchers. Students in doctoral programs in nursing include nurses and non-nurses. Graduates commonly obtain postdoctoral training in nursing and other fields.

The funding for nursing research grows in concert with its relevance and interdisciplinary ties. The discipline of nursing is known for its perspective and knowledge rather than identification of a group of nurses. The word *nursing* refers to a partnership model of health promotion rather than just the profession. Non-nurses seek nursing research opportunities and expand them in funding agencies.

## STRATEGIES FOR NURSING INTERDISCIPLINARY LEADERSHIP

Nursing needs to return to its interdisciplinary collaborative roots to be successful in the future. The unique perspective of nursing will ensure its identity, but the impact depends on nursing bringing that perspective to the general research community.

Nursing has the potential and the resources to make changes that will guarantee usefulness and significance of nursing research, knowledge, and researchers. The approach must be bold and assertive and in an interdisciplinary arena. This is not the image or persona of nursing, but if nursing believes that the nursing perspective—that of partnering with clients to assist them in achieving health—is essential, then nursing will change its approach and market its research ideas and concepts beyond nursing. The marketing must be in research, academic, professional, and public realms. Nurses with interdisciplinary knowledge, skills, and linkages will be critical in this endeavor. The goal should be to have the largest possible number of interdisciplinary collaborators working with nurse researchers to build nursing knowledge.

## Rewards

A first critical step in redirecting nursing to a more productive path is that of structuring rewards to enhance interdisciplinary collaborations, non-nurse researcher participation in nursing research, and communication of nursing research and knowledge beyond nursing. Academic deans and leaders in nursing need to change promotion, tenure, and advancement criteria to fully recognize interdisciplinary appointments, research collaborations, contributions to the research enterprise (e.g., review committees, editorships), and research programs. Nurses who create the interdisciplinary bridges need to be rewarded rather than chastised for not contributing more to nursing activities. These researchers have not "sold out" but rather offer the linkages requisite for the survival and growth of nursing research and knowledge.

## Communication

The second critical step for nursing is to foster research communication and exchanges between nursing and other disciplines. Nurse researchers need to develop common language and skills for interacting and communicating across disciplines and should seek non-nurse collaborators. Doctoral students in nursing need experiences with interdisciplinary teams and exposure to the core knowledge of other disciplines. Given that survival of our future researchers depends on their interdisciplinary skills, doctoral students need immersion in environments where ideas and knowledge generation are of greater importance than socialization in a specific discipline. The latter will shape but must not limit the former. To ensure that a focus on the needs of nursing as a discipline or profession are not preeminent in doctoral programs, non-nurse students should be encouraged to enter doctoral programs and postdoctoral training programs in nursing. Every doctoral program in nursing needs a defined core of course work and research experience to be offered to students pursuing PhDs in other fields and postdoctoral fellows in other disciplines. Offering these research cores and experience will facilitate interdisciplinary communication and collaboration and force an emphasis on nursing knowledge and research rather than nursing identity and professional growth.

## Interdisciplinary Research Teams

The third critical step is that nurse researchers with interdisciplinary communication and research skills and linkages should be prized as being the most culturally competent in the world of researchers, and they should be given resources to create or join interdisciplinary research teams. At the very least, nurse researchers need to take a leadership role to generate the complex, coordinated body of knowledge needed for care delivery by the care-provider teams. Nurse researchers need to participate in interdisciplinary research teams that study outcomes of health care to ensure that outcomes such as quality of life, patient comfort, patient satisfaction, and social role recovery and potential are weighted properly along with measures of cost reduction, disease parameter functional performance, and health care system performance. Fortunately, nursing has researchers with backgrounds and skills to span a range of research from molecular studies of basic biologic processes to epidemiologic studies of population health. In all areas nursing needs to make sure that individual human behavior and responses are included in the study of the biology of diseases and medical treatment and included in the conceptualization of health promotion and restoration.

## Needs of Individuals

Nursing must be the champion of individual humans, including their experiences, needs, and behavior, in the arena of outcomes research, because this is not the primary orientation of medicine or public health. Incorporation of the nursing perspective in outcomes research will ensure that health care is planned with the patient, family, and community included as active participants in health promotion and disease treatment. Nursing also adds a unique perspective to that of medicine and public health and other disciplines conducting outcomes research. Nursing asks questions as to how group interactions and interventions can be used to meet the health needs of individuals, including coping with chronic illness, preventing disease, and complying and benefitting fully from medical therapies. Nursing views disease and disease therapies primarily as human biobehavioral experiences and responses and can simultaneously measure these in individuals and groups. It thus creates the intact human counterpart to human disease processes at the molecular and the population of levels of analysis. In addition, nursing places an emphasis on health promotion and disease prevention through partnership with clients that optimize client autonomy.

Research expertise of nursing in the realm of human behavior will become more important as managed care seeks knowledge, strategies, and outcomes to reduce the costs of illness and promote health. However, nurse researchers must work in an interdisciplinary collaborative mode to make their work relevant, usable, and visible. It is the responsibility of nursing to make this happen. The good news is that managed care has created a requirement of evidence-based practice and the knowledge has yet to be generated. This shift in health care delivery and management thus creates the first real opportunity for nursing to interject its perspective and research as a dominant component.

## Getting Direction

In addition to seeking and treating interdisciplinary research opportunities, nursing needs to participate fully in the research priority setting, review, and funding activities of the interdisciplinary health care research organizations. Nurse researchers have been and need to continue to serve on funding agency and NIH panels, review committees, and councils to interject the nursing perspective. Nursing has been active in the Agency for Health Care Policy Research, and this has brought high visibility to the nursing perspective and the body of nursing research-based knowledge. Similarly, nurse researchers with leadership roles in non-nursing health organizations and foundations such as the American Cancer Society, American Heart Association, Institute of Medicine (National Academy of Sciences), Robert Wood Johnson Foundation, and Kellogg Foundation serve in critical roles that have become more critical to the growth and visibility of nursing research. Nursing needs to continue and expand its leadership role in these organizations and also in role as editors, editorial board members, and contributors to non-nursing and interdisciplinary research publications.

# CONCLUSION

Nurse researchers must shed the cocoon that insulates them from interdisciplinary research collaborations. The new approach should be to actively seek involvement with researchers in other disciplines and to invite non-nurses into the discipline of nursing. Nursing's insular behavior and preoccupation with identity, boundaries, and process belie either insecurity or, perhaps, the misguided ulterior motive of using the discipline primarily to build the stature of the profession of nursing. The latter will be achieved only through nursing fulfilling its societal mandate to improve human health and the experience of humans. Toward that end, nursing needs knowledge that is interdisciplinary in scope and breadth and researchers capable of extensive interdisciplinary, collaborative research.

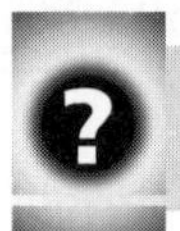

## Discussion Exercises

1. What are the advantages of preparing nonnurses with doctorates in nursing? What arguments could be posed in opposition to nonnurses obtaining nursing doctorates? Do you agree?
2. What specific strategies should be taken by universities and organizations (e.g., professional associations, government agencies) to encourage interdisciplinary collaboration among scientists?
3. You are a senior scientist in nursing interested in promoting collaborative research between nursing and scientists in other disciplines. What strategies would you use to encourage such collaboration?

## References

Donaldson SK, Crowley DM: The discipline of nursing, *Nurs Outlook* 26:113, 1978.

Kasper CE: Going through the motions: the ethics of process, *J Cardiovasc Nurs* 9(3):62, 1995.

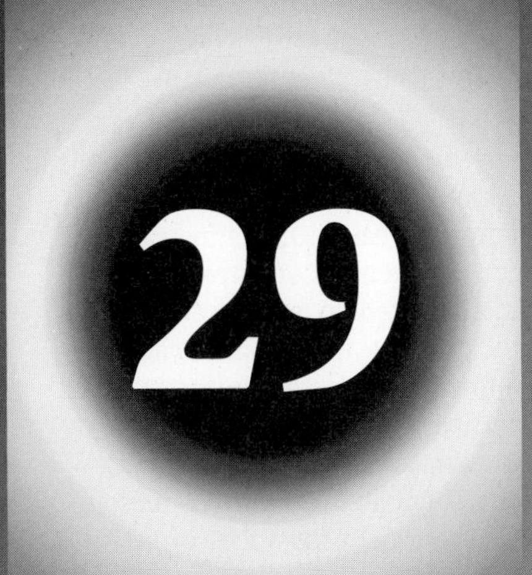

# 29 Preparing Future Researchers

**Virginia P. Tilden**

*If we don't know where we are going, we don't know where we are.*

**Edward Cornish,**
Futurist

## CHALLENGES IN PREPARING NURSE RESEARCHERS

A preferred future of affordable, accessible, cost-effective, and high-quality health care for people in the United States depends on a foundation of multidisciplinary scientific knowledge (NIH, 1993). Nursing has joined medicine and the basic sciences in creating this foundation, as evidenced by the high national regard nursing enjoys at the National Institutes of Health (NIH) and in the U.S. Congress. However, leadership in clinical scientific research depends on the ability of present and future nurse scientists to establish significant and rigorous programs of research.

Preparing future nurse researchers requires planning to ensure success. If left unplanned and allowed to occur accidentally rather than intentionally, programs that prepare nurse researchers will suffer from competition with other priorities that tend to be better understood by the general public and therefore enjoy more public support. For example, as state legislators look for programs where cost cutting will have a less negative impact on the mood of the voting public, they are more likely to cut doctoral program funding than associate or baccalaureate degree program funding because the public poorly understands the need for nurse scientists. Good planning requires a multifaceted approach with simultaneous activities in a number of directions, including educating the public about the importance of preparing nurse scientists, educating nurses bound for graduate education about the advantages and exciting opportunities of a research career, and educating present faculty in schools of nursing about the essential characteristics of successful research programs.

To achieve the preparation of future researchers critically needed to create the preferred future, two main areas of programmatic activities are examined: those related to formal educational programs (doctoral and postdoctoral research training) and those related to the support and development of nurse faculty in schools of nursing. Both avenues rest on a foundation of scientific integrity—high ethical standards, high-quality mentoring and socialization into scholarly behaviors, respect by scientists for diversity and cultural pluralism, and collegiality and encouragement for multidisciplinary collaboration. Thus, we look first at this foundation because it undergirds all aspects of preparing future researchers.

## Scientific Integrity

Traditionally, science has enjoyed a reputation of integrity and the embodiment of such characteristics as honesty, objectivity, collegiality, and service to the public good. The public's faith in science was first seriously damaged by the medical experimentation of Nazi scientists in World War II. The outcome of those events led primarily to a global mandate to the sciences for self-monitoring and self-correction.

The U.S. federal government developed and monitored extensive regulations regarding the use of human and animal subjects in biomedical research, but it left the training of scientists and the standards for scientific integrity up to the private sector and to the sciences. Then, public revelations in the 1980s and 1990s showed remarkably widespread occurrences of research misconduct (Macrina, 1995; National Academy Press, 1995), including numerous instances of scientists' intentional falsification and fabrication of data, widespread plagiarism and conflicts of interest, misappropriation of research funds, and other serious and intentional misconduct. Many of these instances involved reputable and established scientists at such major universities as Harvard, MIT, Stanford, and the University of California.

Careful analysis of contributing factors showed two main causes: a lack of grounding in ethics and an intense pressure for success. Pressures included increased competition for scarce financial support, major scientific breakthroughs in reproductive technologies and genetic engineering, financial incentives connected to some scientific discoveries, rapid advances in communication technologies that allow instant communication of scientific events and research findings, and the hazards associated with computer data storage. Nursing as a science is subject to many of these pressures and has had its own instances of serious misconduct (NIH, 1995; NIH, 1996).

Preparing future researchers not only must emphasize the methodologic and administrative expertise to establish significant programs of research but also must foster scientific integrity, avoiding scientific misconduct. By 1990 the U.S. government began mandating that programs supported by federal dollars must actively teach and promote scientific integrity (National Academy Press, 1995). Universities responded quickly with policies on detecting instances of possible fraud, procedures for managing allegations of misconduct, and levying sanctions when misconduct occurred.

Training programs for scientists began developing methods for prevention, primarily teaching future researchers how to manage the pressures that breed scientific misconduct and how to understand what behaviors constitute misconduct. This represents a fundamental change in society from assuming that scientists naturally embody scientific integrity to acknowledging that scientists, like all humans, are susceptible to pressures, distractions, and moral failures, and therefore benefit from training in the ethical conduct of science. Now all academic health sciences' educational programs that receive federal support must comply with federal regulations to have a formal policy to promote scientific integrity and prevent scientific misconduct and to provide both formal (i.e., course work) and informal methods (e.g., mentoring opportunities) for research trainees to learn about the ethical conduct of science and the pressures on scientists that can encourage sloppy science, misbehaviors, or outright fraud.

## Mentoring

Mentoring is a key process in preparing future researchers. In fact mentoring is the heart and soul of preparing future researchers, for it is more in role modeling than in the acquisition of specific knowledge or technical skill that the preparation of future researchers lies (Macrina, 1995). Mentoring encompasses all of the formal and informal socialization activities that a senior scientist does on behalf of a junior scientist. A mentor guides, instructs, informs, encourages, and promotes the protégé and through this relationship demonstrates the commitment, focus, and grantsmanship activities necessary to establish and maintain a research career. Mentor relationships often begin during a formal education program such as during doctoral or postdoctoral education but sometimes extend well beyond and may last for many years or even endure throughout an entire career.

The mentor relationship lays a foundation for scientific integrity. The mentor can set high ethical standards for scientific conduct by role modeling fairness, collegiality, attention to detail, integrity in dealing with human and animal subjects (and research assistants), and in managing research data. On the other hand, mentors may directly or indirectly signal that integrity in the data, for example, is less important than the number of publications that result from the data. In such subtle ways mentors have tremendous influence over the scientific integrity and behavior of future generations of scientists.

Selecting a mentor usually is an informal process, and mentors commonly are sought because of an active publication record, a record of success in extramural funding, national recognition in their field, evidence of the success of prior protégés, and recognition for student accomplishments, such as joint publications. Whether doctoral students, postdoctoral research trainees, or junior faculty, all beginning researchers should find a mentor or mentors who can serve this socialization function and who will support and promote the new researcher.

Another frequent context in which mentoring occurs and influences future researchers is in the employee relationship of student research assistants employed by faculty investigators (Gift and others, 1991; Sheehan, 1993; Oberst, 1996). It is common for doctoral students to work as research assistants on the faculty member's research, with the employment serving multiple purposes, including financial support and hands-on experience for the student and a ready work force for the faculty. This employee-research relationship provides one of the best opportunities for preparing future researchers. Students in the role of research assistants have the opportunity to observe at close range all of the attributes of a research program and to gain supervised experience in different activities of the program. Close supervision of research assistants sometimes is missing, however, and research assistants may yield to workload pressures by cutting corners or outright misconduct, thus jeopardizing the integrity of the study, the reputation of the investigators, and their own careers. Principal investigators bear important responsibilities to carefully orient and supervise graduate research assistants on their projects.

## Research in a Pluralistic Society

Traditional methods of science tend to be based in large part on assumptions of cultural uniformity (Becker and others, 1992). Scientists typically do not understand well, or adequately account for, variance in scientific data resulting from ethnicity, language, race, culture, and religion. Yet, the United States has always been a "melting pot" society with more racial, ethnic, and cultural pluralism than any other Western country in the world. Demographers predict that by the year 2050, whites will comprise only 53% of the population (Morganthau, 1997). Already, federal officials are field-testing a new census questionnaire that will allow millions of "hyphenated Americans" (those of mixed racial heritages) to check some version of the "other" box on census polls.

### Ensuring Diversity in Sampling

To counteract a tendency to overstudy the most accessible populations, the federal government requires that federally funded studies meet guidelines to ensure proper ethnic and gender representation. This federal mandate, although an honest attempt to ensure diversity, falls short of true and effective sampling because ensuring that representative proportions of ethnic minorities are included in study samples is only one, fairly superficial, characteristic. Too often, sampling is done on ethnicity only, rather than other, more relevant but harder to access variables such as culture, religion, geographic location (e.g., rural), and socioeconomic status.

Danger does lie, however, in undersampling on the basis of ethnicity. For example, African-Americans experience twice the incidence of certain cancers than do European-Americans and experience a 32% higher mortality rate yet have very low rates of participation in cancer research. Paradoxically, danger also lies in mandates to oversample ethnic minority populations, sometimes called *race science*. For example, clinical trials usually contain certain risks to subjects; thus oversampling may place a disproportionate amount of the risk on ethnic minorities. Also, population statistics can be misleading. For example, 12% of the U.S. population is African-American, yet having 12% of an elderly sample be African-American is an inaccurate proportion because only 8% of those over age 65 are African-American (NCI, 1997).

## Barriers to Diversity

Future scientists need training in understanding and overcoming the barriers to appropriate inclusion of diverse populations in research. Without training in how to make sampling and data collection methods more culturally sensitive, study designs are often inadequate to the task and may be seriously flawed. Focus group data (NCI, 1997) repeatedly indicate many barriers to including minorities in study samples. These include the following:

- Mistrust of the dominant culture
- Language barriers
- Economic problems that complicate logistics (e.g., paying for child care or bus fare)
- A sense of fatalism in some cultures
- Prescriptive behavior of some cultures (e.g., wives not being culturally authorized to give informed consent)
- Suspicion of federal regulations
- Intimidating informed consent forms

Often, disempowered groups view biomedical research as a thinly disguised exercise whose main agenda is to improve the careers of the investigators.

Training programs for scientists must include both formal and informal mechanisms to prepare researchers to overcome these barriers. For example, doctoral and postdoctoral research training programs should include courses specifically on research methods appropriate for underserved populations. Dissertation seminars should be led by faculty who are experienced in sampling hard-to-reach populations and whose own research is considered culturally sensitive.

## Multidisciplinary and Interdisciplinary Collaboration

Agencies that fund research, such as the National Institutes of Health and private philanthropic foundations, are sending clear signals that multidisciplinary research projects are preferred over those proposed by single disciplines (see Chapter 28). The environment of science has long fostered competition rather than cooperation—competition between individual scientists, between disciplines, and between schools and universities. Funding agencies are tired of noncollaborative attitudes because so many of the central research questions in health care are shared and can be better informed by studies done from a multidisciplinary perspective. When generated and disseminated by multidisciplinary research teams, findings are relevant to a wider audience and thus can be used more efficiently and thoroughly. Socializing future researchers into both the mentality and the methods necessary for collaboration requires planning. Trainees need to be introduced early to both the importance of, and the steps necessary for, collaboration. In addition, they need help in overcoming some of the natural obstacles to collaboration, such as promotion and tenure criteria that tend to overvalue the contributions of the principal investigator at the expense of others on the investigative team and the issues related to publishing findings in the journals of more than one discipline.

## FORMAL PROGRAMS OF EDUCATION FOR FUTURE RESEARCHERS

### Doctoral Education

Although research is taught at both the baccalaureate and the master's level of nursing education, the concerted focus on preparing future researchers occurs at the doctoral level (ANA, 1989). The number of U.S. doctoral programs in nursing increased dramatically in the last decades of the twentieth century (Jacox, 1993). This rapid expansion led to serious questions about the quality of some programs, especially those without (1) an adequate base of doctorally prepared faculty; (2) faculty experienced in mentoring new scientists through master's theses and doctoral dissertations; (3) faculty engaged in serious, significant, and funded research programs of their own; and (4) administrators who have done research and therefore are experienced in and sympathetic to the process.

Doctoral programs that do the best job of preparing future researchers embody the following characteristics:

1. They have a significant number of senior faculty who are nationally recognized researchers.
2. They maintain the expectation that faculty will mentor students into research through both informal and formal mechanisms, including employment as research assistants under close supervision.
3. They provide mechanisms that appropriately support new faculty to promote success in the research aspects of the faculty role.
4. They develop promotion and tenure criteria that require visible products of research, such as publication in peer reviewed journals, presentations at national and international meetings, and extramural funding.
5. They value multidisciplinary collaboration and foster a climate that promotes it. For example, their promotion and tenure criteria accommodate team work, and their position descriptions of distinguished professorships or endowed chairs specifically address multidisciplinary linkages and collaboration.

In addition to the formal, organized, and prescribed structure and process of doctoral education, doctoral programs are most effective at preparing future researchers when the general environment of the doctoral program is scholarly. Ideally, that environment includes up-to-date technology, frequent scholarly colloquia, distinguished visiting professors, exchange programs with other schools, and other infusions of new ideas and cutting-edge debates that serve to stretch the thinking of faculty and students alike.

Recent rapid advances in the technologic infrastructure of research have the capacity to change dramatically how research is conducted and how findings are disseminated. Doctoral programs will need to adapt quickly to keep pace with the training needed to prepare future researchers to keep up with these advances. Traditionally the dissemination of findings is a methodic process of peer review followed often by a lengthy period of revisions, additional reviews, and, finally, publication. Computer technology now allows rapid electronic dissemination of findings with or without a prior peer review. If future researchers ignore computer-disseminated findings as being of questionable validity, they may lag behind other scientists who will appear more up-to-date to funding agencies. On the other hand, if future researchers use computer-disseminated findings that have not had rigorous peer review, the merit of the work may later be open to question. This is just one example of the many technology-based changes that doctoral programs must consider as they prepare future researchers.

### Postdoctoral Research Training

In the past decade, postdoctoral research training in nursing has changed from exotic to common, which is due in large part to funding by the National Institute of Nursing Research (NINR) for postdoctoral research training (Grady, 1996). In keeping with its commitment to prepare future scientists, NINR has committed significant funding to both institutional and individual postdoctoral research training awards (see Chapter 27). The institutional mechanism allows research-intensive schools to compete for these 5-year awards, which, if funded, provide the school with the resources to select and train highly qualified doctorally prepared nurse scientists.

The individual mechanism allows an individual applicant to submit a proposal for a proposed postdoctoral training experience with a faculty mentor. In both mechanisms the underlying purpose of postdoctoral research training is for beginning nurse scientists to acquire the necessary methodologic and substantive expertise and hands-on experience in a funded, ongoing program of the sponsor's research to become successful researchers in their own right (Lev and others, 1990).

Postdoctoral research training usually focuses on grantsmanship skills that include grant writing, administering a funded program of research, hiring and supervising research assistants, preparing reports, managing budgets, and disseminating findings. The mentorship model is crucial to the postdoctoral research experience because typically the postdoctoral program is based on an individually negotiated plan between a senior scientist and a protégé, with the protégé working in the senior researcher's funded program.

Postdoctoral research programs should have a research environment rich in well-developed resources that include experienced nurse scientists and support personnel, such as statisticians, methodologists, and computer specialists. Ideally, postdoctoral research trainees have private offices, preferably in a research environment such as within the school's office of research. They need the same state-of-the art equipment as faculty to conduct research. The best training environment is one in which peer review, multidisciplinary collaboration, and high ethical standards prevail. Postdoctoral research trainees should be actively involved as participant-observers and junior scientists during peer review sessions for faculty as faculty prepare their own research proposals. Through such mentoring and acculturation processes, postdoctoral trainees learn the essential skills of peer review, as well as improve their own grantsmanship abilities.

## SUPPORT AND DEVELOPMENT OF FACULTY

Although specific training to be a researcher occurs during formal training programs, both doctoral and postdoctoral, the environment in which postgraduate nurse scientists work has a lot to do with whether their research flourishes. Schools of nursing with the highest research productivity generally address the research mission within the school's strategic plan, thus designating resources and making strategies and outcomes explicit. For example, a school might set a strategic goal to increase the amount of research funding by a certain percent within a given time frame and to allocate specific support to faculty to achieve this, such as release time from teaching, additional help with preparing proposals, or by consultant visits. A particular area of faculty research strength might be identified and extra resources allocated to build a "Center for Excellence" or to lay the foundation for a future postdoctoral research program.

The most successful research environments have an organizational structure and process that explicitly fosters an environment that is supportive of research. For example, designing a position within the organizational structure of the school for an associate dean for research and having that individual administer a research unit of support personnel (e.g., statisticians, computer specialists, grants management staff), indicates the school's commitment to the research mission and to supporting faculty in that research mission.

Preparing future researchers includes attending to faculty assignments to encourage research productivity. The associate dean for research usually has the job of working with other administrators to make teaching assignments and other workload considerations so that faculty ready to move their research forward can be protected from excessive teaching assignments.

New faculty, fresh from doctoral or postdoctoral training, must be mentored into the faculty role with an eye toward their programs of scholarship. They may need an explicit message that manuscripts from their doctoral and postdoctoral research need to be published without delay. Teaching and committee assignments should be adjusted for new faculty, specifically and explicitly in recognition of planned research projects. One mechanism that facilitates this kind of planning is the "faculty activity plan," which is simply an annual negotiated agreement about assignments and planned products, such as developing a proposal for a pilot study that is needed in preparation for a major research grant application. In this way systematic planning can occur that will make faculty's short- and long-term research goals achievable.

## CONCLUSION

Preparing nurse researchers for the future requires planning in the present. A major responsibility of nurse educators and program planners is careful analysis of factors that can bring about the preferred future in the discipline of nursing. In nursing science and research, those factors relate to ensuring high ethical standards in research, preparing for the nation's ethnic diversity, and recognizing the importance of multidisciplinary collaboration. Doctoral education, postdoctoral research training, and support for faculty development are the three main avenues in which the preparation of future researchers occur.

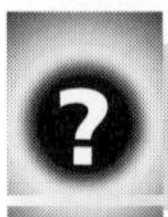

## *Discussion Exercises*

1. A friend asks you why nursing research is important. What would you say?
2. What are the challenges a faculty member faces in implementing a program of research?
3. What suggestions do you have for improving the preparation of nurse researchers? Be bold.

## References

American Nurses Association (ANA): Education for participation in nursing research, position statement, 1989.

Becker DM and others: *Health behavior research in minority populations: access, design, and implementation,* PHS, NIH Pub No. 92-2965, 1992.

Gift AG and others: Utilizing research assistants and maintaining research integrity, *Res Nurs Health* 14:229, 1991.

Grady PA: Landmark anniversary for nursing research at the National Institutes of Health, *Image J Nurs Sch* 28(1):4, 1996.

Jacox A: Estimates of the supply and demand for doctorally prepared nurses, *Nurs Outlook* 41(1):43, 1993.

Lev E and others: The postdoctoral fellowship experiences, *Image J Nurs Sch* 22(2):116, 1990.

Macrina FL: *Scientific integrity,* Washington, DC, 1995, American Society for Microbiology.

Morganthau T: Face of the future: America 2000, *Newsweek* 58, January 27, 1997.

National Academy Press: *On being a scientist: responsible conduct in research,* ed 2, Washington, DC, 1995, The Academy.

National Cancer Institute (NCI): *Minority health strategies: increasing participation in clinical cancer research,* Pacific Northwest Regional Conference, Portland, Ore, April 18-19, 1997.

National Institutes of Health (NIH): *Investment for humanity: a strategic vision for the National Institutes of Health,* Bethesda, Md, 1993, The Institutes.

National Institutes of Health (NIH): *Guide to grants and contracts,* 24(25), July 14, 1995.

National Institutes of Health (NIH): *Guide to grants and contracts,* 25(10), March 29, 1996.

Oberst MT: Student research assistants: an ounce of prevention, *Res Nurs Health* 19:259, 1996 (editorial).

Sheehan J: Issues in the supervision of postgraduate research students in nursing, *J Adv Nurs* 18:880, 1993.

# 30 Career Trajectory of a Nurse Scientist

**Ada Sue Hinshaw**

*Far and away the best prize that life offers is the chance to work hard at work worth doing.*

**Theodore Roosevelt**

A career trajectory for the nurse scientist has evolved in the past two decades. Such a career trajectory for the nurse researcher is a new tradition for the nursing discipline (Hinshaw, 1994). A career trajectory consists of a lifetime commitment to the learning and relearning required during a scientific career. Staying on the "cutting edge of science" demands strong basic research preparation plus a continual renewal of both methodologic and content knowledge in the chosen field of study. In nursing, research capability is built on a solid base of clinical knowledge and skills that is constantly updated in terms of being sensitive to the major issues of the clinical area.

The basis for a nurse investigator's involvement in a lifetime career trajectory is a major commitment to the need to build a strong base of knowledge to guide nursing practice, the excitement and creativity of the scientific inquiry process, and the discovery process involved in research. There are both frustrations and disappointments, as well as new discoveries and "break-throughs," in such knowledge-building endeavors (National Academy of Sciences, 1995). Long-term research programs encompass both experiences, but ultimately progress for the discipline is "predicated on the development of a community of scholars who have a passion for substance" (Meleis, 1992). Such a community of scholars provides intellectual stimulation, constructive criticism and review, as well as collegial support and encouragement. These community attributes facilitate commitment to a long-term career trajectory in science.

## STAGES OF A SCIENTIFIC CAREER

A career trajectory in research involves a series of stages of educational development in scientific preparation that are overlapping and not totally exclusive (Hinshaw, 1994). These include a predoctoral stage, postdoctoral stage, mid-career stage, and senior investigator stage. The *predoctoral stage* includes 3 to 5 years of study culminating in an earned doctorate. *Postdoctoral study* refers to 1 to 3 years of independent research experience with a senior mentor in a specific, chosen field of nursing research. The *mid-career* stage involves a concentration in research study after the successful beginning of an investigators' research program to learn new methodologic and/or content knowledge and skills. The *senior investigator* career stage involves a period of reflection to review a long-term research program and to redirect such a program, possibly including the acquisition of new knowledge and skills. This chapter primarily addresses the predoctoral and postdoctoral programs of study, as well as the environment needed to ensure quality experiences for individuals in these early stages of their scientific careers.

## PREDOCTORAL CAREER STAGE

Acquiring an earned doctorate is the first step in a long-term career in nursing research. However, the understanding and valuing of research begins in the baccalaureate and master's program for nursing professionals. Realizing the importance of research in providing the body of knowledge needed to guide nursing practice is part of the initial socialization of nurses into the profession. Research courses emphasizing the critique and application of research-based findings in practice are an integral part of the these early professional degree programs. The master's program also provides the strong clinical specialization for nurses that is the basis for the conduct of relevant, scientifically rigorous practice research as a nurse scientist.

Doctoral study is the period of socialization into the basic characteristics of being a scientist. The core values of the "enterprise" are instilled during this period: "honesty, skepticism, fairness, collegiality, and openness" (National Academy of Sciences, 1995). Meleis (1992) suggests that doctoral study involves becoming both a scientist and a scholar.

> A difference exists between becoming a scientist and a scholar. A scientist deliberately and systematically pursues the development or testing of knowledge; the scientist finds answers for significant disciplinary questions. A scholar is a thinker, one who conceptualizes the questions as well as pursues the answers. A scholar is able to see the questions as parts of the whole of the discipline. A scholar has a sense of history, a vision of the whole, a commitment to a discipline and an understanding of how scientific work is related to the discipline's mission.

These values and attitudes toward scholarship and science are imparted during 3 to 5 years of full-time study toward an earned doctoral degree. Many nurses in doctoral programs are nontraditional students, for example, returning to school at a later stage of their lives with varying degrees of clinical and research experience. Data from the American Association of Colleges of Nursing (AACN) show that the average doctorally prepared nurse starts his or her academic career at 46.5 years of age. Although their maturity and experience brings a richness to their scientific careers, it is extremely difficult to build their research programs and to be able to use the results in practice and health policy in the time frame allowed by this career pattern. Hinshaw and Ketefian (1996) recommend a "fast tracking" of certain students who are research oriented from the beginning of their nursing careers. This means moving individuals through the baccalaureate to master's, to doctoral, to postdoctoral programs with very few or limited interruptions.

### The PhD and the DNS

In nursing two types of doctoral degrees are most prevalent: the Doctor of Philosophy (PhD) and the Doctor of Nursing Science (DNS) (see Appendix B). In theory the PhD is a doctoral research degree, which prepares the individual to generate knowledge and conduct original research for nursing, whereas the DNS is a professional doctoral degree, which enables the individual to conduct research with an emphasis on its application and usability in practice. Starck and her colleagues (1993) argue that the professional program is critical for the preparation of clinical leaders in nursing. Farren (1991) suggests that, to date, the type of degree is not as predictive of ultimate research productivity as the involvement of doctoral students in faculty research programs. This role modeling and immersion into research is the most important factor in doctoral students being socialized successfully into the scientific investigator role (see Chapter 29).

## Program Content

The doctoral programs in nursing focus on the content or substance of the discipline; theory, research methodologies, and analysis methods; and cognate courses. The substance, or content, of the discipline can be organized in a variety of ways. Ziemer and her colleagues (1992) studied 44 doctoral programs in nursing. The content of nursing was often organized according to clinical program areas of specialization such as medical-surgical nursing, pediatric nursing, or psychiatric nursing. According to Ketefian (1993) the essential content of nursing in doctoral programs can be organized around three foci: health promotion and risk reduction; acute, critical, and long-term care; and nursing/health systems. In some doctoral programs the role content of the profession is one of the foci (e.g., the educator or administrator role). A small number of doctoral students prepare for the role of a nurse researcher in a clinical agency, usually a hospital (Dennis, 1991).

Other content focuses on the theories that describe the major concepts of interest to the discipline and their interrelationships (e.g., Roy's Adaptation Model). A survey of 434 deans in 1993 suggested that five foci would be the most important in the future for program development and funding capability: "psychosocial processes, biophysical processes, health care delivery systems and administration, education, and methodology and instrumentation" (Sherwen and others, 1993).

All the doctoral programs include an emphasis on theory construction, research methodologies, and/or analysis methods. These courses may be taught within the nursing program, or in related interdisciplinary fields, especially the research and statistics courses. The nature and number of cognate courses varies by program; however, three to four are usually required and are often in the social or biologic sciences, depending on the research interest of the student. Dissertations are required in all of the programs, but dissertation seminars are offered only in about a quarter of the programs (Ziemer and others, 1992).

## Mentoring

Mentoring is the process most critical to successful socialization into a scientific career and to ensuring quality in a doctoral program. In *Mentoring: The Tao of Giving and Receiving Wisdom*, Huang and Lynch (1995) define *mentoring* as an interactive process of learning in which the reward is twofold: reaching one's goals and professionally growing together. Both mentor and mentee gain in ideas, collegial support, and achievement of their mutual objectives. The mentoring process empowers both participants, instilling courage and a passion for discovery. The process involves openness, self-reflection, and a sharing of ourselves.

Fields (1991) suggests that nursing has a long history of mentors and mentoring. She defines a *mentor* as a "wise and faithful advisor/tutor" and a *mentee* as "one who is under the care and protection of another who is interested in his or her career or future." Meleis (1988) has emphasized the importance of the mentoring relationship to the socialization of nurse scientists since the blossoming of doctoral and postdoctoral programs in nursing. In 1994 she and two colleagues (Meleis and others, 1994) addressed the essential characteristics of a collaborative mentorship experience: "negotiated relations, mutual interactions, facilitative strategies and empowerment."

A critical characteristic of scientific mentoring is the involvement of the mentee in the long-term research programs of the faculty. This allows for the immersion of the mentee into the systematic inquiry process with a strong element of reality in terms of the field decisions. Field decisions often require some adaptation of the research process in a manner that does not compromise the integrity of the data or interpretation of the study results. The values and ethics of research are acquired primarily through the mentoring process with faculty.

## POSTDOCTORAL CAREER STAGE

Postdoctoral education provides a window of opportunity for the nurse scientist to lay the foundation for a successful research career. It is the time for contemplation, for regrouping after the doctoral dissertation experience, and for considering the directions that are important for the initial phase of a long research career. The postdoctoral research experience usually builds on an individual's predoctoral area of study.

Reed's (1988) developmental perspective of the early postdoctoral years provides an analysis of the first phase of a research career trajectory. Of the several basic principles she cites, one in particular is important during more formal postdoctoral education—the rhythmicity principle. Borrowing from Alfred Whitehead, who proposed the rhythm of learning philosophy, there are three aspects: romance, precision, and generalization. *Romance* refers to the love affair that develops between the scientist and the attachment to science and its generation. The excitement of discovery, the fondness and daring for creating new ideas, and the delight in tracking answers to riddles and finding more questions is the essence of the romance of science. *Precision* entails bringing to bear the various methodologies and systematic inquiry principles to track the data and answers sought within the context of the existing body of knowledge specific to the area of study. *Generalization* refers to the ability to withdraw and see the romance and precision in relation to one another and grapple with applying directions and goals to the discovery process that has been unleashed.

This exciting process needs the opportunity to be savored, to be facilitated, and to be modeled with those who are seasoned and experienced. Postdoctoral preparation provides novice researchers with the role models; research-intensive environment; and time to discover their own directions for study, develop "state-of-the-art" methodologies for the area of research, and formulate the ties needed for the scientific communities related to their area of study.

From the broader scientific perspective, postdoctoral preparation is a critical tradition for nursing to establish. Ensuring excellence in the evolving science base for the discipline requires building depth in areas of knowledge and being able to shape the cutting edge of science (Hinshaw, 1989). Basic to ensuring such excellence is the existence of a well-prepared cadré of nurse researchers. The concept of "well prepared" involves not only initial predoctoral preparation but a commitment to a lifetime of maintaining the "cutting edge" of a substantive and methodologic field of science. The postdoctoral stage of a research career is crucial because it is the point of commitment and of decision about the program of research to be pursued. In addition, scientists are able to invest the time and thought needed to initiate their line of investigation and experience early successes that reinforce the career commitment when they move into demanding multidimensional positions in later stages.

### Formal Programs

Formal programs for postdoctoral education are those offered by specific schools of nursing in a particular content/research area based on single faculty expertise or a critical mass of faculty in a field of study. Often federal training or private foundation funds are available for such programs. Three features of these programs are important to consider: content focus, timing, and individual vs. institutional funding opportunities.

## Content

From a content or substantive focus, the doctoral and postdoctoral experience needs to be linked. The postdoctoral program obviously needs to build on the predoctoral program in terms of the specific content focus the individual wishes to pursue, as well as in terms of the strengths and selective gaps of the doctoral education. Selective gaps are those areas that, by choice, the individual could not acquire in doctoral study but that will be important to obtain during the postdoctoral experience. These may be substantive or methodologic.

Given the complexity of the clinical and research problems with which nursing deals, it is desirable to build a strong interdisciplinary component into the doctoral/postdoctoral training. This will facilitate the ability to synthesize other sciences as desired from the nursing perspective and decrease the possibility of "reinventing the wheel" in the evolution of nursing science.

There are four alternative models that can be considered for doctoral and postdoctoral education that build on a master's degree in nursing (Table 30-1). In Model 1 nursing is the discipline in both the doctoral and postdoctoral education. This will provide a strong perspective for development of science from nursing's philosophic stance but will not foster the interdisciplinary understanding or networks. Such experience must be carefully cultivated through either minor areas of study or through independent study and research activity.

**TABLE 30-1 Disciplinary Content in Doctoral and Postdoctoral Programs**

| Model | Doctoral Program | Postdoctoral Program |
|---|---|---|
| 1 | Nursing major | Nursing based |
| 2 | Interdisciplinary major | Interdisciplinary based |
| 3 | Nursing major | Interdisciplinary based |
| 4 | Interdisciplinary major | Nursing based |

In Model 2 the nurse's doctoral and postdoctoral education may be primarily in an interdisciplinary field that is appropriate for the area of research interest (e.g., psychology, sociology, biology, physiology). The value of this model is that the nurse researcher brings to nursing a strong focus and application of one of the basic sciences. However, this model requires special emphasis on acquiring the nursing perspective and integrating that experience with interdisciplinary education. For example, from 1962 through the mid 1970s (Gortner, 1991) the Nurse Scientist model was a valuable but problematic type of education whereby students were essentially divorced from nursing during their doctoral programs. Some of the nurse scientist programs were very successful in bridging the basic science discipline and nursing, whereas others were not. Such integration would be critical in this model if the predoctoral/postdoctoral experience is to ultimately build science in nursing and from the nursing perspective.

Models 3 and 4 allow for the integration of nursing and an interdisciplinary experience in either the predoctoral or postdoctoral program. The blending of the experiences would be an important aspect of either program, with seminars or mentors functioning to facilitate the merger of ideas and philosophic perspectives. These models would seem to have the advantage of providing nursing and a basic science interdisciplinary perspective that involves the individual in several important networks for their chosen area of study. It also role models for nursing the development of basic science and clinical or applied science, both of which are important for nursing's evolving knowledge base.

## Timing

The timing of postdoctoral education for nursing may differ from that of other sciences. Currently, many individuals engage in postdoctoral study at the mid-career professional stage. Most postdoctoral individuals are successful professionals either in educational, administrative, or clinical positions. They are mature in terms of life experiences and are goal directed. Will this pattern continue or will more nurses pattern their predoctoral/postdoctoral education similar to the basic sciences and medicine? Because nursing is predominantly female, will the selection of postdoctoral education continue to be later in the career trajectory? Certainly, there are professional, as well as personal, benefits from such a pattern (e.g., the goal directiveness enhances the individual's productivity in the science). In addition, the clinical experience of the individual may well enhance the relevance of the research programs developed. Thus, it will be important to value several patterns of postdoctoral study in these early years while the tradition of such education is being established.

### Funding

The models for postdoctoral education cited above will also vary according to whether the nurse chooses to conduct the experience independently or within an institutional postdoctoral program. This issue does not relate to the type of funding mechanism as much as to the type of environment available for the experience. Individuals may select a program based on a single expert or faculty member. Although the scientific expertise may be available, the isolation or feeling of "neither-norness" may be more prevalent. Individuals selecting an institutional program may have more access to a cadré of postdoctoral students, but ensuring the presence of the faculty expertise specific to the area of study will be needed. For either the individual or institutional choice, the presence of a research-intensive environment is critical for a successful postdoctoral experience.

Several characteristics are essential for the success and scholarly productivity of the postdoctoral study experience. These characteristics include the opportunity to establish an independent research program, the availability of a senior mentor or mentors, the existence of a research-intensive environment, and the ability to achieve initial integration into the appropriate scientific communities and networks.

## Establishing an Independent Research Program

Establishing an independent research program requires that the postdoctoral experience be carefully tailored to the individual's strengths and the areas that need to be developed further. This may or may not require formal course work. Major experiences should include independent research study and possibly research work with the chosen mentor, with the focus on facilitating the independent endeavors of the postdoctoral individual. Hopefully, the ultimate outcome of the experience will be the submission of a proposal for funding so the transition into a faculty, administrative, or clinical position will encompass support for the individual's research. The postdoctoral experience should also involve scientific presentations at scholarly conferences, as well as publishing in refereed research journals in collaboration with the mentor and independently. Developing such a track record is valuable in obtaining positions in research-intensive environments because they show strong potential for continued initiative, creative ability, and scientific productivity. Obtaining such positions are important in terms of future development of an individual's research career.

## Senior Mentors

A postdoctoral experience is generally selected on the basis of a specific mentor or faculty member who is an expert and senior scientist in the field of interest of the postdoctoral individual. Sometimes, because of mobility issues for the individual, the match with the senior investigator may not be as consistent as desired. However, the presence of a senior mentor is usually considered the major criteria for selecting a postdoctoral site.

One assumption about the mentor/mentee conceptualization needs to be questioned: Is the concept of only one mentor reasonable given the complexity and diversity of the research problems studied by nurses? It might be better to consider a team of mentors or one central person but a clear relationship with a number of experts in the content and methodologic area of the postdoctoral individual. The concept of one mentor has been successful in a basic science model, but because the science of nursing is different, the mentor relationship may also differ.

A number of lessons are learned with a mentor(s). Not only does the postdoctoral individual acquire the principles for conducting independent research but also other behaviors are role modeled. Values such as scientific integrity and systematic, cautious rigor with research are difficult to convey in doctoral/postdoctoral programs—such values are better inculcated through interactive work and example. Learning to juggle multiple roles and responsibilities in faculty, administrative, or clinical positions is very problematic. Balancing these activities is basic to being able to continue scholarly productivity in later roles. These are examples of a few of the important lessons that are provided as part of the mentor(s) experience for the postdoctoral individual.

### A Research-Intensive Environment

Conducting the postdoctoral experience within a research-intensive environment is basic to having independent scholarly role models. In addition, understanding with regard to being a part of, or a leader in, a scientific community often begins with the institutional community. Alternative models for the research process and the grantsmanship process can be viewed and evaluated by postdoctoral individuals as they make their own choices concerning the issues involved with the processes. Most importantly, the excitement, creativity, and joy of discovery that is a part of a research-intensive environment cannot be simulated or experienced except within such conditions.

### Entering the Scientific Community

The postdoctoral experience provides the opportunity for building the networks needed with the scientific communities that are appropriate to the individual's area of research. Learning to share scientific ideas, to provide and receive critique, and to engage in constructive competition can be undertaken in more protected conditions with time to invest in such endeavors. Mentors of postdoctoral individuals usually view sponsorship into the scientific communities as part of their responsibility. Forming these networks both in nursing and in other sciences is crucial in allowing the postdoctoral individual to maintain such relationships in the future.

## ENVIRONMENT FOR RESEARCH PREPARATION

Basic to doctoral and postdoctoral preparation for scientific careers is the existence of a strong research-intensive environment for the programs (see Chapter 29.) Quality doctoral education and postdoctoral study depends on the support of such an environment. *The Indicators of Quality in Doctoral Programs in Nursing,* developed by AACN (1993), provides the guidelines for a research-intensive environment. The characteristics of such an environment include:

- A critical mass of senior faculty with long-term research programs
- Senior faculty with strong productivity (e.g., funded extramural, peer-reviewed grants and publications)
- An infrastructure that provides resources for research such as Offices of Nursing Research or Center of Excellence
- A university commitment and infrastructure for facilitating research for schools of nursing

The National Institute of Nursing Research (NINR) at the National Institutes of Health (NIH) also developed a model for estimating research-intensive environments of doctoral/postdoctoral programs. The three components used were type of university or institution, existence of a critical mass of well-prepared faculty, and the presence of multiple NIH extramural grants awarded to faculty. These characteristics were operationalized by Hinshaw and Berlin (1997) as a Research I or Carnegie I institution—75% or more of the graduate faculty are doctorally prepared and the school of nursing faculty have been awarded three or more NIH grants. These are important benchmarks for estimating the quality of a doctoral/postdoctoral program in nursing.

## A SCENARIO FOR FUTURE DOCTORAL/POSTDOCTORAL PREPARATION

In the future the doctoral student seeking a PhD or DNS with a major in nursing will enter the master's program directly from the baccalaureate or within 2 to 3 years to obtain their clinical specialization. On completion of the master's degree the student will enter a doctoral program preferably at a different school than previously attended so that different ideas and perspectives can expand horizons. On finishing the doctoral degree the individual will elect 2 to 3 years of postdoctoral study, having successfully applied for a federal or private foundation fellowship.

The doctoral program will be selected on the basis of the area of clinical research that interests the student. The student will immediately become immersed in the long-term research program of a faculty member who is funded in the area of the student's interest. This will provide a second research experience for the student, because one was also possible in the master's program. However, the methodology is different, because in the master's program the faculty member was using grounded theory, and the one in the doctoral program is using causal model testing of a middle-range practice theory.

There are several faculty conducting research in the general area of the student's interest, which allows for multiple opportunities for depth and for focusing the student's research. One mentor is outstanding and the chemistry between mentor and mentee is excellent, so many discussions, agreements, and disagreements occur, each more exciting and challenging than the last, given the practice/research possibilities. Several other faculty are available for consultation and creative discussions.

The student finishes the doctoral program with several publications from the involvement in faculty research and an original dissertation study that wins the doctoral student a prize at the regional research conference in the final year of study. Firmly committed to research, the student's mentor facilitates her or his introduction to one of the top scholars in the country in the student's area of science to enhance the opportunity for postdoctoral study with this well-known nurse scientist.

The student submits and is awarded an individual National Research Service Award (F32) Postdoctoral Fellowship to study with the top scholar at a school of nursing at a Research I institution. The school of nursing is among the most prestigious in the country. Two years are spent on the fellowship, and during the third year the student serves on the mentor's latest funded study as the project director, completing the experience with a series of publications, some of which are first authored. The student has also submitted a First Independent Research Support and Transition (FIRST) research application, received a high-priority score, and is awaiting notification of possible funding. An assistant professor position has been offered to the student by two excellent schools of nursing with strong doctoral, masters, and baccalaureate programs. Where the student selects to go will depend on where the best resources can be obtained for continuing the research program and where the strongest mentors will be available on the faculty.

## CONCLUSION

New traditions have been established in nursing research, including the concept of a career trajectory and the experience of postdoctoral study. The career of a nurse scientist now encompasses a lifetime of study and immersion in long-term research programs. Investigators primarily in academia, as well as in some clinical settings, invest their entire career in the pursuit of knowledge for nursing practice. These individuals are committed to the creative discovery process of science and to the perusal of relevant, scientifically rigorous research to improve the health of individuals, families, and communities.

The career trajectory opens opportunities and possible resources for pursuing long-term research programs working with nursing colleagues and colleagues from other disciplines. Each stage of the trajectory provides new horizons and new challenges as nurse scientists move from being a mentee to becoming a mentor, as well as from junior to senior faculty or investigator status. The basic doctoral and postdoctoral education provides the foundation for the multiple contributions that will be made by the nurse researcher to the science of nursing, to the professions' practice, and to the advancement of the health of the people in the United States.

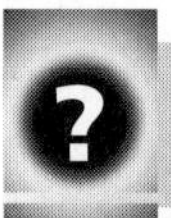

## Discussion Exercises

1. What are the advantages and disadvantages for individual nurses and for the nursing profession if the career trajectory described in the chapter is widely adopted in nursing?
2. What steps should nursing take to promote the suggested career trajectory in the profession?
3. What is your career trajectory? Are you interested in being a nurse scientist? Explain.

## References

American Association of Colleges of Nursing: *Indicators of quality in doctoral programs in nursing,* position statement, October, 1993.

Dennis KE: Components of the doctoral curriculum that builds success in the clinical nurse research role, *J Prof Nurs* 7(3):160, 1991.

Farren EA: Doctoral preparation and research productivity, *Nurs Outlook* 39(1):22, 1991.

Fields WL: Mentoring in nursing: a historical approach, *Nurs Outlook* 39(6):257, 1991.

Gortner SR: Historical development of doctoral programs: shaping our expectations, *J Prof Nurs* 7(1):45, 1991.

Hinshaw AS: Nursing science: the challenge to develop knowledge, *Nurs Sci Q* 2(4):162, 1989.

Hinshaw AS: Developing a research career: a trajectory for career development. In Nursing research and its utilization: international, *International State of the Science,* New York, NY, 1994, Springer.

Hinshaw AS, Berlin L: *The future for quality doctoral nursing programs—are the resources there?* Paper presented at the American Association of Colleges of Nursing 1997 Doctoral Conference, Sanibel Island, Fla, 1997.

Hinshaw AS, Ketefian S: A missing research tradition, *J Prof Nurs* 12(4):196, 1996.

Huang AC, Lynch J: *Mentoring: the Tao of giving and receiving wisdom,* New York, NY, 1995, HarperCollins.

Ketefian S: Essentials of doctoral education: organization of program around knowledge areas, *J Prof Nurs* 9(5):255, 1993.

Meleis AI: Doctoral education in nursing: its present and its future, *J Prof Nurs* 4(6):436, 1988.

Meleis AI: On the way to scholarship: from master's to doctorate, *J Prof Nurs* 8(6):328, 1992.

Meleis AI and others: Scholarly caring in doctoral nursing education: promoting diversity and collaborative mentorship, *IMAGE: J Nurs Sch* 26(3):177, 1994.

National Academy of Sciences: *On being a scientist: responsible conduct in research,* Washington, DC, 1995, National Academy Press.

Reed P: Promoting research productivity in new faculty: a developmental perspective of the early postdoctoral years, *J Prof Nurs* 4(2):119, 1988.

Sherwen LN and others: Educating for the future: a national survey of nursing deans about need and demand for nurse researchers, *J Prof Nurs* 9(4):195, 1993.

Starck PL and others: Developing a nursing doctorate for the 21st Century, *J Prof Nurs* 9(4):212, 1993.

Ziemer MM and others. Doctoral programs in nursing: philosophy, curricula, and program requirements, *J Prof Nurs* 8(1):56, 1992.

# VI

# Expanding the Boundaries

# 31 Alternative and Complementary Health Care Practices

**Nancy Rainville Oliver**

*Our visions of health and healing can become a reality only to the extent that we begin to make them real for ourselves.*

**Peggy Chinn**
1991

There once was a world without nurses and physicians, a world where individuals were the primary providers of health care for themselves and their families. Health care practices, influenced by culture and ethnicity, were shared and passed from generation to generation. Many of these healing practices continue today.

People define health care practices in many different ways. This may include home remedies and/or treatments from nonmedical practitioners. These same practices are frequently referred to as unconventional, alternative, or complementary by medical personnel who, in turn, consider acceptable health care practices as those grounded in science and the Western biomedical model.

Attitudes toward alternative or complementary health care practices were challenged when Eisenberg and others (1993) published their research on the prevalence, costs, and patterns of use of unconventional medicine in the United States. Of particular significance was the finding that one out of every three people in the United States saw an alternative health care practitioner, and the estimated cost related to utilization of unconventional therapies for a 1-year period was more than $13 billion (Eisenberg and others, 1993). Their research also drew attention to the creative and unique abilities of consumers to design their own health care regimens that included alternative or complementary therapies and demonstrated to the health care community that consumers were relieving symptoms and conditions through the use of unconventional therapies. This is a new challenge for consumers and health care professionals alike.

## ALTERNATIVE/COMPLEMENTARY HEALTH CARE

In today's world, activities and practices that individuals engage in for relief or treatment that are beyond medical and nursing practice are called by many different names depending on the perspective of the defining body. The distinction between complementary and alternative will necessarily reflect the position of the current state of acceptability by consumers and providers. Health care providers refer to *alternative* practices as those that are used in place of generally prescribed medical regimens. *Complementary* therapies refer to the use of nonmedical modalities in conjunction with medical protocols. Health care providers may or may not be aware of their patients' use of these therapies.

### Medical Science

The essence of what constitutes complementary and alternative medicine (CAM) is directly related to the current state of medical science and research. The National Institutes of Health (NIH) Office of Alternative Medicine (OAM) was founded in 1992, with a budget of $2 million, and given the responsibility for the study of alternative medical practices. The scope of this responsibility is reflected in their mission statement (NIHOAM, 1997):

> The Office of Alternative Medicine (OAM) identifies and evaluates unconventional health care practices that maintain or induce healing processes that, in turn, promote wellness and alleviate suffering, illness, and disease. The Office supports and conducts research and research training on these practices and disseminates the information on their clinical usefulness, scientific validity, and theoretical underpinnings.

Alternative medicine, as defined by the OAM (NIHOAM, 1994), includes "any medical practice or intervention that: (a) lacks sufficient documentation in the United States for safety and effectiveness against specific diseases and conditions; (b) is not generally taught in U.S. medical schools; and (c) is not generally reimbursable by health insurance providers."

### Classification of Alternative Care

A major contribution from the OAM is the classification system that provides a categorization of therapies into seven areas: alternative systems of medical practice; bioelectromagnetic applications; diet, nutrition, and lifestyle changes; herbal medicine; manual healing; mind/body control; and pharmacologic and biologic treatments. Each category includes related practices, for example, "community-based health care practices," commonly known as "folk medicine," falls under the category of alternative systems of medical practice.

OAM focuses on research such as revision of classification systems and research methodologies to facilitate the continued funding of OAM research. In 1997 the OAM used their $12 million budget to fund 10 OAM research centers designated to evaluate complementary and alternative treatments related to the following: addiction; aging; AIDS; asthma, allergy, and immunology; cancer; pain; women's health; and stroke and neurologic disorders.

A major concern for health care providers is that people are using therapies that have no scientific base and also may be potentially harmful. Data from OAM-funded research studies and from the research centers are needed as health care professionals become better informed about their patients' unconventional health care practices.

### Scientific Assumptions

It is important to reflect on the assumption that has driven and advanced health care in the United States. With the adoption of the scientific method and commitment to reductionistic philosophy, health care professionals embarked on a quest to explain and treat disease and illness. Scientists focused on finding causes and cures and, in many cases, have been successful. Treatment protocols, drugs, and technology have been refined and expanded to combat symptoms and treat our oldest and newest diseases and illnesses. Prescriptions are written, treatment protocols are developed, and medical regimens are designed to provide patients with the best possible opportunities for therapeutic responses.

All of these activities are based on the assumption that patients will comply with written and verbal directives. In an analysis of the principles and assumptions related to complementary medicine, Bratman (1997) reaffirms, "Most prevention and wellness lie under the control of the patient, not the doctor."

## Holistic Medicine

The holistic perspective was recognized and embraced by the physicians who founded the American Holistic Medical Association (AHMA) in 1978. Holistic medicine is described as "a philosophy of medical care that emphasizes personal responsibility and participation in your own health care. It encompasses all safe modalities of diagnosis and treatment while emphasizing the whole person—physical, mental, emotional and spiritual" (AHMA, 1994).

The AHMA publishes a referral directory of holistic practitioners, which also includes general information for the public. Holistic practitioners include physicians in addition to all state-licensed holistically oriented practitioners (e.g., chiropractors, naturopaths, nurses, psychologists, dentists) who may provide alternative therapies such as nutrition, herbal medicine, spinal manipulation and body work, mind-body medicine, energy medicine, spiritual attunement, relaxation training and stress management, biofeedback, and acupuncture. The practitioner (1) views the patient as being ultimately responsible for his or her well-being; (2) fosters and maintains a partnership with the patient, using therapies with which both feel comfortable; and (3) evaluates and recommends treatment options that address the cause of an illness, as well as the symptoms (AHMA, 1994).

Alternative therapies defined by the AHMA are similar to those included in the classification by the OAM.

# WHO USES UNCONVENTIONAL THERAPIES?

In the past it was assumed that alternative or complementary practices would most frequently be associated with culture and ethnicity. Latin American rural practices, Native American practices, Tibetan medicine, traditional Oriental medicine, and shamanism, for example, are all categorized as "alternative systems of medical practice" by the OAM (NIHOAM, 1997). The clinical importance of understanding and recognizing traditional beliefs about health and disease has long been a concern of health care providers. There are major resources that describe cultures, beliefs, and health practices for most of the ethnic groups now residing in the United States.

## Acculturation

Acculturation has been identified as an important influencing factor in decisions to use what U.S. health care providers refer to as unconventional practices. Patcher (1994) developed six categories to consider when attempting to identify people from different ethnic or cultural backgrounds who may be using their own traditional health practices. The categories of people include those who

1. Are recent immigrants to the mainland United States
2. Live in ethnic enclaves
3. Prefer to use their native tongue
4. Were educated in their country of origin
5. Migrate back and forth to the country of origin
6. Are in constant contact with older individuals who maintain a high degree of ethnic identity

These categories are important considerations, but as Hufford (1997) points out, if the focus is only on ethnic or cultural diversity, a large number of people who have adopted different health beliefs and practices (people who use unconventional, alternative, or complementary therapies) will be ignored. This group includes "American-born, English-speaking, middle-class people with college educations" (Hufford, 1997). These characteristics are consistent with the findings from the study of unconventional therapies in the United States in which the use of unconventional therapies was significantly more common among people 25 to 49 years of age; significantly less common among blacks than among members of the other racial groups (white, Hispanic, Asian, other); and significantly more common among persons with some college education and among people with annual incomes above $35,000 rather than with lower incomes (Eisenberg and others 1993). Jonas (1997) helps dispel myths about people who use alternative and complementary therapies when he concludes:

> Patients do not appear to seek out alternative practices because they are disillusioned with conventional medicine in general, or harbor increasing anti-science sentiments, or have a general attraction to CAM (Complementary and Alternative Medicine) philosophies and health beliefs, or represent a disproportionate number of uneducated, poor, seriously ill, or neurotic patients. Patients use alternative practices because it is part of their social network, or they are not satisfied with the process or results of their conventional care.

## Compliance Revisited

People experience symptoms, diseases, and traumatic injuries; their decisions to seek medical care are influenced by factors that are diverse and complex. There are barriers to health care over which individuals have no control. People may use many different health care techniques in addition to adapting medical regimens to meet their economic, social, cultural, spiritual, and environmental needs. Individuals who modify medical recommendations are frequently categorized by health care personnel as noncompliant patients. Recognizing the use of nonmedical therapies provides an opportunity to reconceptualize noncompliance because the individual's "informed decision not to adhere to a therapeutic recommendation" (McCloskey and Bulechek, 1997) may have additional meaning.

Many people have complete trust in health care professionals and believe that all physical problems can be treated, that tests will explain all, and that medications will cure illness and disease. People with these beliefs are usually compliant patients; however, it cannot be assumed that alternative practices are not used as well.

# WHY ARE ALTERNATIVE AND COMPLEMENTARY THERAPIES USED?

Health care providers are more confident than ever before in their ability to diagnose and treat acute bacterial infections, handle trauma, and manage medical and surgical emergencies. The management of viral infections, chronic degenerative disease, allergy and autoimmune disorders, many cancers, and mental illness, however, continue to challenge the scientific community. It is the essence of this challenge that provides some explanation for recognizing and understanding the emerging pattern of people caring for themselves through the use of alternative, complementary, or unconventional therapies or practices. Eisenberg and others (1993) found that the 10 most frequently reported conditions for which the respondents used unconventional practices were, in descending order:

Back problems
Allergies
Arthritis
Insomnia
Sprains or strains
Headache
High blood pressure
Digestive problems
Anxiety
Depression

The types of unconventional therapies identified in the study included imagery, spiritual healing, commercial weight-loss programs, lifestyle diets (e.g., macrobiotics), and those listed in Box 31-1.

Communities are often rich resources for health care practices offered by highly competent practitioners who have not traditionally been affiliated with mainstream medicine. People want health care for themselves and their families and are often willing and able to pay for it, much like families contracted with private duty nurses in the early twentieth century. Specialized magazines and books provide information across all age groups and health conditions. Health professionals have been leaders in providing the public with information about health care. Examples of publications related to general self-care include the following: how to use your mind to stay healthy (Sobel and Ornstein, 1996), wellness (Benson and Stuart, 1992), mental fitness (Butler and others, 1995), relaxation and stress reduction (Davis and others, 1995), and mind body medicine (Goleman and Gurin, 1993).

It is estimated that the average person has about 48 new medical symptoms each year and yet consults a physician only four times (Sobel and Ornstein, 1996). This means that 80% to 90% of the medical symptoms people experience are self-diagnosed and self-treated. These behaviors serve as the foundation for health care that might require professional intervention. Nursing is presented with an opportunity to assist people as they develop their own unique health care plans.

**Box 31-1**
***Alternative/Complementary Therapies***

Relaxation techniques
Chiropractic care
Massage
Herbal medicine
Megavitamin therapy
Self-help groups
Energy healing
Biofeedback
Hypnosis
Homeopathy
Acupuncture
Folk remedies
Guided imagery
Music therapy
Exercise
Prayer

## LEARNING FROM OUR PATIENTS

If our patients are using alternative or complementary health care practices, how do we help them to design the best and safest plan of care? We must learn about health practices from our patients, who will be our teachers as they guide us through their life stories. This means that we will need to be patient and attentive, genuine and open, inquisitive but nonjudgmental. We must listen without challenging or directing.

Storytelling is an ancient art and a newly recognized research methodology. We must assess our learning styles so that we can assist our teachers who perhaps will write books about what they want us to know. Imagine publications with patients as coauthors. We must be good students because the lessons are so valuable. This concept offers wondrous opportunities to integrate the art and science of nursing.

Nurses can learn transcultural information from the texts of, for example, Andrews and Boyle (1995), Giger and Davidhizar (1995), and Spector (1991). Contributions to transcultural nursing will evolve as patients and nurses work together to provide explanations for various health practices used in diverse cultures. Patients are rich resources of information, and we can learn to access that information. Patients can assist in developing assessments to measure nurses' knowledge of culture and ethnicity and nurses' ability to deliver culturally sensitive care. Imagine patients being given the opportunity to monitor the nursing care, just as nurses monitor patient care.

Nurses' responsibilities for knowledge development, dissemination, and utilization would move into new dimensions as nurses develop partnerships with people and these stories are shared. For example, Young-Mason (1997) has published a book of autobiographic stories about experiences of illnesses. Critical thinking activities to facilitate interpretation and understanding are provided at the end of each of the chapters. Books such as these, which are insightful and pragmatic, can help health care providers, patients, families, and the general public understand the illness experience.

Interdisciplinary partnerships could include patients along with health care providers. Values and beliefs steeped in the structure and sterility of the medical model could be replaced by a humanistic approach. The holistic perspective embraced by both the American Holistic Nurses' Association (AHNA) and the AHMA offers a framework for health care that transcends other models. Founded in 1980 by Charlotte McGuire, the AHNA has evolved and developed so that today standards of holistic nursing practice and a certification program in holistic nursing (CHN) have been established. A core curriculum for holistic nursing provides nurses with the scientific knowledge base and nursing practice guidelines consistent with the AHNA objectives (Dossey, 1997). These objectives are as follows:

1. To encourage nurses to be models of wellness
2. To improve the quality of health care by
   a. Promoting education, participation, and self-responsibility for wellness
   b. Interacting with other health-related organizations
   c. Encouraging and reporting the research of holistic concepts and practice in nursing
3. To function as an empowering network for persons interested in holistic nursing
4. To explore, anticipate, and influence new directions and dimensions of health care, especially within the practice of nursing

The AHNA Standards of Practice are based on the philosophy that nursing "is an art and a science that has as its primary purpose the provision of services that strengthen individuals and enable them to achieve the wholeness inherent within them" (Dossey and others, 1995). Holistic nursing provides a framework for explaining and exploring the patterns of health care that have been referred to as unconventional, alternative, or complementary.

## ALTERNATIVE THERAPIES OR NURSING INTERVENTIONS?

The commonalties between nursing interventions and the OAM classification of alternative or complementary therapies are important to note. Agreeing on definitions of nursing interventions was never a simple task, and it is even more complicated today. Clarification between the treatments initiated by nurses and physicians is ongoing, with nursing taking the lead in delineating practice areas. Nursing interventions also are being defined with consideration for interdisciplinary collaboration, international collaboration, and reimbursement for nursing service issues (Snyder and others, 1996). Other perspectives would include nurse/patient collaboration or consumer/nurse collaboration.

In *Nursing Interventions Classification (NIC)* McCloskey and Bulechek (1997) define nursing interventions as "any treatment, based upon clinical judgment and knowledge, that a nurse performs to enhance patient/client outcomes." McCloskey and Bulechek have classified nursing interventions and developed a standardized database for nursing. Comparison between the OAM classification of alternative or complementary therapies and NIC reveal that counseling, imagery, humor, hypnosis, music, and relaxation are included in the category of mind/body control; these also are included in NIC as nursing interventions. Similarly, massage and therapeutic touch are included in the category of manual healing and are also in the NIC classification of nursing interventions. It is anticipated that as research develops, therapies will be moved from the OAM list into general medical practice.

The challenge for nurses is to increase the research and utilization of these nursing interventions. The excerpt from a publication for primary care physicians (Wender, 1996) illustrates the profound nature of nursing contributions and their potential.

> . . . despite the humor explosion in medical care, little literature specifically examines humor in primary care. The nursing profession has led the study of humor including developing techniques to increase its use in clinical settings. There is no surprise here; no health care professional deals with stress, suffering, and loss as routinely and consistently as the hospital nurse. Efficiently functioning nursing teams weave humor through all aspects of their work. Hospice care, intensive care units, and critical illness have all served as foci for humor, which helps staff and patients alike cope with stress and fear.

## MEASURING PATIENT BEHAVIOR

People choose to use alternative or complementary therapies for many different reasons. When patients choose therapies to control symptoms, the behavior is classified as *symptom control behavior* in *Nursing Outcomes Classification (NOC)* (Johnson and Maas, 1997). This behavior is defined as "personal actions to minimize perceived adverse changes in physical and emotional functioning." The indicators used to measure the *patient's behavior* in decisions about symptom control include assessing activities related to the characteristics and experience of the symptoms (onset, persistence, severity, frequency, variation) and use of preventive and relief measures. The relief measures may be classified as alternative or complementary by the OAM. The important consideration is that nursing has developed a way of assessing information about the behavior patterns that patients use for symptom relief. This information is vital to understanding how people develop their own unique health care plans.

Similarly, actions taken to promote wellness, recovery, and rehabilitation are defined as *adherence behavior* in NOC (Johnson and Maas, 1997). The indicators focus on patient behaviors related to activities used to develop potential health care strategies and the decision making related to choices in terms of risks, unhealthy behavior, maximizing health, and self-monitoring.

The systematic use of these patient outcomes provides a common language to begin assisting patients and helps other health care professionals manage the complexities of health care practices. Dissemination and utilization of outcomes classifications can be advanced through consumer participation and nurse/patient partnerships.

## PROBABLE FUTURE OF ALTERNATIVE AND COMPLEMENTARY HEALTH CARE PRACTICES

People will continue to develop their own patterns of health care with or without direction or assistance from health care professionals. Television, magazines, and the Internet provide the general public with information about health care, and individuals make choices depending on all of the variables that affect their day, their lives, and their world at that particular time, in addition to other considerations such as access and availability of resources. It has been predicted that by the year 2010 there will be a 124% increase in the number of alternative practitioners, specifically chiropractors, naturopaths, and practitioners of Oriental medicine (Cooper and Stoflet, 1996). For those who do have access to alternative or complementary therapies, the OAM will continue to provide scientific data to ensure that the practices are safe.

The reductionistic approach will continue to guide medical science and practice, although the number of medical schools offering courses on alternative and complementary therapies will expand (Jonas, 1997). Physicians will learn more techniques such as acupuncture and homeopathy, but the philosophy that grounds the techniques will, for the most part, be ignored by the medical establishment. People will continue to challenge the health care team and insurance companies to provide alternative care. There may even be a health insurance revolution (Goodwin, 1997). The 1997 director of the OAM (Jonas, 1997) offers these thoughts about the future:

> Complementary and alternative medicine is likely here to stay. With increasing patient demand and the search for lower cost health care, insurance companies, health maintenance organizations, hospitals, and other groups will begin to provide these services. Family physicians, as the leaders in primary care, can use the current interest in CAM to help bring common sense and science together with compassion and service in the alleviation of human illness.

Nursing will continue to provide safe care to all persons. Nurse researchers will investigate the relationship between alternative health care behavior and the efficacy of nursing interventions. There will be continued attention to cultural diversity and culturally competent nursing care. Relationships between cultural care and alternative care will be developed, and creative health care patterns will emerge; however, utilization may be limited. Collaborative relationships with health care providers will be efficacious. Nursing practice will continue to develop and reflect advances in nursing science; however, nursing's energy to meet the needs of the nations' people may be at risk.

## PREFERABLE FUTURE OF ALTERNATIVE AND COMPLEMENTARY HEALTH CARE PRACTICES

Lessons from the people will be heard. The patterns of health care developed by individuals will be honored, and nurse/people collaboration will provide unlimited opportunities and challenges for nursing practice, standards of care, and scope of practice. Safe health care practices will be ensured by attention to legal and practice issues related to alternative practices. Geddes and Henry (1997) suggest that: "Nurses have a long history of providing alternative care and must remain vigilant to assure that their right to practice is both protected and appropriately expanded within nursing regulation. A concurrent imperative is to collaborate in the development of the knowledge base for the practice of alternative medicine."

Research methodologies will include therapeutic techniques such as storytelling and focus groups that will expand our understanding from the people's perspective. People who do not have opportunities to share their stories will not be forgotten.

Holism will run rampant, and nursing theories will be revitalized. Nursing education will provide opportunities to learn and study alternative and complementary health care practices. Required reading for undergraduate students will include self-help books and consumer-driven, health-related best sellers. Nursing practice will be energized through the collaborative efforts of health care providers and consumers.

## CONCLUSION

The potential of alternative and complementary health care practices to affect the health and well-being of people in the United States has barely been tapped, but the future holds promise for the proliferation of these practices. Cost consideration, lack of access to traditional providers, easily accessed information through the media and over the Internet, and the desire by individuals to retain control over their own health and treatment will encourage expansion of nontraditional practices. Nurses, whose practice encompasses alternative and complementary therapies, will have the opportunity to be active participants with their patients in designing and providing such care.

Alternative and complementary therapies and self-care activities will have new meaning as nurses learn to care for themselves. Energy will come from nurses assuming the position of role models for health. Nurses are the general public; we are who we care for.

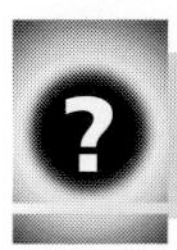

## *Discussion Exercises*

1. What has fueled the recent and growing interest in alternative and complementary therapies? Draw your answer from societal realities, as well as health care.
2. What forces are impeding the widespread use of alternative and complementary therapies?
3. Have you or anyone you know used alternative or complementary therapies? What was your/their experience?

## References

American Holistic Medical Association: *American Holistic Medical Association referral directory,* Raleigh, NC, 1994, The Association.

Andrews MM, Boyle JS: *Transcultural concepts in nursing care,* ed 2, Philadelphia, 1995, JB Lippincott.

Benson H, Stuart, EM: *The wellness book: the comprehensive guide to maintaining health and treating stress-related illness,* New York, 1992, Birch Lane Press.

Bratman S: Alternative medicine: how well does it live up to its own ideals? *Alternative Therapies* 3(6):128, 1997.

Butler M and others: *Managing your mind: the mental fitness guide,* New York, 1995, Oxford.

Cooper RA, Stoflet SJ: Trends in the education and practice of alternative medicine clinicians, *Health Aff* 15:226, 1996.

Davis M and others: *The relaxation and stress reduction workbook,* Oakland, Calif, 1995, New Harbinger Publications.

Dossey BM: *American Holistic Nurses' Association: core curriculum for holistic nursing,* Gaithersburg, Md, 1997, Aspen.

Dossey BM and others: *Holistic nursing: a handbook for practice,* ed 2, Gaithersburg, Md, 1995, Aspen.

Eisenberg DM and others: Unconventional medicine in the United States, *New England J Med* 328:246, 1993.

Geddes N, Henry JK: Nursing and alternative medicine: legal and practice issues, *J Holistic Nurs* 15:271, 1997.

Giger JN, Davidhizar RE. *Transcultural nursing: assessment and intervention,* ed 2, St. Louis, 1995, Mosby.

Goleman D, Gurin J, editors: *Mind body medicine: how to use your mind for better health,* New York, 1993, Consumer Reports Books.

Goodwin J: A health insurance revolution, *New Age J,* p 95, March/April, 1997.

Hufford DJ: Cultural diversity, folk medicine, and alternative medicine, *Alternative Therapies* 3(4):78, 1997.

Johnson M, Maas M, editors, *Nursing outcomes classification (NOC),* St. Louis, 1997, Mosby.

Jonas WB: Alternative medicine, *J Fam Pract* 45(1):34, 1997, (editorial).

McCloseky JC, Bulechek GM, editors: *Nursing interventions classification (NIC),* ed 2, St. Louis, 1997, Mosby.

National Institutes of Health Office of Alternative Medicine: *NIH Office of Alternative Medicine fact sheet No. 4,* Washington, DC, 1994, The Office.

National Institutes of Health Office of Alternative Medicine Clearinghouse: *Classification of complementary and alternative medical practices,* Washington, DC, 1997, The Office.

National Institutes of Health Office of Alternative Medicine: *Complementary alternative medicine at the NIH, IV*(1), Washington, DC, 1997, The Office.

Patcher LM: Culture and clinical care, *JAMA* 271(9):127, 1994.

Sobel DS, Ornstein R: *The healthy mind healthy body handbook,* New York, 1996, Patient Education Media.

Snyder M and others: Defining nursing interventions, *IMAGE J Nurs Sch* 28(2):137, 1996.

Spector RE: *Cultural diversity in health and illness,* ed 3, Norwalk, Conn, 1991, Appleton & Lange.

Wender RC: Humor in medicine, *Prim Care* 23(1):141, 1996.

Young-Mason J: *The patient's voice: experiences of illness,* Philadelphia, 1997, FA Davis.

# 32 Interdisciplinary Practice and Education

**Eileen Zungolo**

*You must do the thing you think you cannot do.*

**Eleanor Roosevelt**

This chapter forecasts the probable and preferred future in nursing with respect to the development of interdisciplinary education and practice. An assessment of the current state of affairs is presented within the framework of possible ways in which health professionals can and do work and learn together. Recommendations to enhance and foster interdisciplinary endeavors is offered in the hope that the preferred outcomes for nursing, health care, and our clients will occur.

## CURRENT ENVIRONMENTAL FORCES

At present, prestigious, as well as powerful, forces are challenging the health professions to find new ways of educating neophytes to foster interdisciplinary models. The literature related to interdisciplinary or multidisciplinary efforts abounds with recommendations for increased attention to interdisciplinary approaches in education and practice (AACN, 1996; Brickell and Cole, 1996; Watson, 1996). A significant example is found in the series of reports supported and published by the Pew Foundation (Pew Commission 1991, 1993, 1995). Multiple and interrelated factors existing in the health care system and the higher-education sector are analyzed in these documents. As a result recommendations are made regarding the education, regulation, and person-power resources needed for the future.

These studies and others cite the complexity and acuity of problems that confront the human service professions and the inability of any single discipline to respond to them comprehensively. In addition, the very complexity demands that health professionals work as team members to provide services that are integrated to meet the needs of patients/clients (Pew,

1995). Hence, the stage is set to forge a future characterized by genuine collegial partnerships between health professionals. There appears to be near unanimity that interdisciplinary practice is desirable and that it should be built on educational approaches that ensure that the neophyte acquires interdisciplinary-oriented skills. However, to date systematic investigation of interdisciplinary practices is limited to anecdotal experiences with minimal documentation of improved outcomes for patients, students, faculty, or health professionals.

The disparities between and among the health professions, particularly the maldistribution of power and influence, are so great they cannot be ignored. They cannot be ignored in planning for interdisciplinary work or in open discussion with students from the various professions. Nursing clearly lacks the financial resources and power base that go with the economic advantage that medicine has. Reimbursement issues go far beyond mere payment for professional work and encompass more than issues of fair trade and fair access to trade. Without the leverage of economic influence, nursing's role will not be fully actualized.

The historic development of the health professions indicates considerable overlap between and among them, yet despite, or perhaps because of, this entwining, the health professions generally spend more time differentiating themselves than in exploring commonalties. Each advancement or step forward in interdisciplinary efforts seems to end with a return to point of origin (Baldwin, 1996). Although all the health profession groups aim to improve the health of the citizens, they go about achieving that goal in very different and often competing ways.

## DEFINITIONS

An impediment to the establishment of a body of literature that enhances interdisciplinary efforts is the confusion that prevails in the way in which different terms are used. The current terminology with respect to interdisciplinary effort is imprecise, and various words are used interchangeably or without clarity as to meaning or usage in a particular context.

In recognition of the importance of interdisciplinary endeavors, the National League for Nursing has created an Interdisciplinary Health Education Panel charged to develop consensus related to interdisciplinary education and practice. Among the elements to be addressed are core competencies, quality indicators for interprofessional education, possible initiatives for pilot demonstrations, and a glossary to establish a common way of addressing shared efforts (Fitzpatrick, 1997).

The following definitions are used in this chapter:

*Multidisciplinary*—Two or more disciplines collaborating to enhance the practice, education, or service of each discipline (Modified from AACN, 1996)

*Interdisciplinary*—The integration of contributions from several disciplines to enhance the practice, education, or service of each discipline (Meeth, 1978)

*Transdisciplinary*—Relates to those outcomes of inter/multidisciplinary work that lead to new approaches (Watson, 1996)

*Interprofessional* care—Collaboration between and among health professionals in the clinical practice arena (Fitzpatrick, 1997)

## CONCEPTUAL MODEL FOR INTERDISCIPLINARY PRACTICES

In addition to defining the elements of interprofessional work, it is also necessary to assess the ways in which health professionals work together. The conceptual model developed by Ivey and elaborated on by Huff and Garrola is useful in providing an overview of the range of ways in which disciplines can and do work together, as well as what level of development could occur in the future (Ivey, 1987; Huff and Garrola, 1995). This framework suggests five types of practice placed on a continuum beginning with parallel practice and extending to interdisciplinary health care team as shown in Figure 32-1. In progressing from one level of practice to the next, personal autonomy decreases as shared expertise increases and the interdisciplinary health care team is approached. The key ingredients of the model relate to control, information sharing, attention to overlap of responsibilities or areas of concern, and structuring interventions.

Although Huff and Garrola see parallel practice as the weakest form of collaborative interaction wherein personal autonomy is primary and professionals share little, in actual practice there appears to be an even weaker form, which is some sort of "taking turns." In taking turns there is sequential attention to disciplines, but no genuine interaction. A good example of this kind of "team" is found in nursing education where faculty claim they are "team teaching" when, in fact, they are taking turns in presenting the content; those not lecturing are frequently not even present for the previous or subsequent presenter.

At the other end of the continuum there is a higher level of disciplines working together than multidisciplinary. When the parameters of the disciplines merge, transdisciplinary work becomes achievable. Incorporating these elements to the concepts of Ivey and Huff and Garrola leads to the configuration presented in Figure 32-1.

## Parallel Practice

Parallel practice is a common form of interaction between health care providers and educators at this point in our respective developments. A number of health professionals may be working in a given setting or classroom, but the actual sharing of information or exchange of knowledge that might occur is serendipitous, and the mode of functioning is essentially one of isola-

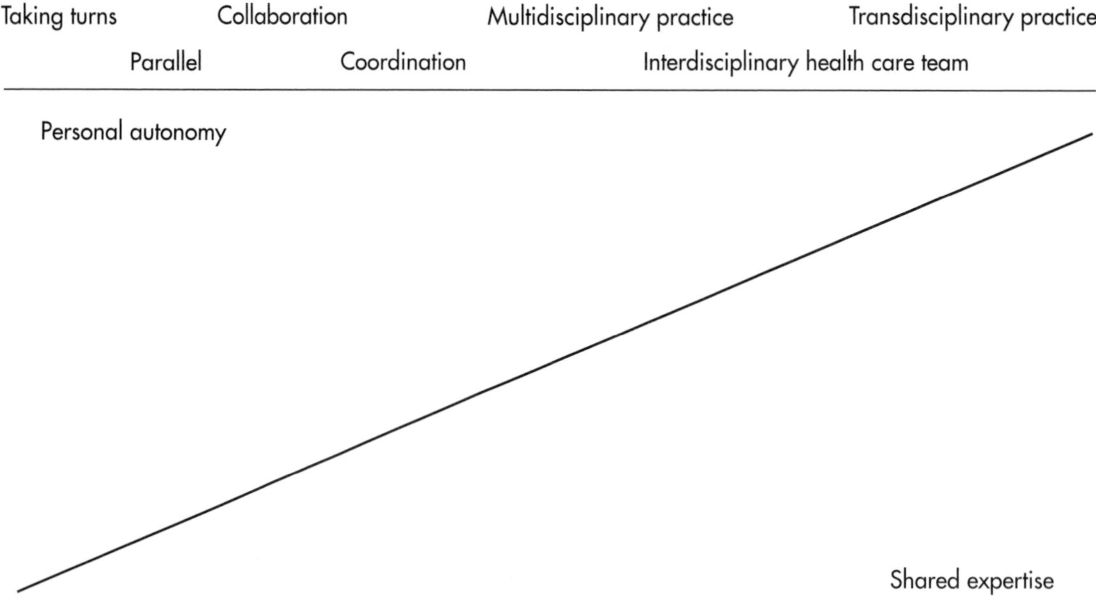


**Figure 32-1** Continuum of interdisciplinary practice (Data from Huff F, Garrola G: Potential patterns, *J Allied Health* 25:359, 1995; Ivey SL: A model for teaching about interdisciplinary practice in health care settings, *J Allied Health* 17(3):189, 1987).

tion. The establishment of opportunities to engage in parallel practice appears to be the primary mode of providing students with interdisciplinary experiences in nursing education. The assumption appears to be that if the students from various health disciplines are in the same arena, they are bound to interact and learn from each other.

## Collaboration and Coordination

There appears to be efforts to develop and engage in collaborative projects or systems of health care delivery. Collaborative research in nursing and other health professions literature report success stories and high-quality research as a result of these efforts (Bergstrom and others, 1984; Hagle and others, 1987). In addition, certain clinical areas appear to lend themselves to the enhancement of collaboration more than others.

Successful collaborative efforts among practitioners in gerontology and long-term care have been reported (Bennett and Miller, 1987; Gitlin and Corcoran, 1991; Clark, 1994). Coordination where services interact and create comprehensive care plans can facilitate patient progress (Clay and others, 1996). Each discipline incorporates the input and plans for the other professional groups engaged in the patient's team. Progress has been made in coordinating activities to avoid duplication and minimize redundancy, and reports suggest that professionals support the work of other disciplines and complement individual efforts as well. Attention must be directed in other clinical areas to developing the one comprehensive plan that integrates the expertise of each discipline rather than a sequential presentation of care as visualized by each discipline.

## Interdisciplinary and Multidisciplinary Education

The distinction between interdisciplinary and multidisciplinary education represents a quantum leap in differentiation. Nursing has been very successful working with two or more disciplines in teaching students and in planning the care for complex clients. We have been less successful in integrating the efforts of those disciplines to achieve positive outcomes for clients. Furthermore, we have rarely operationalized the concept of transdisciplinary care or provided significant learning experiences to the elements of transdisciplinary approaches. The highest form of professional sharing occurs when professional groups transcend the boundaries of their individual disciplines and blend to emerge with new approaches to patient needs.

The future of interdisciplinary health care depends on the degree to which the interdisciplinary approach is advocated and operationalized in the education process. Despite considerable attention to the need and importance of interdisciplinary education for the health professions, only pockets of activity are evident. For example, in a recent study of half of all the health science centers where nursing and medicine were present, only 5 of 35 respondents offered even one interdisciplinary course (Larson, 1995).

# DEVELOPMENT OF INTERDISCIPLINARY EDUCATION

Interdisciplinary education evolved because some educators believed that interdisciplinary approaches foster and enhance learning (Grady, 1994). The matrix of subject matter and content that students need to master as they travel through the educational system has been likened to a jigsaw puzzle (Furner, 1995). Hence interdisciplinary education is associated with organizing and integrating content so that various topics or themes can be transmitted to students in a coherent fashion.

Interdisciplinary study is most commonly associated with the general education component of the undergraduate experience. Usually no prerequisites are required before registering in a core interdisciplinary course; the assumption is that each interdisciplinary course will teach the student what is needed about the various disciplines on which it draws. Outcomes of interdisciplinary course work have been identified as including enhanced respect for differences between and among students and faculty and an appreciation for perspectives other than one's own, including an enlarged capacity for creative and unconventional thinking (Newell, 1994).

The most important component stressed in interdisciplinary education is learning about the way in which a given discipline views a phenomenon. The very heart of interdisciplinary work is the incorporation or integration of disciplinary perspectives into a larger, more holistic perspective. Although interdisciplinary approaches use concepts and methods from various disciplines, their distinguishing feature is the diverse perspectives from which those concepts, methods and paradigms, for example, emerge. It takes years to learn a discipline, yet it takes much less time and effort to begin to understand how that discipline characteristically looks at the world.

## Application in Health Professions

Unfortunately, when courses that claim to be interdisciplinary in content but lack a true interdisciplinary approach are offered, very little genuine sharing occurs. A course developed around the theme of death provides an illustration of what happens when faculty from various disciplines provide a different perspective about death. The goal of this course was to enable the student to "see a relationship among those differing views" (Morgan, 1987). However, each of the 26 faculty members who participated in the course was present only for that portion of the course that he or she taught (i.e., taking turns).

The faculty quickly identified that the learners were being expected to integrate a number of perspectives with limited guidance and assistance and, essentially, no role modeling. Consequently, the faculty added a requirement for students to keep a journal in which they were to integrate the information presented in the lectures (i.e., parallel teaching).

Although this was a good-faith effort to approximate an interdisciplinary approach, the students failed to learn what would happen if they actually worked together to derive something new from the diverse perspectives and observations they brought to the total project. How much more innovative and progressive it would have been had the faculty made a commitment to learn with the students and develop a more comprehensive way of visualizing phenomenon. If the faculty had attended each session, they, too, would have learned to integrate numerous perspectives, perhaps even develop a new view of the phenomenon (i.e., transdisciplinary education). Thus it appears that the commitment to interdisciplinary education may be limited to revising the students' view of the world, not the faculty's.

Unfortunately this scenario reflects a number of concepts in health professions education whereby the faculty believe they are providing interdisciplinary education; however, there is barely parallel practice. Typical are interdisciplinary efforts that attempt to articulate the values and focus of one's own profession to the other members of the interdisciplinary team and describe the expertise of each other's discipline (Lough and others, 1996). This orientation seems to emphasize the differences within the professions.

The continued emphasis in nursing education and other health professions on the centrality of their own discipline focuses on the independence of each profession rather than on their shared goals. An example of this is the practice of requiring students from different disciplines to independently assess and plan for a client and then compile a single case report. As a result the student is generally thrust into the role of advocating for a particular course of action for the client—usually one that chauvinistically advances that individual's discipline. On the framework shown in Figure 32-1, such an approach fosters work at the collaborative level in professional isolation.

Compare this approach with the notion of working together that emanates from the improvisation of artists. What might have been in the outcome if a team of students delegated portions of the data collection to appropriate members of the team and then compiled a single report, noting the interdependence of the work of each in achieving success for the patient. The ideal is epitomized in the work of artists creating something together. As Schoen (1983) notes: "When good jazz musicians improvise together they feel the direction of the music that is developing out of their interwoven contributions, they make new sense of it and adjust their performance to the new sense they have made." This is the nature of the interaction our preferred future should hold for health professionals working together.

In the final analysis we are all striving to find the best approach to patient problems. It is not enough that we listen or incorporate ideas from other disciplines, we need to fully use the insights and ideas of others and learn from them. We will not move on the continuum of shared expertise into the domain of transdisciplinary practice and education until we have set a goal to develop new knowledge stemming from genuine discovery in the integration of the knowledges and perspectives from all others involved in health care (Box 32-1).

## Box 32-1
### *An Example of Interdisciplinary Education*

The College of Nursing at Northeastern University had a unique opportunity to foster interdisciplinary education and operationalize it in practice through a community partnership. Beginning in 1990 with funding from the W.K. Kellogg Foundation Health Professions/Community Partnership Initiative, this project pioneered a new coalition. This partnership, known as *CCHERS* (Center for Community Health, Education, Research, and Service), included Boston University, School of Medicine; Northeastern University, College of Nursing; the Boston City Department of Health and Hospitals*; and 10 neighborhood health centers. Their goal was to find new ways to educate health professions students, redirecting education to the primary care sector.

The design of the community-based educational program was formulated by a large group of community partners, educators, and health care providers and stressed interdisciplinary learning experiences. Considerable thought was given to having the nursing students and medical students learn together. First-year medical students and nursing students in their first clinical courses engaged in shared clinical learning experiences and clinical conferences. Although strong collegial relationships and authentic efforts to advance primary care initiatives occurred, interdisciplinary learning has not advanced as far as was originally hoped. Barriers included problems of professional socialization; inherent, fundamental differences between medical and nursing students; comprehensive, immutable differences in medical and nursing education; and the respective place of medicine and nursing in higher education (Zungolo, 1994).

What was particularly frustrating was that all the parties verbalized a commitment to see the students from medicine and nursing work together in more collaborative ways.

*As a result of mergers and reconfigurations this entity no longer exists and has been replaced with the following: Boston Medical Center (formerly Boston City Hospital and University Hospital), Boston Department of Public Health.

## What Makes Interdisciplinary Efforts So Difficult?

Many elements impede the achievement of a health care environment characterized by innovative, interprofessional care teams who function in a transdisciplinary fashion. Edwards (1997) notes the impact that differences in socioeconomic class, professional hierarchy, gender, and educational patterns have on increased segregation between and among the various health professions, for example.

### Ways of Knowing

One of the primary reasons to organize interdisciplinary studies is to enable students to see the view of the other. If we are to achieve those dimensions of transdisciplinary practice so essential to our patients in the future health care environment, we must carefully assess those elements that impede our progress. We can no longer be like Alice in Wonderland and hopelessly unable to see the world of the other (Gunby and others, 1991). We must develop insight into the ways other disciplines view their contribution to health services. For example, we have the medical intervention plan but rarely see or appreciate how it was derived. Because the medical model is grounded in a pathophysiologic paradigm, it is little wonder that nursing's more holistic orientation fails to coalesce with it (Rowe, 1996).

Clark (1994) describes the impact of these different orientations to patient problems and the profound effect this has on the way in which we function in the clinical arena. He suggests that the approach of medicine, replete with a central decision-making role for the physician, would fundamentally fly in the face of nurses who conceptualize their role in empowering patients to remain in control of their health.

## Language

In addition to conceptualizing nursing care differently from care provided by other health professionals, different language and tools are used to describe and implement our work. Although on the surface there appear to be more areas of similarity than differences among the health professions, we convey information about ourselves in dissimilar ways and talk with our students and patients in various vernaculars.

Furthermore, nursing is handicapped in a society that makes extensive use of linear thinking, which is communicated in our language. As Senge (1990) notes: "We see what we are prepared to see." He suggests that because language shapes perception, the world is commonly viewed in linear terms when, in fact, interactions and interrelationships flourish within a language of circles. These considerations focus on differences in a basic frame of reference. When that is coupled with differences in content, serious areas of disagreement occur. For example, pharmacists advocate for pharmacologic interventions; nutritionists suggest dietary solutions; occupational therapists recommend exercise-focused approaches; and nurses might consider a combination. All of these approaches might be used to address a relatively simple problem such as constipation; all might be effective.

## Conceptual Interactions

An even bigger problem may be, however, that too much attention is given to content and not enough attention is given to the components related to the interface or to the interaction of different perspectives. Faculty may spend considerable time developing the course or clinical experience content from the perspective of their discipline but far less time in examining how this perspective interfaces with the notions of others. As a result the student is expected to do the integration, not the faculty. Because faculty lack information about the relative interface of concepts from the different professional groups, there is no reference point from which students can determine the validity or potential contribution of their perceptions. For transdisciplinary education to occur, faculty must look at the overlap between the professions and the ways in which these elements can be strengthened and developed.

## Professional Identity

Most of the advocates of interprofessional practice emphasize that the student must develop a strong professional identity before engaging in interdisciplinary learning experiences. As a result genuine efforts to engage in interdisciplinary experiences do not occur until late in the student's education. This orientation among health profession faculty, especially nursing, smacks of professional insecurity or immaturity. There is little evidence related to how and when a student develops a professional identity, and we have less reason to believe that developing this view of the world is productive. Exposing students to the ideas and framework of other disciplines creates the opportunity for the student to develop an *interdisciplinary identity.* Such an orientation would appear to be better directed to the desired outcome for the patient rather than one limited to a single professional perspective.

### Team Building and Group Dynamics

Consistent attention to health-related content in interdisciplinary teaching and practice is common, but little attention is given to the dynamics of the team itself. Literature on the nature of groups, elements of team building, and phases of development within teams and groups point to certain features that must be considered in forming successful interdisciplinary learning or practice teams. Some authors identify faculty limitations with regard to information on team development to be a serious impediment to creating the conditions under which their students' education in an interdisciplinary rubric could flourish (Toner and others, 1994). For example, a basic element of team formation is time. For a student to be able to function as part of a team, sufficient time must be provided for members of the group to work together. This does not ordinarily happen in a typical semester or term (Gersick, 1988).

Factors that must be present in a group for learning to take place include a feeling of security with the group, a healthy degree of disequilibrium whereby disagreement is viewed as an inevitable part of working together, and a sense of challenge to explore issues and solutions. Strategies to handle conflict must be developed and role modeled for students. Faculty from different disciplines are likely to minimize differences of opinion in front of students, denying students the opportunity to learn about conflict management directly.

## FUTURE DIRECTIONS

### Faculty Development

The future of interdisciplinary education and practice is faculty development and commitment to teaching students to be members of a functioning collaborative team. Currently faculty lack role models, just as they did as students in earlier phases of their careers. Many faculty are trying a variety of approaches to create an environment in which learning with other disciplines can flourish. Lacking a systematic view or data about how students actually formulate impressions, faculty strive to maintain the impression that everyone is getting along even in situations in which there is tension and obvious discomfort. This is an erroneous approach because students are astute observers of the interactions between faculty in the classroom and in the clinical area.

### Examples of Emerging Work

At Northeastern University, the College of Nursing is committed to interdisciplinary work and is moving toward it in new directions, most recently by establishing a relationship with a discipline not commonly associated with nursing—law. The College of Nursing received a grant from the Massachusetts Medical Security Division to address domestic violence in the community. As part of this funding nursing students became engaged in the legal system of the community, which was developing a comprehensive "round table" approach to managing domestic violence. Faculty from nursing, law, and the Center for Community Health, Education, Research, and Service partnership (mentioned earlier) jointly developed a proposal to the federal Centers for Disease Control that was focused on violence in intimate relationships. This grant provides $2.6 million to implement a comprehensive plan to prevent and treat intimate relationship violence in the community.

The College of Nursing is actively engaged in this project with students, following the progress of victims in the community and in the neighborhood health centers and employing and working with violence prevention advocates. Relationships between and among professionals involved in this project are expanding rather than retracting. In addition, the group is in the process of defining new ways of working with groups in the community.

The Community Partnership project has expanded to focus on developing residency programs in the primary care sector, as well as enhancing the role of the advanced practice nurse in primary care. Although this is a continuation of work that has been in progress for more than 5 years, as new players come into the system, new orientations and ways of working together must be established and integrated into existing efforts.

The accelerated shift from the acute care sector to community-based services provides unique opportunities for a recommitment to interprofessional care. The very nature of community-based care demands collaboration from diverse health care providers to meet client needs. Although there are many challenges, there are also many windows of opportunity to work with and learn from various community-based agencies. Engaging students from the beginning of their clinical education in work with community-based social services, religious groups, and consumer advocates enables these students to develop a much broader vision about the role of health professionals. Students who have initial clinical learning experiences outside of the hospital environment perceive recipients of nursing services far beyond the parameters traditionally associated with the patient role. A natural extension of this broadened viewpoint is a far more comprehensive perception of health itself. As a result of such expanded perceptions, these students demonstrate an openness to create roles for nurses functioning within new partnerships. It is to these students that we turn for the implementation of our mounting commitment to transdisciplinary education for interprofessional care.

### Working at the Boundary

For the future of interdisciplinary education and practice to change radically, an appreciation of the shifting pattern of organization seems essential. Drawing on the work being done in systems analysis, it is evident that the system of health profession education and practice is undergoing maximal change with a genuine blurring of lines between and among multiple functions. It may be the time to begin to focus attention on those very areas of overlap that we have been avoiding because ownership of those elements at the fringe is not clear, especially those areas that currently create ambiguity and dissension.

As traditional organizational maps disappear, old boundaries defining the hierarchy and functions of groups within the organization change as well. To capitalize on this movement, health professionals must be prepared to work within highly ambiguous settings with a sufficient sense of self to function well in a diverse array of roles. It has been noted that in emerging organizations "subordinates must challenge in order to follow while superiors must listen in order to lead" (Hirschhorn and Gilmore, 1992). We must challenge our students with a new sense of investment with others and to listen with full attention to the ideas and examples of their colleagues.

## CONCLUSION

Major changes in the quality of sharing of expertise or in the origination of new and innovative approaches to clinical problem solving depends on the degree to which nursing and other health care professionals make a concerted effort to understand each other's disciplines. Nursing can and should take the lead in bringing an end to the era of chauvinistic protection of one's occupational group. The explosion of knowledge and the diversity of needs that our patients present demand that we develop new ways of responding to those needs and to optimizing the work of other health professionals.

The preferred future for interdisciplinary education, practice, and service is one based on a strong educational core of students from the health professions learning together from their first day at school. Faculty from the respective disciplines will learn and work together in preparing students to assess process, as well as grasp content. In carefully fostered and conducted seminars, students and faculty together will analyze the elements of patient problems and, like improvising jazz musicians, will find new and creative ways to work with patients to resolve problems. In clinical settings health care teams will work together on the basis of talent, interest, and expertise, with less regard for disciplinary affiliation than for competence, clinical judgment, and creative problem-solving ability. When this day arrives, we will emerge as practitioners of transdisciplinary health care services. In addition to enhancing the professional satisfaction such an organization will facilitate, the people we serve will be a lot happier too.

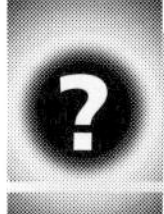

## *Discussion Exercises*

1. What have been your experiences with interdisciplinary education and practice? Have they been positive or negative? Explain.
2. What steps can a school of nursing take to foster interdisciplinary education and practice activities? Be specific.
3. Transdisciplinary practice is defined in the chapter. Using the example in Box 32-1, describe some hypothetical outcomes that could have occurred?

## References


AACN: Interdisciplinary education and practice, position statement, *J Prof Nurs* 12(2):119, 1996.

Baldwin DC Jr: Some historical notes on interdisciplinary and interprofessional education and practice in health care in the USA, *J Interprofessional Care* 10(2):173, 1996.

Bennett R, Miller P: Interdisciplinary approaches to graduate health sciences education in geriatrics and gerontology. In Lesnoff-Caravaglia G, editor: *Handbook of applied gerontology,* New York, 1987, Human Services Press.

Bergstrom N and others: Collaborative nursing research: anatomy of a successful consortium, *Nurs Res* 33(1):20, 1984.

Brickell JM, Cole CM: Using a problem-based learning format to teach CLS students interdisciplinary health care practice, *Clin Lab Sci* 9(1):48, 1996.

Clark P: Social, professional, and educational values on the interdisciplinary team: implications for gerontological and geriatric education, *Educ Gerontol* 20:35, 1994.

Clay JC and others: Patient and family education: an interdisciplinary process, *Med Surg Nurs* 5(5):333, 1996.

Edwards J: Collaboration between nursing and medicine in community-based settings. In McCloskey J, Grace H, editors: *Current issues in nursing,* ed 5, St. Louis, 1997, Mosby.

Fitzpatrick J: Building community: developed skills for interprofessional health professions education and relationship-centered care, Unpublished document, 1997.

Furner J: Planning for interdisciplinary instruction: a literature review. Paper presented at annual meeting on Effective Classroom Teaching, Tuscaloosa, Ala, April 26, 1995.

Gersick CJ: Time and transition in work teams: toward a new model of group development, *Acad Manag* 31(1):9, 1988.

Gitlin LN, Corcoran M: Training occupational therapists in the care of the elderly with dementia and their caregivers: focus on collaboration, *Educ Gerontol* 17:591, 1991.

Grady J: Interdisciplinary curriculum development, paper presented at Midcontinent Regional Educational Laboratory, March 20, 1994.

Gunby SS and others: Alice in wonderland: a metaphor for professional nursing education. In *Curriculum revolution: community building and activism,* NLN Pub No. 15-2398, p. 63, 1991.

Hagle M and others: Research collaboration among nurse clinicians, *Oncol Nurs Forum* 14(6):55, 1987.

Hirschhorn L, Gilmore T: The new boundaries of the "boundaryless" company, *Harvard Bus Rev* reprint No. 92304, p 104, May-June, 1992.

Huff F, Garrola G: Potential patterns, *J Allied Health* 25:359, 1995.

Ivey SL: A model for teaching about interdisciplinary practice in health care settings, *J Allied Health* 17(3):189, 1987.

Lam R, O'Neil EH: *Critical challenges: revitalizing the health professions for the 21st century,* San Francisco, 1995, Pew Health Professions Commission, University of California at San Francisco Center for Health Professions.

Larson E: New rules for the game: interdisciplinary education for health professionals, *Nurs Outlook* 43(4):180, 1995.

Lough MA and others: An interdisciplinary education model for health professions students in a family practice center, *Nurse Educ* 21(1):27, 1996.

Meeth LR: Interdisciplinary studies: a matter of definition, *Change 10* (6):10, 1978.

Morgan MA: Learner-centered learning in an undergraduate ID course about death, *Death Stud* 11:183, 1987.

Newell WH: Designing interdisciplinary courses. In Kleig JT, Dopy WG, editors: *Interdisciplinary studies today,* San Francisco, 1994, Josses-Bass.

Pew Health Professions Commission: *Critical challenges: revitalizing the health professions for the twenty-first century,* San Francisco, 1995, UCS Center for Health Professions.

Pew Health Professions Commission: *Health professions education for the future: schools in service to the nation,* San Francisco, 1993, UCS Center for Health Professions.

Pew Health Professions Commission: *Healthy America: practitioners for 2005: an agenda for action for U.S. health professional school,* San Francisco, 1991, UCS Center for Health Professions.

Rowe H: Multi disciplinary teamwork: myth or reality? *J Nurs Manag* 4:93, 1996.

Schoen D: *The reflective practitioner: how professionals think in action,* New York, 1983, Basic Books.

Senge P: *The fifth discipline: the art and practice of the learning organization,* New York, 1990, Doubleday Dell.

Toner JA and others: Conceptual, theoretical, and practical approaches to the development of interdisciplinary teams: a transactional model, *Educ Gerontol* 20:63, 1994.

Watson MJ: From discipline specific to "inter" to "multi" to transdisciplinary" health care, education and practice, *Nurs Health Care Perspectives Community* 17(2):90, 1996.

Zungolo E Interdisciplinary education: the challenge, *Nurs Health Care* 15(6):288, 1994.

# 33 Achieving a Multicultural Nursing Profession

**Eleanor J. Sullivan**
**Jacqueline F. Clinton**

*We must not, in trying to think about how we can make a difference, ignore the small daily difference we can make which, over time, adds up to big differences that we often cannot foresee.*

**Marian Wright Edelman**

Since the beginning of recorded history, human beings have opposed people who were different from themselves. Appearance and behavior were the first attributes to separate groups; race, religion, nationality, culture, lifestyle, class, and gender divide us today. In the past such differences existed, but many of the world's peoples were relatively unaware of them. They had neither the means to explore the world themselves nor the ability to explore it technologically. Excursions for war or exploration provided brief glimpses of the world beyond one's tribe or region.

Today, advances in communication technology have eliminated those barriers and shrunk the world into one global village. The mass media, television especially, brings every corner of the world into millions of homes. Computer technology enables vast amounts of information to be sent down the hall or around the world. Telecommunication networks allow simultaneous interactions among participants in distant locations, and air transportation offers overnight delivery nearly anywhere in the world. Worldwide, diverse human groups have become linked by complex, impersonal, technologically driven systems of social interaction.

Knowledge and understanding of and respect for different cultures, values, beliefs, traditions, behaviors, and patterns of living, however, have not kept up with technology. Ethnocentrism encourages using oneself as the standard for others who are culturally different; for example, those of a different ethnicity, gender, religion, or nationality. The world is far behind in recognizing, accommodating, and valuing human diversity, and the nursing profession is no exception.

## DIVERSITY AND ASSIMILATION

The spectrum of diversity and assimilation among and within different groups around the world varies from country to country. In some parts of the world uniformity of certain beliefs and practices is required by law or religious dictates, which may be one and the same. Other nations allow for and protect individual freedoms and have been more open to the foreign born and their traditional patterns of living. Historically, before the 1924 National Origins Restriction Act, United States' liberal immigration policies led to the rich cultural diversity of the U.S. population that exists today.

### Demographics Today

With the exception of Native Americans, few Americans have original ancestors born in this country. The United States was a haven to many who suffered persecution because of their religious beliefs, cultural traditions, or generations of unrelenting poverty. The United States had vast natural resources, developing industries needing workers, and unexplored territories. Many immigrants imagined that streets in the United States were paved in gold. Hence, U.S. immigration policies before the twentieth century, the enslavement of Africans, and the perseverance of Native Americans ensured the diverse population in this country today; it is the most culturally diverse nation in the world.

The population of the United States of approximately 250 million is three-fourths (72.3%) European-American, 12.5% African-American, 10.6% Hispanic-Latino, 3.7% Asian/Pacific Islander, and a scant 0.9% Native American (U.S. Department of Commerce, 1996). Ethnic groups in the United States are far from being culturally homogeneous. For example, the Hispanic-Latino population is composed of many different cultures and national origins, including those with cultural roots in Puerto Rico, Cuba, Spain, El Salvador, Nicaragua, the Dominican Republic, Mexico, and other Central and South American countries. The Asian-American population is also diverse and includes people from Japan, China, Korea, India, the Philippines, Southeast Asia, and the Pacific Islands. The Native American population totals 1.4 million and constitutes more than 500 federally recognized nations (U.S. Department of Health and Human Services, 1988) speaking no less than 150 different languages.

### In the Future

In the twenty-first century the United States will undergo a dramatic shift in the cultural makeup of its population. Those currently classified as ethnic minorities will become the emerging majority. For example, by the year 2000 Hispanic-Latinos will become the largest ethnic minority population in the United States. Relative to within their own ranks, the Asian-American population is the fastest growing minority in the country. By the year 2050 groups currently classified as "minority" will constitute 52% of the American public; European-Americans will become the minority population (Day, 1996).

Inherent in these changing demographics for the United States in the next century are a number of salient implications. First, over the past two centuries it has become clear that health indices in this country vary according to the ethnic factor, including infant and maternal mortalities, chronic morbidity and disability rates, life expectancy at birth, and access to and use of professional health resources (Clinton, 1997). Ethnic minorities do not yet enjoy the same level of health as the general population. Second, the emerging majority is and will be in the next century considerably younger than the majority population in the United States in this century, which suggests an even greater emphasis on health promotion and prevention strategies will be important in the future. Third, nursing and other health professions are insufficiently prepared to address the health needs of the increasingly diverse public in the next century. This includes knowledge generation, research, innovative practice, and curricula change, as well as professional personnel who reflect the diversity and diverse needs of the public (Clinton, 1997).

## Uniformity Versus Diversity

### Uniformity

At least two different explanations of how different cultural groups interact with each other are uniformity and diversity. Uniformity, or the "melting pot" approach, originated in nineteenth century social theory called *assimilationist ideology.* The ideology suggests that immigrants and minorities should be encouraged to assimilate or become more like the predominant culture. Both formal and informal means are used to encourage uniformity and to discourage those not in the mainstream from retaining their cultural heritages and traditions. For example, job opportunities often require the ability to speak the predominant culture's language. Another example is not having access to resources and facilities to continue and pass on one's religious practices to the next generation.

### Diversity

In contrast, the diversity explanation, sometimes called the "salad bowl" orientation (Airhihenbuwa and Pilneiro, 1988), suggests that groups' different ethnic and cultural heritages should maintain their unique identities and traditions in complex societies. This explanation is most commonly known as the *cultural pluralism theory* and first emerged in the twentieth century in the United States. U.S. citizens with many different origins and cultures have kept their beliefs and practices alive in spite of policies and economics that encourage assimilation into the dominant Anglo-Saxon, Protestant, mainstream U.S. culture.

Many other factors besides national origin and culturally shaped traditions divide groups. Skin color, religion, and other characteristics, regardless of how many generations may have lived in close geographic proximity, continue to create animosity, discrimination, persecution, and even genocide. Racism and ethnocentrism remain the cause of the most recalcitrant problems facing today's world. Gender and sexual orientation still provoke hostilities from subtle discrimination to outright violence. Health professionals have remained marginal to many of these social issues, and little is reflected overall in their curricula, research, and practice that specifically addresses these issues (e.g., research on the effects of racism on health).

### Similarities

Acculturation is directly related to similarity, especially visible characteristics. The more people share the same physical characteristics, the more they are likely to assimilate into the predominant culture, including intermarrying. This explains why Irish, German, and Russian immigrants, for example, are the ancestors of many European-Americans today. Conversely, Americans of African or Spanish descent continue to be segregated, in varying degrees, from the Americans of European descent.

### Language

In addition to geographic and social segregation, language can also segregate people. Anyone who has traveled to a foreign country and cannot speak the language knows how isolating language can be. Imagine immigrants' experiences. Every encounter is unknown, unfamiliar, and unexpected. Tremendous effort is needed to learn the language well enough to be able to communicate adequately and be successful in a new country.

## Diversity Versus Multiculturism

The word *diversity* reinforces the differences between and among people. *Multiculturism,* on the other hand, implies neutrality, at the least, and embraces our differences, at best. Multiculturism acknowledges that there are diverse cultures included in the population, but it does not try to assimilate newcomers or minorities into the predominant culture. As the world continues to shrink, as business becomes multinational, and as communication technology allows exploration and interaction between people from any place in the globe, acceptance of the world's multiple cultures becomes more imperative.

Diversity describes where we are today; multiculturism is where we need to be (Tyler-Wood,

1997). Denial, defensiveness, and attack characterize interactions at the diversity stage. Differences are emphasized and used to separate people. Conflicts result in a win for one side and a loss for the other (i.e., win-lose) or both sides lose (i.e., lose-lose). In the multicultural stage there is an appreciation for what each individual brings to the circumstances and environment. Respect characterizes the relationship, and communication is direct, unambiguous, nonconfrontational, and based on awareness, acceptance, and data. Relationships and decisions are made based on mutual understanding of data, and each party is willing to hear and listen to the other's point of view. Affirmation and fairness characterize the multicultural stage (Tyler-Wood, 1997). Regardless of the terminology used, nursing falls far short of accepting minorities as colleagues or patients.

## DIVERSITY IN NURSING

In contrast to the total U.S. population in 1996, the nursing profession is extremely underrepresented in its makeup of minority nurses (Figure 33-1). This exists in all areas of the profession, including clinicians, educators, administrators, and scientists. This underrepresentation of minority nurses is now at a critical stage and will become more so in the next century, with the emerging majority population growth. People in the United States require professionals who understand the links between culture and health, racism and health and know how to build on the strengths of our ethnic communities for health promotion. Access to health care is particularly problematic for ethnic minorities; an important aspect of access is having a professional you can trust. Some believe that this is more likely if the professional is one who shares your heritage and you believe in good faith will act on your best interest.

To provide appropriate care to an increasingly diverse public, additional numbers of nurses must be recruited from all of the populations served by nurses. What better way to learn which health issues concern African-Americans or Native-Americans, for example, than to have their participation and leadership in the profession. If current downward trends persist, however, mi-

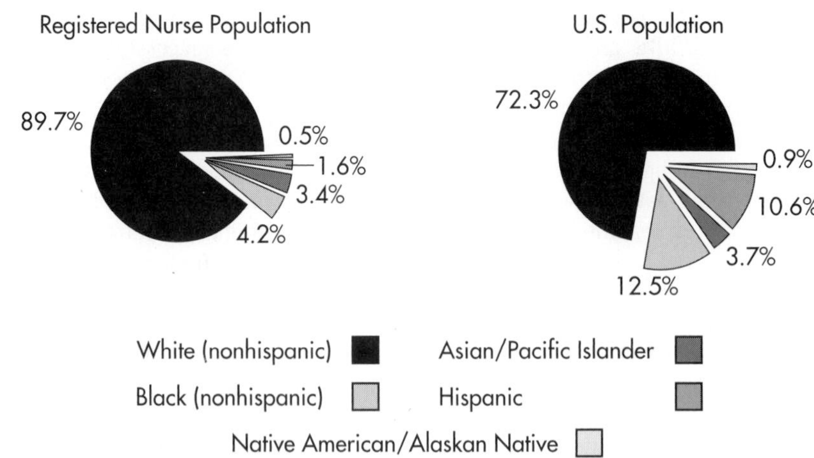


**Figure 33-1** Distribution of nurses by racial/ethnic group. (From U.S. Public Health Service, Health Resources and Services Administration, Bureau of Health Professions, Division of Nursing: *The 1996 registered nurse population: finding from the national sample survey of registered nurses,* Washington, DC, 1996, The Administration; U.S. Department of Commerce, Bureau of Census: *Current population survey,* Washington, DC, 1996, U.S. Government Printing Office.)

nority populations will continue to be underrepresented in nursing as more of them retire or leave the profession and little effort is made to recruit, retain, and advance current minority nurses within nursing. This underrepresentation of minority nurses is occurring at a time when they are needed more than ever before.

Nursing is a microcosm of society and reflects its attitudes and behaviors. Discrimination and racism occur in nursing just as they do throughout the nation. Numerous incidents of discrimination against minority nurses, including faculty and students, have been reported (Tullmann, 1991; Campbell and Sigsby, 1994). Unless these long-established patterns of practice are changed, subtle, as well as overt, discrimination and racism against minority nurses can be expected to continue. As a result nursing will be chosen as a profession by fewer minorities in this country. Ultimately, it is the general public who will bear the burden of our inability to recruit, retain, and promote minorities.

## Gender Differences

The nursing population also does not have the numbers of females and males proportional to the population. As shown in Figure 33-2, the percentage of men in nursing is increasing but still remains small (U.S. Public Health Service, 1996). Many reasons have been proposed for this, including historic roles for women as domestic caregivers. Nursing was seen as an extension of this traditional female role for many centuries. Even after years of nursing as a profession, it continues to be considered by the vast majority of the public as a female profession.

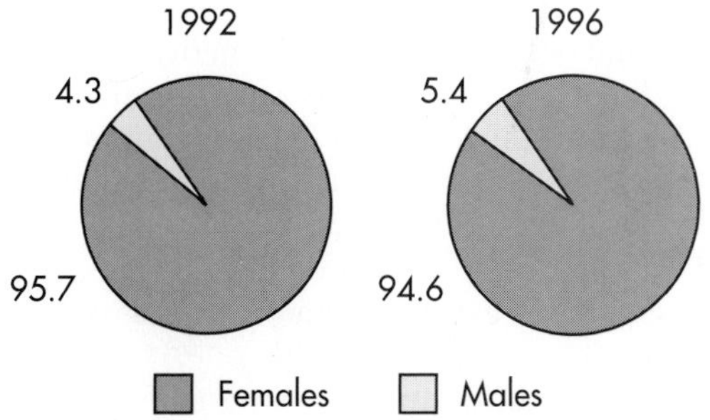


**Figure 33-2** Distribution of nurses by gender. (From U.S. Public Health Service, Health Resources and Services Administration, Bureau of Health Professions, Division of Nursing: *The 1996 registered nurse population: finding from the national sample survey of registered nurses,* Washington, DC, 1996, The Administration.)

Men's roles in nursing are "acceptable" if they work in high-technology or high-intensity care or administration where men are overrepresented. Men are often viewed negatively if they prefer a more relational role with patients and are professionally satisfied by rendering good patient care (Porter-O'Grady, 1995). That there is an "old girls club" in nursing cannot be disputed by anyone who has worked in nursing for long. Unacknowledged, unspoken, and often unintentional, it perpetuates reverse discrimination against men as surely as women are excluded from the "old boys club." Just as racial and ethnic minorities are uncomfortable and often unwelcome in predominantly white schools and health care organizations, so are men who enter a female-dominated profession. For example, how often do you hear the nurse referred to as "she"? How many times do our books, journals, and symbols appear feminine? Not only are we telling male nurses that they are not included but we are also perpetuating a feminine image to others.

Today, when nursing must take its place among the decision makers for the future, we must, more than ever, be viewed as serious, savvy, and professional players in the larger arena of health care policy. Gender neutrality is essential to the future health of the public and the survival of the profession.

## Impact of Lack of Diversity on Nursing Research

The generation of nursing knowledge is affected by characteristics of the individuals who create it. With fewer minorities entering nursing, there are fewer minority nurse scientists and scholars. Although researchers are free to study a wide range of topics, some health problems of certain populations may be of greater interest to those affected by them (e.g., sickle cell anemia for African-American researchers).

Furthermore, interest in and awareness of the appropriateness or inappropriateness of existing nursing interventions with specific cultural groups is less likely if the researcher lacks the experience with the target population. For example, research on conditions specific to females, such as breast cancer, was woefully underfunded until concerted efforts by afflicted women and their families forced increased appropriations targeted to breast cancer research. Another example of sorely lacking scientific knowledge about health was the extensive study of white males with conditions that affect both men and women (e.g., heart disease). Public attention to the fallacy of this reasoning generated a change in policy at the National Institutes of Health, requiring grant applicants to either use both male and female subjects or explain why female subjects were not appropriate.

More recent work has revealed that, not unexpectedly, studies using female subjects often reveal quite different results from those using male subjects. Without efforts to recruit nurse scientists across the broad spectrum of the population, nursing research on specific health issues of some groups and on the effectiveness of nursing interventions in various cultures will lag behind the studies already done on health problems of the current majority. This pattern of public funding for health research diminishes the potential to correct the serious health disparities among U.S. minority populations.

In addition to the population it serves, the nursing profession also suffers if individuals from diverse populations are not included. The influence of any group is related to its ability to generate interest and support from the wider public. The more often the group includes members from various segments of the population, the more likely that population is to be supportive. Legislation and funding are related to visibility and positive appreciation from the public. This is more likely to be achieved when the profession considers the needs of the entire population. For that, the profession needs representatives from all segments of the populations they serve.

## WHAT THE FUTURE MAY HOLD

### A Worst Case

If current conditions of discrimination, recrimination, and alienation prevail or escalate in the future, the advantages of multiculturism will elude us. These conditions include:

- Continued or escalated lack of understanding and appreciation of cultural, racial, and ethnic differences
- Continued disparities in mortality, morbidity, disability, and other health indices for minority populations
- Intensified anti-immigrant fervor
- Legislation aimed at reducing immigrants' opportunities and services expanded across the United States
- Persisting erroneous, stereotypic attitudes, leading to discriminating practices (e.g., Muslims labeled terrorists)
- Urban decay with concomitant loss of business and increased drug use, crime, homelessness, and violence
- Poorly subsidized inner-city schools, resulting in high dropout rates and teen pregnancy
- Lack of concern and support from surrounding suburban areas, further eroding cities
- More crime that results in a backlash of crackdown on criminals, especially minority and poor defendants
- Escalating tension between races (e.g., African-Americans versus Asian-Americans) and religions (e.g., Christians versus Muslims)
- Declining public health (e.g., sanitation, housing) and the personal health of economically disadvantaged individuals.

Nursing could experience the following results:

- Fewer minorities will choose nursing as a profession. Those who do will be quickly driven out by lack of opportunities, racism, and hostility.
- Individuals from diverse backgrounds will find a lack of understanding when they encounter health care providers and, as a result, will avoid contacting the health care

system until their conditions become more serious; thus the cost of care will increase.

Nursing will continue to be divided along gender lines.

Women will continue to find that opportunities in nursing stop at the boardroom door.

Men in nursing will experience discrimination and hostility from female nurses but will enjoy some rapport with male physicians and grudging respect from female physicians.

## A Better Case

On the other hand, conditions may improve. We may learn to value our differences and accept each other for our various contributions, skills, and talents. A serious attempt to understand other cultures and people who are different from ourselves may occur. Opponents to the civil rights legislation in the 1960s argued that the state cannot legislate attitudes and that no law can really improve behavior. Sitting in restaurants in the south today with people of many different races and colors proves that change can happen, albeit slowly and painfully. How might nursing become multicultural?

# MULTICULTURAL PRACTICE

As the world becomes more diverse, so does nursing's client population. How does nursing accommodate cultural diversity? What mechanisms are in place, for example, to communicate with clients who speak a language that is different from one's own? Religious practices and restrictions, holiday celebrations and symbols, views on health and illness, and family roles and relationships are some of the areas of difference that can affect our ability to give individualized nursing care. In fact, being oblivious to differences in others is a hallmark of racism.

Felder (1995) suggests that culturally competent care requires movement from ethnocentrism to ethnorelativity. Ethnocentrism must be reduced from a unicultural perspective to a multicultural one. DeSantis (1988) states that nurses must temporarily step out of their own cultural traditions to perceive situations from a client's perspective and strive to incorporate the client's perceptions into a mutually agreed on plan of care.

## Becoming Culturally Competent

In 1997 the Division of Nursing held its third Minority Congress. Entitled "Caring for the Emerging Majority: A Blueprint for Action," the goal was to implement a nursing action agenda to enhance the health care of the nation's emerging majority. One objective was to develop and refine proposals geared toward preparing all nurses to provide culturally competent care.

All nurses can and must become sensitive to, knowledgeable about, and skilled at creating interventions specific to cultural differences. These skills are necessary for providing safe, ethical care for now and in the future. Individual lifestyles (e.g., sexual orientation), class, religion, race, gender, and culture must all be considered within the context of care. How can nurses learn to give such individualized care?

Awareness, appreciation, and accommodation are three steps necessary for providing culturally specific care.

### Awareness

To understand another culture, individuals must first understand themselves and their own culture and how they are influenced by it (Cassetta, 1983). Families are the center of most cultures and determine how members interact with each other and with people outside the family; expectations of different family members according to their talents, their age, and their gender; and customs that are considered sacrosanct (holidays, e.g., often have immutable customs). Community influences play a large part in forming and maintaining a culture. Schools, teachers, and peer groups exert extraordinary influence in most cultures and determine how children are treated and behave. Adults are shaped by these influences and may adhere to them or rebel against them and behave contrary to expectations; however, individuals continue to be affected by their cultural heritage.

### Appreciation

The second step is to appreciate and accept individuals with different values, lifestyles, religions, and ethnic backgrounds. Nurses must move out of their own traditions to perceive and understand a culturally different environment (Lindquist, 1990). Becoming aware that a world exists beyond one's neighborhood, city, and country is the beginning to appreciating the world's rich diversity.

### Accommodation

The third step is to develop sensitivity and respect for individuals who are members of different cultures and to accommodate those differences into the nursing plan of care. Attitude and the willingness to respond to and respect individual differences cannot be overemphasized. Genuine interest and sincere human compassion go a long way in conveying concern for fellow human beings.

Madeline Leininger (1995), known as the founder of transcultural nursing, states that there are three ways of maintaining the integrity of the client's belief system and accommodating diverse practices. One is to preserve the beliefs and practices that have a beneficial effect. Acupuncture, for example, is known for its pain relief in China and could be incorporated into Western nursing practice.

Another way to accommodate clients' belief systems is to adapt or adjust neutral or indifferent practices. Various religious ceremonies that do not interfere with the client's care, for example, are basically neutral so there is no need to interfere with them as long as we give the needed care.

The third way to preserve clients' beliefs while providing care is to repattern practices that have the potential to interfere with the client's recovery or may be harmful. For example, the Muslim practice of fasting (no food or drink) during the daylight hours during the month-long observation of Ramadan could have serious consequences if frail, elderly, or undernourished clients followed this restriction. Explaining the health hazard of strictly adhering to the practice at this time and asking the client to discuss with a Muslim clergy the possibility of lifting some of the restrictions would be a way to accommodate a client's religious beliefs and protect the client's health (Grossman, 1996).

Nurses also have a responsibility to those who work for them and with them to help these colleagues recognize and adapt nursing care to individual client differences. There is no doubt that it is easier to work with and care for clients who are much like oneself. But that is neither the reality today nor will it be in the future.

It is imperative that nurses become culturally informed and committed to giving culturally sensitive care to clients from diverse racial and ethnic backgrounds. This is not easy. It requires high-level commitment in organizations and from individuals and a willingness to change. It means setting aside long-held prejudices and viewing our clients as individuals and not "the Jewish woman in 321."

## Making Nursing Education Multicultural

Another way to influence care is to educate future nurses to give it. For such cultural diversity and internationalization efforts to be successful, faculty and administrators must be committed to improving the environment for students from diverse cultures, for integrating cultural diversity into the curriculum, and for teaching culturally specific care. The educational program; faculty recruitment, retention and promotion; and student recruitment, selection, and policies all can be designed to maximize this goal.

### Curriculum Content

Meticulous attention to the inclusion of information about cultural differences in our own countries and internationally is essential in designing curriculum content, selecting textbooks, developing lectures, deciding classroom activities, and choosing clinical experiences for students. There are a number of strategies that can be used.

Faculty and other nurses who have worked with clients in various cultures and countries can be both advisers and classroom teachers. Both theory and practicum courses on cultural aspects of health should be required at all levels of the nursing curriculum. Foreign students can be invited to visit class or, better yet, can be recruited to attend the school. Faculty and student exchanges and study abroad programs offer in-depth opportunities to learn about the culture and lifestyles of people in another country.

### Student Recruitment and Retention

Student recruitment, selection, and retention is critical to success in implementing a diversity program. A sustained effort to develop a sensitive and supportive environment and implement a proactive recruitment plan is required. "They don't apply" is not an excuse. Encouraging individuals to prepare for and apply to nursing school who might not otherwise have done so must be a priority. Nurses and community leaders from minority populations can help. They know what will work and what will not in that community. They can serve as liaisons with minority communities, encouraging potential students. However, too often the recruitment of minority students is viewed as the job of only minority faculty. This is all faculty members' responsibility. These young individuals respond very positively when they can see that others in the school reach out and welcome them.

### Faculty Recruitment

Faculty recruitment requires similar efforts. Promising minority nursing students can be identified early, encouraged to consider teaching as a career goal, and helped with entry to graduate school. A critical mass of minority faculty is necessary to influence the organizational culture, to help enlighten others about diverse cultures, to encourage new faculty to join the school, and to provide a welcoming environment to minority students. Nothing is more discouraging to potential students or employees than entering an institution and seeing no one who looks like them.

Sometimes schools may have to "grow their own" cadré of ethnically diverse faculty. Work-study programs, research and teaching assistantships, scholarships, and traineeships can be tied to an agreement for return of service, thereby increasing the likelihood that minority faculty will be retained. Regardless, the school will have increased the pool of minority faculty so acutely needed in nursing education today.

## CONCLUSION

The world of the twenty-first century will be more, rather than less, diverse than today's, and nursing must be proactive in preparing for this diversity. Nursing must embrace these differences and celebrate individual uniqueness. Diversity in our profession and among the patients who depend on us for their care must be recognized and appreciated. Nursing must be committed to improving health worldwide by removing barriers to good care both in this country and beyond. It is a moral imperative.

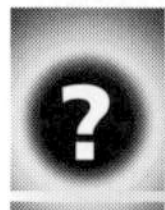

### *Discussion Exercises*

1. What did you learn about cultural differences in your nursing educational program? Did it prepare you adequately to care for patients who are culturally different from you? How would you change nursing education to be more responsive to cultural differences?
2. What are your personal experiences with discrimination? Have you been discriminated against because of your gender, race, religion, or ethnic heritage? Have you observed others being discriminated against for any of the same characteristics? How did you feel in either situation? Did that experience change how you treat people who are different from you?
3. What is your cultural and ethnic heritage? How were your attitudes toward diversity shaped by your heritage? Have your beliefs changed?

## References


Airhihenbuwa CO, Pineiro O: Cross-cultural health education: a pedagogical challenge, *J Sch Health* 58(6):240, 1988.

Campbell DW, Sigsby LM: Increasing minorities in higher education in nursing: faculty consultation as a strategy, *J Prof Nurs* 10(1):7, 1994.

Cassetta RA: Emphasizing cultural diversity to improve nursing education care, *Am Nurse* 25(8):15, 1983.

Clinton JF: Cultural diversity and health care in America: knowledge fundamental to cultural competence in baccalaureate nursing students, *J Cultural Diversity* 3(1):4, 1996.

Day JC: Population projections of the United States by age, sex, race and Hispanic origin: 1995 to 2050, U.S. Bureau of the Census, *Current Population Reports,* p. 25, Washington, DC, 1996, U.S. Government Printing Office.

DeSantis L: A profile of cultural diversity in nursing practice, *Cultural Connections* 8(2):1, 1988.

Felder E: Integrating cultural diversity theoretical concepts into the educational preparation of the advanced practice nurse: the cultural diversity practice model, *J Cultural Diversity* 2(3):88, 1995.

Grossman D: Cultural dimensions in home health nursing, *Am J Nurs* 96(7):33, 1996.

Leininger M: *Transcultural nursing: concepts, theories, research and practice,* New York, 1995, McGraw-Hill.

Lindquist GJ: Integration of international and transcultural content in nursing curricula: a process for change, *J Prof Nurs* 6(5):272, 1990.

Minnick A and others: Ethnic diversity and staff nurse employment in hospitals, *Nurs Outlook* 45(1):35, 1997.

Porter-O'Grady T: Reverse discrimination in nursing leadership: hitting the concrete ceiling, *Nurs Adm Q* 19(2): 56, 1995.

Tullmann DF: Cultural diversity in nursing education: does it affect racism in the nursing profession? *J Nurs Educ* 31(7):321, 1991.

Tyler-Wood I: *Critical leadership skills for organizational survival: moving from conflict to consensus.* Paper presented by Trustee Leadership Development, Indianapolis, Ind, April 25, 1997.

U.S. Department of Commerce, Bureau of Census: *Population projections of the United States by age, sex, race and Hispanic origins: 1990-2050,* Washington, DC, 1993, U.S. Government Printing Office.

U.S. Department of Commerce, Bureau of Census: *Current population survey,* Washington, DC, 1996, U.S. Government Printing Office.

U.S. Department of Health and Human Services: *Indian health service chart series book* (0-218-547:QL.3), Washington, DC, 1988, U.S. Government Printing Office.

U.S. Public Health Service, Health Resources and Services Administration, Bureau of Health Professions, Division of Nursing: *The 1996 registered nurse population: finding from the national sample survey of registered nurses,* Washington, DC, 1996, The Administration.

# 34 Encouraging Risk Taking and Entrepreneurial Approaches

**Joyce J. Fitzpatrick**
**Victoria J. Larson**

*Whatever you can do or dream you can, begin it. Boldness has genius, power and magic to it.*

**Goethe**

The chaos and change expected in the health care system creates an opportunity for the entrepreneurial nurse. Widespread attention has been paid to the current and future expectations of crises within the health care system. As attempts are made to deal with escalating demands at a time when there is a concerted effort to reduce costs, there is an incredible opportunity for entrepreneurship. The nurse, because of his or her education and experience, is well suited for business.

The nursing process: assess, plan, implement, and evaluate is of itself a formula for business success. Who better than a nurse can assess the needs of the clinical practice environment and current practice methods to facilitate change. Throughout the world the same outcomes are desired: improved health care results for individuals and communities, at a lower price, and with knowledgeable health care providers. Such goals set the stage for entrepreneurial/intrapreneurial behavior.

It is likely that without attention toward creative solutions such as those proposed through entrepreneurial/intrapreneurial approaches, there will be a further increase in the management-driven health care system rather than a clinician-driven system. As the business component of health care becomes more dominant, there is more opportunity for creative challenges but also more risk.

## SHAPING THE FUTURE

As leaders in nursing we have a responsibility to shape the future of the discipline. How better to shape the future of health care than from the perspectives of a nurse entrepreneur, creatively and with calculated risk? Our challenge in the midst of a health care crisis is to embrace the opportunity inherent in the crisis and mediate the threats. While the debate continues about whether entrepreneurs and leaders are born or created, we know for certain that there are identified characteristics of leaders, entrepreneurs, and intrapreneurs that can be encouraged, supported, and taught.

This chapter describes the essential components for entrepreneurial development, includes characterizations of an entrepreneur, and a brief discussion of possible teaching methods for entrepreneurial/intrapreneurial development in educational programs. Examples of entrepreneurship in nursing are described along with the start-up of an actual nurse-run business.

## Characteristics and Behavior

The most essential characteristic of the entrepreneur is vision, not a commonplace or typical vision but rather a creative vision. This creative vision serves as the driving force, the motivation for channeling the aggressive activity and the "I can do it better attitude" that drives the entrepreneur. Very often the characteristic behavior of the entrepreneur is described as "naked aggression," but in reality the entrepreneur is a *facilitator of change.* The entrepreneur thinks of solutions to problems quickly, solutions that are innovative, particularly compared with the solutions offered by others. The entrepreneur demonstrates these behaviors in pursuit of a clearly defined vision. The entrepreneur is driven toward goals, and although it may seem that these goals are narrow in direction, it is often because the goal is clearly defined and clearly articulated in the entrepreneur's mind.

Creative thinking (thinking "out of the box") is a prerequisite for entrepreneurial behavior. The entrepreneur is often described as a loner; autonomy is extremely important in maintaining focus. The entrepreneur is apt to take an idea from one area and transfer it to another place where the idea is novel. The entrepreneur does this outside the established organizational structure, whereas the intrapreneur facilitates the change idea within the organization.

The entrepreneur/intrapreneur is the vehicle for the transfer of the idea, its implementation, and its acceptance. The idea gains credibility and hence is accepted through the entrepreneur's efforts and circles of influence. The autonomy that the entrepreneur possesses and maintains ensures the crystallization of the idea in its entirety, from conception and birth to maturation. The entrepreneur demonstrates leadership and strong negotiation skills, skills that can be further developed and honed as the entrepreneur/intrapreneur progresses.

Other important characteristics of entrepreneurial/intrapreneurial behavior include decision-making skills that are oriented to action rather than continued deliberation; a high tolerance for ambiguity (the "grey zone"); a valuing of transitions, change, and at times even chaos; and a willingness to learn from failure and, in fact, a positive attitude toward the values inherent in failure. Often the entrepreneur is described as a risk taker, but it is important to note that the entrepreneur engages not in high but rather in moderate risk-taking behavior. For the entrepreneur the risks are calculated ones, ones that he or she can control (Box 34-1).

## Entrepreneurship

What would the curriculum for preparing nurse entrepreneurs include? Currently several business schools include courses, and some even include a major program with emphasis in entrepreneur-

**Box 34-1**
***Characteristics of an Entrepreneur***

Creative thinking
Autonomy
Leadership
Facilitating change
Negotiating skills
Action-oriented decision making
Risk taking
High tolerance for ambiguity
Valuing transitions and change
Willingness to learn from failure

ship. Thus, it is possible to learn the basics of entrepreneurship while studying management, including strategic planning, continuous quality improvement, business plan development, marketing, management information systems, leadership, and financial management. These curriculum components provide a foundation on which to establish and nurture the core dimensions of entrepreneurial behavior, but most critical are the characteristics of entrepreneurial behavior previously described and the experiential learning that must take place to develop entrepreneurial thinking. The core curriculum also must contain extensive required outside reading from popular business entrepreneurs, business greats, motivational speakers, and writers.

An effective teaching/learning strategy includes student placements with successful entrepreneurs in the business community. Student projects and class assignments must be focused on the development of entrepreneurial/intrapreneurial approaches to real or hypothetical problems. Projects that stretch students' creativity and tolerance for ambiguity are important for developing entrepreneurial skills. All of these learning activities can be built into the educational programs at any level, as well as developed through continuing education programs and workshops.

The teaching and learning of entrepreneurial styles and behaviors also could be integrated within programs and courses offered in schools of nursing, at any level and as part of any course. For example, students could be encouraged to dream of new approaches for comfort and care of patients during clinical rotations. They could design new ways of assisting patients with activities of daily living, as well as with complicated care procedures. They could be inventors of health care equipment or devices to improve care. Entrepreneurial behaviors could be introduced in professional issues and management courses. For all educational offerings it is important for both the teachers and the students to grasp the goals of entrepreneurial activity, to engage in the creative thinking and freedom from the constraints that so often characterize professional education and typical corporate structures. Teachers and students can chart new territory by engaging entrepreneurial individuals in dialogue to explore questions and to entertain endless possibilities during this time of change in the health care industry.

## EXAMPLES OF ENTREPRENEURIAL ACTIVITIES

Many ideas exist for innovation in nursing. Entrepreneurial activities can include new product development; clinical consultation services provided to other nurses or health care providers in a specialty area; development of in-service or continuing education of specialized training for nurses; supplemental staffing and contracting with home health agencies, health maintenance organizations, and Medicare and Medicaid for skilled and unskilled services in the home. Personnel might include certified home health aides, skilled nurses, social workers, social worker assistants, occupational therapists, certified occupational therapy assistants, and physical therapists and physical therapy assistants. Services offered could include specialized patient care programs, patient education, healing or complementary therapies, and technology applications. In the face of any existing gap in the health care delivery system, entrepreneurial behavior offers creative solutions. Given the current flux of the systems and the lack of a national plan, it is an opportune time for innovation, entrepreneurship, and intrapreneurship. Examples that follow illustrate the creativity already reflected in education, research, business, and practice. Box 34-2 describes a nurse entrepreneur's journey from idea to success.

### Product Development

Product development holds great potential for nurse entrepreneurs because nurses are most often knowledgeable about the comfort and care needs of patients and their families. Although it has not been commonplace for nurses to patent their "inventions," we can expect more interest in ideas for product development, particularly in

## Box 34-2

### *Business Development of Ackley Home Health, Inc., San Diego, California*

**Vicki Larson**

I started my own business because of the autonomy it afforded me in professional practice. I wanted to be my own boss. I wanted to take the risk; I felt that I had little to lose and much to gain. I placed the following anonymous quote on my big white refrigerator in the kitchen, exemplifying my desire to start, own, and operate my own business and to keep me motivated: AN ENTREPRENEUR IS A SELF-EMPLOYED PERSON WHO WILL WORK 16 HOURS A DAY JUST TO AVOID HAVING TO WORK 8 HOURS A DAY FOR SOMEONE ELSE. I had an idea that I gleaned from my work experience over the years, and I believed I could make it work.

My idea was not anything new except in where I implemented the idea. I took the idea of supplemental staffing and specialized it in the provision of a niche service: psychiatric nursing. I identified that experienced, trained staff were needed for the burgeoning psychiatric facilities of the 1980s. I was sure I could fill the many shifts available because of the shortage of qualified personnel and do it faster. Even better, I was more cost effective than any other staffing service. This is the first essential ingredient to success in business: the formulation of the idea through the understanding of the current clinical environment. It is the identification of the need and subsequent timely plan development for meeting the need that enables the nurse entrepreneur to succeed.

There were no entrepreneurial programs at the time I started my business, but a new organization started by David Norris, RN, was blossoming. It is known today as the National Nurses in Business Association, or NNBA. Through networking I came to know of the NNBA and attended its first annual conference, which was in San Francisco. The speakers, all successful nurse entrepreneurs, were phenomenal and full of recipes—their recipes for success. I was inspired! I learned at the conference that my training in the nursing process of assessing, planning, implementing, and evaluating would ensure my success in my own business. This empowered me.

Networking is the art of making others aware of your business plan and intentions, exchanging business cards, and waiting and listening for desired results or answers, which proved to never be greater than three people away. I learned through reading; I mastered the art of networking through practice. I actively engaged in networking both knowingly and, frankly, sometimes even unknowingly. For example, I contacted a fellow Alfred University alumnus, graduate of the same BSN program, after reading an article in the alumni newsletter outlining his successful company, Sullivan Nursing Services. I discovered in a future issue that his success continued 2 years later. He had passed the start-up phase and had just received financing for his growth phase. He was anxious to share and be validated. Most businesses fail within the first 5 years of starting, so having passed the 2-year mark, we both knew he had done something special and worthy of recognition.

I did not know, when I called with my congratulations, that he would become my mentor. He enabled me to start my business through his kind sharing and support. I unknowingly had networked myself. I mailed out my first letters to local psychiatric units around San Diego County on May 6, 1989 and received my first booking for shifts on Monday, May 9. The doors have been open ever since. The key is simple: train, educate, and empower nurses during their training phase. Alfred University had done this for both my mentor and myself. Nurses can be trained to come up with viable solutions to health care dilemmas not yet occurring and/or not yet known. We can empower future nurses not only to come up with the answers but also to do so in a timely manner. This truly would be a legacy for nursing, ensuring the health and safety of future generations. The nurse entrepreneur, trained in the art of negotiations, networking, and facilitating change, would exert the influence needed for patient advocacy. After all, it was a nurse who studied postoperative infections, concluding that the surgeon must wash his or her hands before operating. This measure alone has saved many lives and is a standard of practice today.

the expanding area of care of persons with chronic health conditions.

Several examples of new product development can be cited. Many ideas for new products arise from nurses' identification of needs in direct patient care. Nurse Susan Skewes redesigned patient bathing with the development of the "Bag Bath," a self-contained prepackaged disposable bathing system. Nurse Michelle Boasten created "Dial-a-Document," a point-of-care clinical documentation system that allows users to phone in information and enter it directly into the patient's electronic chart. Focusing their work on clinical nursing innovations, Wardell and Engebretson (1993) not only describe the development of a pacifier for low-birth-weight infants but also examine the process for technology development and assessment, based on several years of research and product development.

## Innovations in Nursing Education

Partnerships between nursing education and service have attracted the interest of both public and private schools of nursing. Two examples of innovative educational programs recently launched at the Frances Payne Bolton School of Nursing, Case Western Reserve University, illustrate both the local model and the global model of educational initiatives.

## International Initiative

A collaborative course between undergraduate students in nursing at the Bolton School and those at Catholic University in Santiago, Chile, has begun. Students enroll in a shared course "Professional Trends and Issues" to be offered through the Internet. Opportunities for collaborative projects are presented, and students are encouraged to extend the relationships beyond this one course offering. The local initiative is being launched as a partnership model that could be replicated by several schools of nursing partnering with health care agencies.

### Advanced Practice Initiative

The Cleveland Clinic Foundation Health Care Ventures (HCV), a home care agency based in the Cleveland metropolitan area, is supporting a special master's degree adult nurse practitioner program to prepare the majority of their professional nursing staff as advanced practice nurses. The program is offered in a condensed format, weekends and evenings; preceptors are selected from among the current HCV staff, and work schedules are adjusted so that classroom and clinical experiences can be completed.

### Other Innovations

A number of schools of nursing recently have experimented with flexible course offerings and flexible scheduling to tap new markets for nursing education. The recruitment of college graduates into post-baccalaureate nursing education programs, such as the "bridge" program at Vanderbilt University and the doctor of nursing (ND) programs at Case Western Reserve and Rush Universities and the University of Colorado represent other examples of the creative intrapreneurial spirit in nursing education. Most recently the introduction of computer technology into teaching and learning, such as at the University of Kansas, has led to more creativity in program offerings. Within the twenty-first century, creativity within education can be expected to increase dramatically.

## Innovations in Clinical Interventions

Clinical nursing practice offers many opportunities for innovation and change in practice, and there is strong support in the nursing literature for such innovations. Some of these, such as the Kangaroo Care method described by Anderson (1995), are based on continuing programs of research. The Kangaroo Care method, skin-to-skin contact between mother and infant in the newborn period and throughout the breastfeeding experience, has been translated into practice in several countries and has been implemented with populations other than preterm infants.

## Healing and Complementary Therapies

Concomitant with the self-care movement and the beginning globalization of health care there has been an increasing interest in complementary therapies, that is, those not traditionally associated with standard medical intervention. Nursing therapies, such as movement and music, hold much potential for the nurse entrepreneur in practice, education, and research. An excellent example of the current research being undertaken in the area of the complementary therapies of music and relaxation is described by Good (1996). Patients with postoperative pain are being introduced to music tapes; the type of music is chosen by the patient. Patients then are instructed to use the tapes as a relaxation method to reduce their pain.

Another example is the guided imagery tapes developed by nurse entrepreneur Diane Tusek and produced through Guided Imagery, Inc. The program consists of two audio tapes with stories and music that encourages people to work through feelings of fear, anxiety, and negativity. The tapes have been used with postoperative patients and also with others needing assistance with stress management and coping (Tusek, 1997). Current research on complementary therapies, such as music therapy, guided imagery, and relaxation, can provide a springboard for the nurse entrepreneur who wants to apply research to practice and/or education (see Chapter 31).

## Technology Applications

Technologic advances have changed dramatically the manner in which health care is delivered and research is conducted (see Chapters 10, 11, and 12). One of the most promising areas for both nursing education and practice is that of the application of computer technology to the teaching/learning process, such as in distance learning, and the delivery of direct patent care, such as the use of CD-ROMs with health information in patient waiting areas. Although computers are an important component of the administration of the current health care delivery systems, the future holds many challenges and opportunities for use of computer technology in education and practice. An example of an innovative entrepreneurial application is the ComputerLink project.

ComputerLink was designed by Brennan and colleagues (Brennan and others, 1991a; Brennan and others, 1991b; Brennan and others, 1995) as an innovative response to everyday patient and caregiver problems. ComputerLink is a computer-based network designed to answer questions about specific health problems and/or caregiving concerns of those with chronic diseases. ComputerLink contains three functional areas: (1) the electronic encyclopedia, which serves as a clearinghouse for factual information about the disease, the caregiving experience, clinical care, and local services; (2) a decision support system, which uses a decision modeling approach to assist clients; and (3) a communication pathway, which links clients to peers and professionals. ComputerLink has been tested with caregivers of Alzheimer's patients and with AIDS/ARC patients and their caregivers and widely acclaimed as an innovative nursing intervention to patient care.

# CONCLUSION

Tremendous opportunities await the nurse entrepreneur who is creative, visionary, a problem solver, flexible, and committed. Change in health care (or any system) opens the door for innovation. As the momentum of change increases, entrepreneurial possibilities increase. The challenges ahead present a myriad of opportunities for creativity, leadership, innovation, and the new class of nurse: the nurse entrepreneur.

## *Discussion Exercises*

1. What entrepreneurial or intrapreneurial ideas do you have for your school or workplace? List several and describe.

2. What obstacles to nurse entrepreneurship or intrapreneurship exist? How can these be overcome?
3. Name one behavior you can change or enhance to help you become more entrepreneurial, and describe how you can begin developing this characteristic.

## References

Anderson GC: Touch and the kangaroo care method. In Field TM, editor: *Touch in early development,* Mahwah, NJ, 1995, Lawrence Erlbaum.

Brennan PF and others: ComputerLink: electronic support for the home caregiver, *Adv Nurs Sci* 13(4):14, 1991a.

Brennan PF and others: The effects of a special computer network on caregivers of persons with Alzheimer's Disease, *Nurs Res* 44:166, 1995.

Brennan PF and others: The use of home-based computers to support persons living with AIDS/ARC, *J Community Health Nurs* 8(1):3, 1991b.

Covey SR: *7 habits of highly effective people,* NY, 1994, Simon & Schuster.

Good M: Effects of relaxation and music on postoperative pain: a review, *J Adv Nurs* 24:905, 1996.

Peters T, Austin N: *A passion for excellence: the leadership difference,* New York, 1985, Warner Books.

Tusek D: Personal communication, 1997.

Vogel G, Doleysch N: *Entrepreneuring: a nurse's guide to starting a business,* New York, 1988, National League for Nursing.

Wardell DW, Engebretson J: Technology assessment for nursing innovations, *Appl Nurs Res* 6:172, 1993.

# 35 Nursing in the Global Arena

**Connie Vance**

*Do not fear mistakes; there are none.*

**Miles Davis**
Jazz musician

Entering a new millennium presents us with a scenario of massive and accelerated change throughout the world. The new century will be characterized by various interconnections of people, power, and resources. We will be confronted with social, political, economic, environmental, technologic, and communication metamorphoses that cannot be contained by national boundaries. These factors inevitably influence the health of people worldwide and fuel a growing revolution in health care.

Our global village will be confronted with serious health problems that will require global planning and problem solving. "Nations everywhere are grappling with the economic and ethical dilemmas of achieving and maintaining healthy populations, since these are both cause and consequence of true development. Increasingly, the thinking is global, because there are comparisons to be learned from, connections that have implications, obligations to fulfill, and costs that are somehow shared" (Institute of Medicine, 1996). In short, health and nursing concerns are global concerns. In addition, the probable and preferable futures in global nursing are becoming merged; what will be the probable global future is what nurses are in the midst of creating—what they prefer. The preferable, likely future of a global nursing community is being enacted at the edge of the twenty-first century by nurses in practice, policy, politics, education, and research.

## EVOLVING INTERNATIONAL ACTIVITIES

The global goal of "Health for All" was established at the International Conference on Primary Health Care at Alma-Ata in 1978. This conference, sponsored by the World Health Organization (WHO) and the United Nations International Children's

Emergency Fund (UNICEF), developed the key principles of what is known as the *Alma-Ata Declaration.* These principles have continued to serve as the cornerstone for action by professions, governments, and policy bodies worldwide. They are committed to the following:

Universal access to health services, with an emphasis on prevention
Effectiveness and affordability of services
Community involvement, self-reliance, and self-determination in the development of services
Intersectoral action on health-related matters (World Health Organization, 1979)

Subsequent WHO meetings have provided opportunities for recommitment to these principles. Indeed, the Institute for Medicine has made clear that the declaration's principles were "not a passing exercise in rhetoric destined for policy oblivion but, instead, were permanent fixtures in international health policies and programs" (Institute of Medicine, 1996).

Nursing organizations and nurses in various sectors of health care have rallied around these principles, as well as those contained in other major documents, including *The World Development Report 1993: Investing in Health* (World Bank, 1993); successive iterations of the UN *Human Development Reports* (United Nations Development Programme, 1993, 1994); and *The State of the World's Children* (Grant, 1995, 1996). The nursing profession's core values are congruent with the priorities that are contained in these documents. Primary care and disease prevention, development of partnerships, empowerment, and sharing of human and material resources are the values that have driven nurses' global activities.

The global vision and values of the nursing profession are portrayed by a story of worldwide organizational and individual involvement. Nurses, as the largest health care group practicing internationally (Andrews and Fargotstein, 1986), historically have created a bond among their colleagues, transcending national, cultural, language, geographic, and political boundaries. Theirs has been a sustained and vigorous voice on behalf of joining together through strong alliances and partnerships to improve health care and nursing practice, education, and research around the world.

## International Council of Nursing

The visionary action of nurses was responsible for the creation of the International Council of Nursing (ICN)—the oldest and largest international professional organization in the health care field—in 1899. Its constituent member organizations are the nursing associations of 120 countries, with 1.5 million nurses represented worldwide. Since its founding, ICN has carried out its mission through wars and international crises to improve health services and to maintain nursing's vital role in health care. ICN has two major goals for the 5-year period of 1994 to 1999: to influence matters of health and social policy and professional and socioeconomic standards worldwide; and to empower national nurses' associations to act on behalf of nurses, nursing, and the public's well-being (Ghebrehlwet, 1997).

One of ICN's major publications is the *International Nursing Review,* which provides synthesis of the literature on topics that are relevant to nurses around the world. The international nursing community has clearly demonstrated its vision and values of global networking and action through this influential, organized voice. With its growing membership, ICN continues to position itself as a vital presence in the future of global activism in nursing.

## Status of Women

A future in which females enjoy full human rights and fundamental freedoms has become a priority in the global agenda. Women of the world—including female nurses, who are members of a female-dominant profession—have been the driving force in shaping this agenda and moving it forward. In 1946 the UN established the Commission on the Status of Women, which has been a vehicle for mobilizing this agenda. The commission's purpose is to document the status of women's rights in economic, social, cultural, educational, and political arenas and to make recommendations for improvement (Reanda, 1992).

The first United Nations Conference on Women was held in Mexico City in 1975. Nurses' voices were heard at that historic meeting and at subsequent conferences, including the Fourth World Conference on Women, which convened in Beijing in 1995. In addition to nurses' being official national delegates, nursing was represented in the nongovernmental organizational (NGO) forum by ICN President Dr. Margretta Styles. Many nurses also attended the conference as members of various socially active organizations. Both the American Nurses Association (ANA) and ICN have been active in follow-up dissemination and implementation of the Beijing agreements.

Virginia Trotter Betts, former president of the ANA, was appointed to the conference as an official governmental delegate. She says, "Just as professional nurses are increasingly recognized as an invaluable health care delivery resource, the Fourth World Conference on Women reflected nurses' rising prominence in global health policy discussions, as many official national delegations had nurse members. Thus the nursing perspective of health, holism, disease prevention, and attention to family and community systems was discussed and included in the *Beijing Declaration and Platform for Action*" (Betts, 1997).

The Beijing conference called on governments, the international community, and civil society, including nongovernmental organizations and the private sector, to take strategic action in 12 critical areas of concern, including the "inequalities and inadequacies in and unequal access to health care and related services" (United Nations, 1996). Securing improved health care for women and girls is a serious concern that will continue to be addressed by nurses in the twenty-first century. Health information and access, quality of care, environmental hazards and pollution, poverty, violence, economics, and education all have profound implications for health that will require the global involvement and leadership of nurses.

## World Health Organization

The WHO established its *Ninth General Programme of Work: Covering the Period 1996-2001* (1994), making clear the following objectives for the future:

- To reaffirm WHO's commitment to the principles of Health for All
- To set global targets for major health-related problems
- To identify the major policy issues for the world and for the WHO

Collaborative efforts by all health professions around the world will be necessary to realize for the future the policy initiatives that integrate health and human development, ensure equitable access to quality health care, promote and protect health, and prevent and control specific health problems (Institute of Medicine, 1996).

Nurses have assumed a leadership role in these initiatives through the Global Network of WHO Collaborating Centers for Nursing and Midwifery Development. This nursing network is a major force in promoting the ". . . attainment of a level of health for all people that will permit them to lead a socially and economically productive life" (World Health Organization, 1977). The collaborating centers promote this goal of Health for All by education for and provision of primary health care.

The global network consists of 34 nursing schools and universities, hospitals, research institutes, and ministries of public health in six regions—America, Europe, the Eastern Mediterranean, Africa, Southeast Asia, and the Western Pacific; representatives meet every 2 years. The network supports the efforts of participating members to improve primary health care and nursing development toward Health for All through education, research, and service. One collaborating center states: "The global network is unique in that no other nursing network has the potential for such a rich and rewarding interplay of nurse leaders and institutional capacities to respond to relevant nursing development towards primary health care in support of national, regional and global health goals" (George Mason University, 1995).

## Global Initiatives of Nursing Organizations

American nursing organizations have established clear value statements regarding their desire for and understanding of the necessity of global involvement now and for the future. These values are evident through various collaborative initiatives, alliances, and partnerships whose intent is to provide global leadership in education, practice, research, policy formulation, and decision making. Each of the major professional nursing organizations, through its goals and activities, clearly demonstrates that nursing's concerns are increasingly global. Communication technology and modern modes of transportation allow nurses across the world to easily communicate and share information with each other. The future of nursing will undoubtedly include its increased impact on global health affairs because of the global information network. Nurses will assume an expanded and valuable role in worldwide networking and education.

## Sigma Theta Tau International

This involvement is exemplified, for example, in the focus and activities of Sigma Theta Tau International, the second largest nursing organization in the United States and one of the largest international nursing groups. Founded in 1922, it was incorporated as an international organization in 1985 and currently consists of 383 chapters and more than 130,000 members in 75 countries. Sigma Theta Tau International has held international research congresses in seven countries and has demonstrated a sustained commitment to global nursing research and scholarship. One of its stellar achievements is the establishment of the Virginia Henderson International Library, a computerized collection of databases and knowledge resources that are available through Internet or dial-in access. In 1994 the library launched *The Online Journal of Knowledge Synthesis for Nursing,* which gives nurses around the world access to the latest nursing research findings.

## International Nursing Center

The International Nursing Center (INC) was created by the ANA in the early 1990s in response to a *White Paper* prepared by the American Academy of Nursing. This report emphasized the need for strong and sustained support and involvement in international nursing issues (American Academy of Nursing, 1992). The INC advances nursing practice, education, and research by providing funding for American representatives to attend international conferences, facilitating the collaboration of U.S. nurses and overseas colleagues, and assisting undergraduate and graduate nursing students and faculty in their participation in joint educational and research ventures.

The INC also assists in drafting and disseminating resolutions developed by the International Council of Nursing. Dr. Jane Weaver, the director of the International Nursing Center, reports that in 1995 the International Council of Nursing adopted a resolution condemning female genital mutilation and opposing nurses' participation in this practice. In turn, the International Nursing Center distributed copies of that position statement to the media, women's groups, and international governmental agencies. This resolution sent a strong, unified nursing voice that addressed an ethical issue of cultural sensitivity and safety, child protection, and prohibition of violence against women. Dr. Weaver states: "While it is difficult to estimate the impact of this nursing resolution, it should not be underestimated. In fact, in 1996 the U.S. Congress, whose key members were sent copies of the ICN resolution by the Center, passed a law making it a federal felony for anyone in the U.S., including health care providers, to perform female genital mutilation on females under age 18 without a bona fide medical necessity" (Weaver, 1997).

## Tri-Council of Nursing

The members of the Tri-Council of Nursing in the United States—the American Nurses Association, the National League for Nursing, the American Association of Colleges of Nursing, and the American Organization of Nurse Executives—are collectively advancing the preferred future of global nursing influence. They are engaged in innovative activities that transcend national boundaries. These organizations serve an integrative and facilitative role as they join in collaborative partnerships to create new bridges that link geographic, cultural, political, economic, and organizational avenues. Their global agenda includes establishing various mechanisms for dialogue and building relationships that will promote Health for All, primary care, and quality nursing care and education. By capitalizing on the rich resources of human talent and generosity worldwide, they are creating opportunities and generating new approaches to improving the health needs of all people. Their collective activities include assisting nursing schools in meeting the challenges of international students; convening international educational and research conferences; facilitating study and work exchanges and teleconferencing; preparing international leaders for a rapidly changing health care environment; and providing consultation and technical updates in patient care standards (Anderson, 1996; Brooks, 1996; Malone, 1996; Ryan, 1996).

The Tri-Council and other nursing organizations also have linkages with various nonnursing organizations involved in international health, such as the UN, WHO, Project Hope, World Bank, the Red Cross, the Peace Corps, World Vision, and the Institute of Medicine. For example, the ANA is a founding agency of the National Council for International Health; the American Association of Critical Care Nurses and the American College of Nurse Midwives serve as supporting nursing associations. The National Council for International Health, located in Washington, D.C., is a consortium of corporate, governmental, professional, religious, foundation, and private entities dedicated to the advocacy and support of global health issues. Dr. Weaver serves on the Board of the Tri-Council. Collaboration and interdisciplinary involvement provide rich opportunities for realization of complex goals.

## American Academy of Nursing

Another nursing organization advancing the preferred future of global nursing influence is the American Academy of Nursing. Through the establishment of the Expert Panel on International Health, the academy's goal is to improve nursing practice globally, promote and maintain the status of professional nursing worldwide, enhance nursing knowledge and educational programs, and articulate human rights (Donahue, 1996). The academy believes that globalization of economics, politics, and health has enormous implications for the international nursing community. Issues such as violence, HIV/AIDS, access to health care, the provision of culturally sensitive health care, prevention, and primary and managed care are of concern worldwide.

*The International Role of the American Nurses Association and American Academy of Nursing: A White Paper* (American Academy of Nursing, 1992) is a comprehensive document that presents the mission statement, objectives, and 14 recommendations and implementation strategies to guide ANA and the academy in international affairs. It is a compelling statement of nursing leaders' commitment to a likely future of intense global advocacy of the profession. Proceedings from an academy conference, "Health Care in Times of Global Transitions," presents the health implications of global migration (American Academy of Nursing, 1997).

## National Student Nurses Association

Nursing students have established an international presence through the organized efforts of the National Student Nurses Association and by their individual participation in various student exchanges and international projects. Faculty mentors are often the catalysts and supports for student involvement. The first international Student Assembly took place during the 1977 Quadrennial Congress of the International Council of Nurses (Mancino, 1993). The Fuld Fellowship program, sponsored by the Helene Fuld Health Trust, supports nursing students' attendance at international nursing conferences, such as the ICN Congresses and those of the International Society of Nurses in Cancer Care. Convening of students from across the world has continued to provide opportunities for student dialogue and sharing. Dr. Diane Mancino, executive director of the National Student Nurses Association, says "By examining global issues in nursing and health care, nursing students gain a broader perspective and appreciation of their own health and educational systems, as well as those in other countries. For students, a larger world view can foster a lifelong commitment to improve health care globally and promotes a deeper understanding of cultural diversity" (Mancino, 1997).

## PATHWAYS TO FUTURE GLOBAL ACTIVITY

Nurses have increasingly become activists in the globalization of nursing and health. Much of their activity occurs through organizational, governmental, and international agency sponsorship. Other initiatives take place through the commitment of schools and universities, clinical agencies, and individual nurses. Impediments to this involvement range from language, cultural, professional, and educational differences to a lack of clear organizational structures for dealing with international concerns (American Academy of Nursing, 1992). Finding fiscal sources to support projects, travel, materials, and professional costs is a major challenge. Some information about funding for activities abroad is available through the Internet and other sources (Schlachter and Weber, 1996). A vision of nurses, to improve health and nursing around the world, has been a driving force in spite of many constraints. The involvement of nurses in global education, practice, and research initiatives provides glimpses of the future that nursing hopes to create. The dream of Health for All undergirds this involvement. Specific examples of nursing organizations' commitment to international efforts follow.

### Nursing Practice

"The primary health care movement brings to nurses, internationally, the opportunity to share some common goals. At the same time, this approach to health affords nursing a prime opportunity to be a leader in health care policy and delivery systems in the United States and worldwide" (American Academy of Nursing, 1992).

- The monograph *Primary Health Care: Nurses Lead the War—A Global Perspective* (Kim, 1993) highlights the work of 17 nursing partners in the Global Network of World Health Organization Collaborating Centres for Nursing/Midwifery Development. The 22 case studies provide evidence of the nursing profession's success in implementing global networks for promoting primary care. They are a "story of teamwork and leadership in a changing world searching for answers to the attainment of the goal of Health for All" (Kim, 1993).
- Through the American International Health Alliance, sponsored by the U.S. Agency for International Development, nurses in the United States are joining with nurses in Central and Eastern Europe and the newly independent states of the former Soviet Union in more than 40 hospitals, community health, and health management education partnerships (American International Health Alliance, 1997).
- The American Organization of Nurse Executives (AONE), in conjunction with various groups, is sponsoring telenursing conferences, practice and educational exchanges, and technical updates across the global community. The AONE president believes that preparing international leaders through partnerships and collaboration is the key to improving patient care outcomes worldwide (Brooks, 1996).
- Nurses in the United States have joined forces with colleagues in Russia to expand the notion of hospice, first established in that country in 1990. U.S. nurses have been able to assist their Russian colleagues in establishing hospice as an "avenue to raise the standard of care for a particular segment of society" (Cooke, 1995).
- Members of the American Association of Critical Care Nurses (AACN) have joined with the World Federation Societies of Intensive and Critical Care Medicine to assist in disseminating patient care standards and research and in promoting leadership development. The AACN participates in the World Congress on Critical

Care Nursing and in online continuing education packages for global nursing audiences. The AACN president states that the individual and collective nurses' multinational emphasis is on the exchange of ideas, networking, collective support, and problem solving (Krumberger, 1996).

- A Women's Health Education Program in St. Petersburg, Russia, supported by the College of New Rochelle School of Nursing and a Russian midwife and a nurse-midwife consultant from the United States, is providing information and clinical support to childbearing women. Many midwifery leaders and nurses from the United States have contributed to the success of this grassroots women's health and nursing project (Vance, 1996; Cole, 1997; Vance, 1997).

## Nursing Education

Jane Salvage, RN, states: "Nursing education change is a global concern. There is a remarkable similarity in the issues being tackled, primarily curriculum review and reorientation to primary health care at all levels of the educational systems; new program development, especially in higher education; training of nurse teachers; provision of good-quality learning materials; continuing education schemes; closer links between education and service; and, perhaps a more recent trend, the evaluation of outcomes" (Salvage, 1995).

- Through the WHO Regional Office for Europe, Nursing and Midwifery, the LEMON Project (*Learning Material on Nursing*), provides a package of curriculum materials for all nurses, students, practitioners, and teachers in the official language of their country. Salvage states that a well-trained nursing workforce is the backbone of every health service and that this largest health care group needs the best possible basic and continuing education (Salvage, 1995). Other popular WHO nursing publications include the *Health for All Nursing Series* and the HIV/AIDS workbooks. These nursing materials address the compelling educational needs of nurses while strengthening their capacity to become self-sufficient and empowered to improve nursing and health care in their countries.
- The first international conference on nursing education, "Expanding Boundaries of Nursing Education Globally: Focus on Nursing Education Research," was held in Bolzano, Italy in 1993. Nurse educators from 36 countries attended this conference organized by the International Institute of Nursing Research (Padua, Italy), Case Western Reserve University Frances Payne Bolton School of Nursing (Cleveland, Ohio), and the Province Board of Nursing (Bozen, Italy). The conference goals included sharing innovative approaches to nursing education, reporting cross-cultural and collaborative research, and developing collaborative research (Modley and others, 1995).
- The Commission on Graduates of Foreign Nursing Schools (CGFNS) recently announced the opening of a new division, the International Commission of Healthcare Professions (ICHP), to meet the expanding need for international expertise on the education and preparation of health care professionals around the world. Barbara Nichols, president of CGFNS, states: "As the healthcare professions become increasingly global in their outlook, they urgently need dependable information and analysis to understand education and professional practice in different countries . . . we are deeply committed to the nursing profession, and we are delighted to build on our 20 years of experience to help other professions as well" (Commission on Graduates of Foreign Nursing Schools, 1997).
- A Vietnamese health care priority identified by the Ministries of Health and Education is to move nursing education into institutions of higher learning. This goal is being supported through the global linkages of three U.S. colleges (Teachers College, Columbia University, Newman College [Pennsylvania] and the College of New Rochelle [New York]) with three Vietnamese schools of nursing in Ho Chi Min City, (Danang) and Thanh Hoa (Hanoi). The U.S. nursing faculty in this project also has

participated in a multidisciplinary rehabilitation project sponsored by Health Volunteers Overseas and funded by USAID. Activities have included curriculum workshops, a biennial Vietnamese Nursing Conference, obtaining grant monies to purchase laboratory equipment, English lessons, and support of Vietnamese faculty visits to the United States (Moore, 1997). Collaboration and a consortial approach serve as a model of success in Vietnam.

- Dr. Bernadette Curry of Niagara University School of Nursing (New York) is concerned that the percentage of nursing students participating in study-abroad programs is relatively small compared with students in other majors. She states: "Since nursing education routinely incorporates the importance of culture in an era of interactive education and global focus, study-abroad can be a poignant and effective method to expand personal and professional insights" (Curry, 1997). Dr. Curry has designed culture-abroad programs for nursing students, particularly in France, that focus on cultural wellness and lifestyles.
- The second Nursing Academic International Congress sponsored by the University of Kansas School of Nursing and the University of Canberra (Australia) was held in 1996 and drew over 360 participants from 28 countries. The third congress was held in 1998 in Canberra Australia, and the fourth is scheduled for 2000 in Washington, DC, with George Mason University joining as a sponsor. Global collaboration and partnership have made the congress a successful shared educational experience. Patricia Wahlstedt, organizer of the congress in Kansas City, believes the goals of the meeting were accomplished: enhanced global communication, information exchange about various educational technologies and methods, promotion of cultural understanding, and creation of collaborative mechanisms in nursing practice, education, and research (Wahlstedt, 1997).

## Nursing Research

"Setting nursing research priorities has become a trend internationally . . . similarities and differences facilitate international networking among investigators in various countries who share clinical nursing research interests," states Ada Sue Hinshaw (1997), former director of the National Institute of Nursing Research.

- Sigma Theta Tau International sponsored the eighth International Research Congress as part of the International Nursing Congress in Vancouver in June, 1997, and the ninth congress was held in Utrecht, The Netherlands in July, 1998. In celebration of its seventy-fifth anniversary in December, 1997, the theme of its biennial convention focused on global health with the presentation of more than 275 research papers, posters, and symposia by nurses from around the world. The advancement of nursing through global research is a major tenet of Sigma Theta Tau's long-range plan. The Virginia Henderson International Nursing Library offers the *Registry of Nursing Research,* which provides electronic data and research information to nurse scholars all over the world (Sigma Theta Tau International, 1996).
- The North American Consortium of Nursing and Allied Health was formed in 1993 as part of ongoing transatlantic cooperation for international education and research with an existing European consortium. The three initial nursing schools are Pace University (New York), Thomas Jefferson University (Pennsylvania), and St. Joseph College (Connecticut). This consortium's intent is to promote international cooperation in research and education in nursing and allied health. The goals are to facilitate cross-cultural understanding; increase research and educational collaboration; develop student and faculty exchanges; recognize members' curricula; disseminate educational innovations; and promote linkages among members and other public and private organizations (Shortridge-Baggett and Haloburdo, 1997).
- A partnership between the University of Maryland School of Nursing and the Henrietta Szold Hadassah-Hebrew University School of Nursing began in early 1997. This partnership promotes student and faculty exchanges, sharing

of research projects and results, and creation of a graduate program at the Szold School. "Globalization of our research is our ultimate goal," Dean Barbara Heller states. "So many questions could be answered by doing research together, avoiding duplication and using synchronized research methods" (Feldman, 1977).

- The Hunter-Shanghai Research Project began in the late 1980s between the Hunter College-Bellevue School of Nursing in New York and the Department of Nursing at Shanghai Medical University. This research mentoring program evolved into collaborative nursing research activities, which expanded to include multiple sites on four continents—North America, Europe, Asia, and Africa. Faculty at both universities developed a joint research program, honed research skills through active collaborative participation, and published their research findings in international journals. "The mutual desire to teach about and use research as a basis for practice forms a common bond for nurses across continents. The culture of caring that is uniquely nursing can act as a mutual language for mentorship across cultures" (Gioiella and others, 1998).

## NURSING'S GLOBAL VISION

"There are many paths to the future. How well the future evolves will depend on what our vision of the future is" (Bezold, 1996). Nurses' vision of the future of health and nursing care encompasses a strong global perspective of an evolving world characterized by profound change, diversity, and complexity. Nurses' actions in global health affairs reflect their understanding of the need for, and commitment to, a worldwide transformation in health care. The language of this new world substitutes *global* for *international* and *cooperation* for *assistance,* terms more balanced and finely tuned for the "new" reality (Institute of Medicine, 1996).

The scenarios painted by the current global initiatives of the nursing community portray the discipline's vision for the preferred future of nursing and health care. These nursing initiatives are creating a future that is driven by a comprehensive global agenda. This vision is characterized by the following principles.

1. The focus is on the web of human relationships and on people-centered development through the capitalization of human resources and talents.
2. Collaboration through the development of partnerships, alliances, and networks is the key working modality.
3. Education is the pivotal modality for improvement of nursing practice and quality care.
4. Empowerment occurs through a mentoring model, a reciprocal caring relationship in which mutual learning and sharing of ideas and resources occur.
5. The richness of diversity and unity of goals, problems, and solutions is respected and celebrated.
6. Nursing's global vision is enacted by both collective/organizational and individualized/private actions.
7. Cyberspace is the mechanism for expanding cyber-nursing activities.
8. Interdisciplinary and multiorganizational engagement is the modus operandi for global policy formulation, political action, and decision making.
9. Economic issues, such as poverty and lack of fiscal support, are fundamental obstacles to human development and worldwide health for all.
10. The credo of women's rights as human rights (United Nations, 1996) is becoming more prominent in matters of health and nursing, applicable to both health care recipient and caregiver.

## CONCLUSION

Nurses clearly have an opportunity and an obligation to be participants in the historic opportunities that exist on the brink of a new century.

Nurses have the concern, commitment, compassion, and competency to assist policy makers in designing and implementing health care systems to meet the diverse needs of the world's population. Through strengthening the global health and nursing network, the nursing community can play a major role in transforming the world of the twenty-first century.

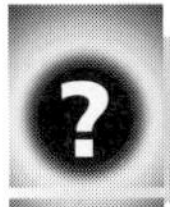

## *Discussion Exercises*

1. Why is it important for nursing to pursue global initiatives?
2. What do you think are the barriers to global collaboration in nursing? What strategies would you suggest to overcome these barriers?
3. Have you had professional experiences with nurses from countries other than your own? If so, what did you learn from them? If not, how do you think your professional work would be enhanced by exposure to nursing in other countries?

## References

American Academy of Nursing: *The international role of the American Nurses Association and American Academy of Nursing: a white paper,* Washington, DC, 1992, The Academy.

American Academy of Nursing: *Global migration: the health care implications of immigration and population movements,* Washington, DC, 1997, The Academy.

American International Health Alliance: American health care partnerships, *Common Health: J Am Health Alliance* 5(1):42, 1997.

Anderson C: Global initiatives: the American Association of Colleges of Nursing, presentation on Panel of Presidents at the Second Nursing Academic International Congress, Kansas City, Mo, September 1996.

Andrews MM, Fargotstein BP: International nursing consultation: a perspective on ethical issues, *J Prof Nurs* 2(5):302, 1986.

Betts VT: Personal communication, June 10, 1997.

Bezold C: Your health in 2010: four scenarios, *Futurist* 30(5)35, September-October 1996.

Brooks AM: Global initiatives: the American Organization of Nurse Executives, presentation on Panel of Presidents at the Second Nursing Academic International Congress, Kansas City, Mo, September 1996.

Cole MR: Woman to woman, *Nurs Spectrum* 9(9):17, 1997.

Commission on Graduates of Foreign Nursing Schools: CGFNS launches new division, *Int Evaluator,* p 1, Winter 1997.

Cooke M: The Russian way of hospice, *Am Hospice Palliative Care* 12(5):8, 1995.

Curry B: Personal communication, May 20, 1997.

Donahue B: Global initiatives: the American Academy of Nursing, presentation on Panel of Presidents at the Second Nursing Academic International Congress, Kansas City, Mo, September 1996.

Feldman HC: Szold on the idea, *Baltimore Jewish Times,* p 1, April 25, 1997.

George Mason University, College of Nursing & Health Science: *WHO collaborating center for health policy, health care ethics and nursing administration,* Fairfax, Va, 1995, George Mason University.

Ghebrehlwet T: Personal communication, April 7, 1997.

Gioiella E and others: The Hunter-Shanghai project: an international cross-cultural experience in research mentorship. In Vance C, Olson RK: *The mentor connection in nursing,* New York, 1998, Springer.

Grant JP: *The state of the world's children,* New York, 1994, 1995, Oxford University Press.

Hinshaw AS: International nursing research priorities, *J Prof Nurs* 13(24):68, 1997.

Institute of Medicine, National Academy of Sciences, Board on International Health: *Global health in transition: a synthesis,* Washington, DC, 1996, National Academy Press.

Kim Mi Ja, editor: *Primary health care: nurses lead the way—a global perspective,* Washington, DC, 1993, American Association of Colleges of Nursing.

Krumberger J: Global initiatives: the American Association of Critical Care Nurses, presentation on Panel of Presidents at the Second Nursing Academic International Congress, Kansas City, Mo, September 1996.

Malone B: Global initiatives: the American Nurses Association, presentation on Panel of Presidents at the Second Nursing Academic International Congress, Kansas City, Mo, September 1996.

Mancino D: American student participation in ICN and international affairs, *Imprint* 40(3):71, 1993.

Mancino D: Personal communication, June 11, 1997.

Modley DM and others, editors: *Advancing nursing education worldwide,* New York, 1995, Springer.

Moore MN: *A consortium approach to international education,* unpublished manuscript, 1997.

Reanda L: The Commission on the status of women. In Alston P, editor: *The United Nations and human rights,* Oxford, England, 1992, Clarendon Press.

Ryan S: Global initiatives: the National League for Nursing, presentation on Panel of Presidents at the Second Nursing Academic International Congress, Kansas City, Mo, September 1996.

Salvage J: Global trends in nursing education: a world health organization perspective. In Modly DM and others, editors: *Advancing nursing education worldwide,* New York, 1995, Springer.

Schlachter GA, Weber RD: *Financial aid for research and creative activities abroad 1996-1998,* San Carlos, Calif, 1996, Reference Service Press.

Shortridge-Baggett LM, Haloburdo E: Report of the North American Consortium of Nursing and Allied Health, unpublished manuscript, 1997.

Sigma Theta Tau International: *Information 1996-97,* Indianapolis, Ind, 1996, Sigma Theta Tau International.

United Nations Development Programme: *Human development reports,* New York, 1993, 1994, Oxford University Press.

United Nations, Fourth World Conference on Women: *The Beijing declaration and the platform for action,* New York, 1996, United Nations Department of Public Information.

Vance C: Project funds women's health education in Russia, *Nurse Pract World News* 1(3)15; 1(6):15, 1996.

Vance C: Women to women: an American and Russian partnership, *Nurse Pract World News* 2(1):14, 1997.

Wahlstedt P: The Nursing Academic International Congress, unpublished manuscript, 1997.

Weaver J: The International Nursing Center of the American Nurses Association and Foundation, unpublished manuscript, 1997.

World Bank: *World development report 1993: investing in health,* New York, 1993, Oxford University Press.

World Health Organization: *World Health Assembly resolution, series 30,* Geneva, 1977, The Organization.

World Health Organization: *Formulating strategies for health for all by the year 2000, series 2,* Geneva, 1979, The Organization.

World Health Organization: *Ninth general programme of work: covering the period 1996-2001, health for all, series 11,* Geneva, 1994, The Organization.

# 36 The Role of Professional Organizations

**Fay L. Bower**

*Organization is the power of the day. Without it nothing great is accomplished.*

**Sophia Palmer**
1897

This chapter is about the future of nursing organizations. It is necessary to look at the past to determine how nursing organizations were established and to examine what nursing organizations do and why they are successful or have problems. This chapter describes the future of nursing organizations using the probable future and preferable future processes (Hancock and Bezold, 1994). Appendix B provides a list of the major nursing organizations.

## DEVELOPMENT OF NURSING ORGANIZATIONS

According to Lewenson (1996), the establishment of nursing organizations was one important way to emancipate nurses in the late 1800s. Because private duty nurses were isolated from other nurses at a time when women were trying to support one another and take their place in social reform, they formed associations. These associations paralleled the development of similar groups within other women's professions and study groups among middle-class matrons who had attended college.

Superintendents of nurse training schools and other nurse leaders between 1873 and 1893 entertained the ideas of association, affiliation, and organization. Graduates of the early nurse training schools, these professionals saw their educational freedom hampered by the attempts of those outside of nursing, such as hospital boards and physicians, to control nursing education (Lewenson, 1996). Box 36-1 lists some of the pioneer nurse leaders who spearheaded the drive for the professional organization of nursing.

### Box 36-1
### *Pioneer Nursing Leaders*

Linda Richards (1841-1930)
Isabel Hampton Robb (1860-1910)
Lavinia Dock (1858-1956)
Adelaide Nutting (1858-1948)
Annie Damer (1858-1915)
Sophia Palmer (1853-1920)
Martha Minerva Franklin (1870-1968)
Adah Belle Samuels Thoms (1870-1943)
Lillian Wald (1867-1940)
Ella Phillips Crandall (1871-1938)
Mary Sewell Gardner (1871-1961)

America's progressive spirit of reform embraced by superintendents of the newly formed nurse training programs was translated into organizational activities. Nursing superintendents created what is believed to be the first national professional women's organization in the United States, the American Society of Superintendents of Training Schools for Nurses in 1893 (Lewenson, 1996). In 1912 this organization was renamed the National League for Nursing Education (NLNE) and is known today as the National League for Nursing (NLN).

The development of the American Nurses Association (ANA) had a similar but slightly different evolution. "As the number of hospital schools of nursing increased, the number of trained nurses rose steadily from 157 graduates in 1880 to 471 in 1890 and more significantly to 3,456 in 1900" (Lewenson, 1996). These working women had unique needs related to job satisfaction, financial security, professional credentialing, and academic accreditation of schools. Because the Superintendents' Society limited its active membership to superintendents, the Nurses Association of Alumnae of the United States and Canada was formed. To incorporate under the laws of the state of New York, it was necessary to drop the reference to another country. In 1901 it was named the Nurses' Associated Alumnae of the United States, and in 1912 the organization became known as the American Nurses Association.

There was a common theme throughout this early organization of nurses and was best stated by Sophia Palmer in 1895 at the annual convention of the Superintendents' Society as a result of a survey she had completed in 1894. Her comments were based on the results of a survey of 164 training schools (144 in the United States and 20 in Canada). "Remember that it is only through organization that individual members can be reached, and their cooperation in progressive movements be obtained, and that without their support and their good influence with the public we lose an immense power" (Palmer, 1897).

A review of what has happened over the last 50 years indicates that there are more than 45 national nursing organizations. An effort in 1952 to restrict the number of nursing organizations was a failure because of the numbers and diversity of nurses. That same issue makes it difficult to reduce the number of organizations in nursing today. The nurse workforce today is the largest occupational group in the health care industry, with more than 2.5 million registered nurses (U.S. Department of Health & Human Services, 1996). Furthermore, nursing is a highly stratified occupation, with nurses prepared in a variety of educational programs and licensed by states at three different levels: practical nurses, registered nurses, and advanced practice nurses.

Although some fear there is a loss of political power because of this proliferation of national organizations and the inability to speak with "one strong voice," several coordinating groups or coalitions have been formed around political agendas. The Tri-Council (which is made up of the ANA, NLN, American Association of Colleges of Nursing [AACN], and American Organization of Nurse Executives [AONE]), sets the major Washington agenda for nursing. The National Alliance of Nurse Practitioners (NANP) brings together 12 nurse practitioner organizations, and the National Federation of Specialty Organizations (NFSO) is composed of approximately 38 specialty organizations (Bullough and Bullough, 1994).

The early purposes for nursing organizations have not changed. There still is a need to support nurses, to improve the health of the world's people, to foster high standards of nursing practice, to promote professional development, and to advance the economic and general welfare of nurses. Accreditation of nursing programs; certification and licensure of nurses; standards of care; and a voice that speaks for nursing when federal, state, and local initiatives threaten nursing continue to be the purposes of nursing organizations. Leadership from nursing organizations has always been important to the development and advancement of the nursing profession.

## SUCCESSES AND FAILURES OF NURSING ORGANIZATIONS

The education and general welfare of nurses and the nursing care delivered to patients have improved as a direct result of nurse organization activity. Accreditation by NLN has improved the required qualifications of nurse educators, the quality of the nursing curricula, and the resources available to nursing programs. The collective bargaining efforts of ANA have improved the working conditions and salaries of nurses, even for those nurses not part of a collective bargaining unit. The practice of nurses, whether basic or advanced, has improved as a result of improved standards of care, and the legislation affecting nurses has been monitored and influenced by many of the 45 nursing organizations.

With these successes, however, there is a growing occurrence of overlapping goals; conflict between organizations; and competition for federal, foundation, and corporate funding. There are even declining memberships in some of the largest organizations. The "one strong voice" of nursing has often been lost, even though there have been efforts to cooperate and collaborate lobbying activities and information dissemination. The most harmful activity has been the internal fighting between organizations, which sends a signal to those outside the profession that nursing is in disarray.

Hegyvary (1994) suggests that these conflicts and fights have surfaced because of the evolutionary nature of organizations. She cites three major themes in the development of organizations: *differentiation*, *integration*, and *interdependence*. Although it is clear that professional organizations need to serve the purposes of self-regulation, representation, and organizational development, the current trend is to focus less on structure and definitive stated purposes. Increasingly, professional organizations are concerned about interorganizational linkages and changing activities in response to changing environments.

Most nursing organizations are organized in the differentiation model, that is, they are large and organized into specified parts. Some organizations are involved in an integration (the collaboration of groups), such as the Tri-Council), but only a few are moving toward the interdependence stage (joint efforts to promote the same goal). As Hegyvary (1994) points out: "The integration of differentiated groups requires linkages based on the type and extent of interdependence." She cites the response of organized nursing to the American Medical Association's (AMA) intent to create three categories of caregivers as an example of an interdependent organizational effort. When nursing organizations came together to ward off the AMA's model of preparing "care givers," nursing was unified and worked together for a common goal. She also states: "When the interests and activities of nursing organizations are in conflict, however, the perception both within and outside nursing may be of trouble within the profession. An example of an issue generating considerable conflict is entry into practice." Nursing's ability to determine the level of preparation and the title for the professional nurse for entry into practice has been an area of contention for nurses all over the nation and has created much disagreement and bad feelings among nurses.

Currently nursing is faced with a conflict between the NLN and AACN regarding accreditation. Both organizations believe accreditation is their purview (see Chapter 24). Conflict also exists between ANA and The National Council of State Boards of Nursing (NCSBN) regarding whether advanced practice nurses should be certified by the profession or licensed by the state and between ANA and nurse practitioner specialty groups about who should certify nurse practitioners and who should establish and monitor standards of practice for nurse practitioners.

It is highly likely that other conflicts will arise as the environment of health care continues in the throes of much change and as nursing organizations find themselves in the position of trying to adjust and respond to those changes. At a time when nursing organizations should appear as a source of power and be able to respond in "one strong voice," there is a splintering of effort and a tendency to compete or duplicate service. Vested interest, historic perspectives, and perceived threats influence nursing organizations' abilities to successfully respond to these changes. Whether they will be able to sustain as they are or be able to change will depend on whether a probable future or a preferred future occurs.

## PROBABLE FUTURE OF NURSING ORGANIZATIONS

The probable future is what will likely happen based on the present situation and an appraisal of current trends (Hancock & Bezold, 1994). Until very recently the probable future of health care was seen as hospital based, physician dominated, and high tech. Ironically, recent changes have proved this vision to be the wrong one. If we had begun our projections based on what was, we would have missed the future entirely. As Hancock and Bezold (1994) state, "Descriptive forecasting based solely on recent trends can preclude futures that are different; they also often turn out to be the future we don't want!"

These limits of probable future predictions have implications for nursing organizations. If we were to predict the future from recent trends, we would see continued goal duplication among nursing organizations, more conflict between and among groups, and repeated attempts to form coalitions. Organizations would continue to seek collaboration but would probably fail, for the trends suggest that collaboration is not enough. Even though the Tri-Council speaks in one voice to legislators, other nursing organizations muddy the dialogue with different viewpoints. Although the National Alliance of Nurse Practitioners has pulled together several nurse practitioner organizations, there is disagreement among them about which one should certify the nurse practitioner. A larger and more inclusive coalition of nurse practitioners is needed; however, one must ask, if a larger coalition is necessary, then why is there a need for so many nurse practitioner organizations?

Furthermore, because many nursing organizations are seeking ways to respond to changes in the health care delivery system and thus have differentiated activities, prediction of a probable future suggests organizational goals will overlap more often and increased conflict about who is to carry the ball forward will likely occur. Ultimately, nursing organizations will lose their ability to respond effectively to changes or to meeting their own purposes. More energy will go into sustaining the organization, in redefining its purpose, and in recruiting members than to meet the organization's purposes. Duplication, confrontation, and decreasing membership will result.

Currently membership in most of the nursing organizations is on the decline; when new graduates are faced with a choice about which organization to join, they often join none. The lack of differentiation between organizations frustrates the nurse so that the decision is not what organization to join but rather whether to join any organization.

The result of declining membership is reduction in resources. Where membership declines and organizational purposes are not distinct, recruitment of new members is very difficult. Ultimately a cyclic activity occurs: decreasing membership means less money for recruitment, and less recruitment means more decline in membership. This cycle over time will result in extinction of the organization. Smaller organizations will fold first, and one by one so will the others.

It is probable that there will not be more than 45 nursing organizations in the future. This decrease in numbers of organizations when considered alone is not, by itself, negative, but what is detrimental is the destruction that will result if the present trend of conflict within and between organizations, which is much more devastating, is not stopped.

The entry to practice issue is a good example of what occurs when members of a profession begin to fight among themselves or cannot agree on an objective for the profession. Nurses disagree in public, hate letters are exchanged, and deep wounds inflicted. The profession becomes weakened and vulnerable to outside attack and to outside decisions that affect nursing. The best action must be a supported action. Although the entry to practice issue must be solved, it cannot be accomplished in a probable future format that suggests that current trends predict future outcomes. Fundamental changes in the way nursing organizations function and the roles they play as leaders must occur, and those changes can only happen if the future is based on a *preferred* prediction.

## PREFERABLE FUTURE OF NURSING ORGANIZATIONS

The preferable future is what we want to have happen and is sometimes called "prescriptive futurism" or "normative forecasting" (Hancock and Bezold, 1994). "Preferable futures are visions that generally begin by identifying and trying to create a future that does not yet exist" (Hancock and Bezold, 1994). It is often helpful to look at the future that is likely to happen (probable) and the one that is preferred to determine which direction to go. The difference is liberating.

Most often we look into the future based on what is likely to occur. If we do this, we are likely to inadvertently disempower people and deny them choice. If the prediction for the future is a probable one, then the only choices we have are how to prepare for it or brace for it and how to deal with it when it arrives. However, when we look at the preferable future we are liberated and empowered. As Hancock and Bezold (1994) state, "This is the future we value and that we want to create. The energy and creativity released in a 'preferable future's' process can be quite astonishing."

The preferable future for nursing organizations must be based on reaching the *interdependent* stage of organizational development. This means that nursing organizations of the future will have the following characteristics and responsibilities:

1. Each nursing organization will have clearly defined goals that do not replicate another organization's purpose.
2. Interdependent activities between nursing organizations and between and with other health care groups will be the norm, not the exception.
3. Systems thinking will be necessary so that the roles and responsibilities of the nurse are not performed in a vacuum. Nurses are but one of the health care worker groups and are part of a huge and complicated system of care, so nursing organizations will approach decisions from a systems perspective.
4. Consensus will be the mode for managing differences, and nursing organizations will provide direction and leadership for nurses.
5. New responsibilities for certification, accreditation, and licensing of basic and advanced nursing practice will be established by nursing organizations. States (through the NCSBN) and the nursing profession will settle their differences and assure the public of safe, quality care from all levels of nurses. This movement will be staged and managed by the nursing organizations, both private and public.
6. Preferable futures thinking will be the framework for solving issues about nursing and that affect nursing.

### Clearly Defined Mission Statement

Originally, nursing organizations had clearly defined mission statements. This was partially the case because the world of health care was smaller and simpler. However, as the health care system became more complex so did nursing organizations. In attempts to address the changes and opportunities, new organizations sprang up and the older organizations took on more without letting go of former initiatives so that today there are many organizations with overlapping missions, activities, and goals.

In the preferred future each organization will have a clearly defined mission that makes it distinct. Sigma Theta Tau International is a good example of a nursing organization that has a clearly defined mission unlike any other nursing organization's.

> Sigma Theta Tau International is the honor society of nursing and it exists to promote the development, dissemination and utilization of nursing knowledge. Sigma Theta Tau International is committed to improving the health of people worldwide through increasing the scientific base of nursing practice. In support of this mission, the Society advances nursing leadership and scholarship, and furthers the use of nursing research in health care delivery as well as in public policy (Sigma Theta Tau International, 1997).

In the future each nursing organization will have a unique and clearly stated mission statement that outlines its direction and makes it clear that one organization is not like another. This means that there will be fewer nursing organizations because only those that can define their mission clearly will survive. Some organizations will meld with others and some will collapse. But it is clear that if the organization cannot define its unique mission, then there is no place for it in the preferred future.

A clearly defined mission statement also will increase the membership of the organization because nurses will be able to determine where they want to specifically direct their allegiances and their energies. This one very important task will clear up a lot of the conflicts that exist in nursing organizations today and thus will provide for member involvement that is absolutely essential if the organization is to be healthy and useful. Nurses, like others, like to belong to organizations that are in "good shape," doing important things, and that provide direction for members. Nurses, as do other professionals, want to belong and contribute in a meaningful way through their organizations.

## Interdependent Linkages

Interdependence, the ability to link with other organizations who have common interests in or a responsibility for a particular issue, will be the mode used to resolve problems or to expand the influence of nursing in the future. Other entities like the Tri-Council will develop to address issues of importance to nursing. Power will emanate from the coalition and not from any one organization. This movement to interdependence will take its leadership from those groups that have been successful in making change as a coalition.

Furthermore, coalitions will be formed between nursing and medicine and nursing and other groups, including consumer groups, because the focus in the future will be on multidisciplinary power to solve health care "system" problems that affect all health care professionals. In the past there has been competition and fighting between health care worker groups. In any fight there is always a loser, and because nursing has had its fair share of "losing," it is preferable to seek models that are win-win. The Pew Health Promotions Commission recommended such a direction in 1995 (Pew, 1995). The importance of interconnected networks between and among organizations will be essential if the approaches to tomorrow's health care needs are to be addressed.

### Systems Approach

Systems thinking is a major part of the future of nursing organizations that will determine their success (Senge, 1995). No longer can nurses and nurse leaders think about what is best for nurses without thinking about the bigger picture—what is best for the public and how the system can provide quality care to keep people healthy. The process of defining health and how health can be maintained and promoted is a process of determining what kind of workers will be needed and what the multidisciplinary organizations can do to promote and support them. The decisions revolve around health at the center. This complex process cannot be accomplished by nursing alone; it is a multidisciplinary process.

Currently, nursing is not at the table when health care system decisions are made, whether they are hospital based, government controlled, or decided by insurance companies. In the preferred future nursing through its organizations will be part of the decision team because multidisciplinary approaches will be used. To accomplish this nursing organizations will have to reach beyond the present discussions and invite others to join the dialogue.

### ARISTA II

Such an attempt was made in April of 1996 when Sigma Theta Tau International sponsored ARISTA II, a think tank that included physicians, nurses, government leaders, hospital administrators, insurance executives, foundation directors, media representatives and health care redesigners, where the preferred role for nurses was discussed. A monograph of the proceedings is available (Sigma Theta Tau International, 1996). More think tanks of this nature will occur in the future as a strategy for solving problems and setting directions that affect health care, health care workers, and the health care system as a whole. Multidisciplinary approaches to health care decision making will be an important aspect of the future.

## Certification, Accreditation, and Licensing

### Certification

*Certification* of advanced practice nursing and basic nursing practice has been available for many years. The American Nurses Credentialing Center, an aspect of the ANA, provides opportunity for individual nurses to be certified. Several other nursing organizations provide specialty certification also. Most states require certification for recognition as an advanced practice nurse (APN) before they will grant a license or designation as an APN. In the future, however, there will be more clarity about the reason for certification and who will provide it. More than one agency will provide certification, and all states will include certification as an eligibility requirement for licensure as an advanced practice nurse. Given the competitive nature of managed care, certification at the basic (RN) level also will occur as a value-added way of promoting quality care (Sponselli, 1997). ANA and other specialty organizations will have this issue on their agenda for a good part of the next 5 years. Working together they will promote certification as a way to measure quality care.

### Accreditation

*Accreditation* for nursing education programs has been the prerogative of the National League for Nursing (NLN) for over a century. Recently the AACN has established an organizational entity, the Commission on Collegiate Nursing Education, to also accredit academic nursing programs (see Chapter 24). In the preferred future these two organizations will work more closely together and in an interdependent way. Both will accredit but at different levels. In fact there will be a closer relationship of accrediting agencies across the health-related disciplines so that in a few years accreditation will also be a multidisciplinary event.

### Licensing

*Licensing* as we know it today will be different in the preferred future. Our national nursing organizations, including the NCSBN will agree on how to provide safety for the public (basic licensing) and quality recognition (certification) for all levels of nursing. Licensure that is recognized by all states and certification that is provided by the profession, in keeping with the way other health care professionals function, will be determined in a joint way by NCSBN, ANA, and practitioner groups. Using consensus, leaders of these groups will set the model that will be used by other professional groups (see Chapter 23).

## Consensus Building and Leadership

It would be a mistake to discuss the preferred future and omit a discussion of the long-term tendency in nursing for internal strife. The entry-to-practice issue is a good example of how internal disagreement has confused the public and other health care workers and weakened the power of nursing. Although it may have been premature in 1965 to suggest two levels of nursing practice, today it is obvious that there are *several* levels of nursing practice and that it is time to determine the educational preparation and licensure for all of them. In the preferred future this unresolved decision will be solved by leadership from nursing organizations. Until recently, the majority of nurses were employed in hospitals and the baccalaureate degree for entry-level practice was feasible but not probable given the limited number of nurses with baccalaureate degrees. Now that health care is more often community based, the decision regarding the appropriate preparation for entry to professional practice is a new one and will take a new direction. Many believe that the advanced practice nurse with a masters degree should be the entry level for professional nursing. Leadership from our nursing organizations will tackle this decision in the future. Clearly a decision will be made.

Because the major purpose of a nursing organization is to provide leadership, whatever decision is made will be done by consensus within and between nursing organizations. Furthermore, the decision will be supported by nurses everywhere because more nurses will be college graduates and thus prepared for the professional role of the future. The past has taught us a lesson. When there is conflict, there is loss of power; with loss of power there is a loss of opportunity to be engaged in higher-level discussions.

Encouraging different opinions is a major strength of a democratic society, so different perspectives about entry to practice or any other issue in nursing will not be discouraged. Difference does not mean, however, that there is no way to resolve an issue and set a direction. Using the principles of "new leadership" as outlined by Prestwood and Schumann (1997), leaders of nursing organizations will guide their organization and membership to do the following:

1. *Know who they are.* "We must understand what we know and what we don't know about ourselves. We must assess our resistance to—and tolerance for—change, our fears, our preferences, and our skills and abilities."
2. *Let go of what they've got hold of.* "We must discover the chains that bind us to our past and prevent us from understanding who we are. Once we understand the chains that bind us, we must let them go. Letting go puts us on a path to new experiences."
3. *Learn their purpose.* "Each one of us has a purpose. Not all of us understand what our purpose is. We learn our purpose through lifelong introspection coupled with interaction with others. It is also important that we develop habits of mind that allow us to filter through interactions and choose the positive ones. Habits of mind are developed from values that we have. As we discover our purpose, we can decide to change our values, allowing us to continue our lifelong process of learning."
4. *Live in the question.* "In the Industrial Age, we learned to analyze a situation, isolate the problem, and administer a quick fix. In the Age of Interaction, we must recognize that everything is tied to everything else. Therefore, we must live in the question long enough to understand the relationships important to a systems solution. Flexibility is required so that we can be open to the potential of the unknown."
5. *Learn the art of "barn raising."* "Barn raising is a tradition of the pioneer culture where people came together to help someone build a barn. Today's emphasis on teamwork recognizes this basic need to work with and through others. A shared purpose motivates individuals to contribute their energy, talents, and abilities."
6. *Give it away.* "A paradox of life is that the

more we try to hold on to something, the more likely we are to lose it. Viewing people as abundant, renewable resources and giving away authority allows the full power of individuals to be realized. This is accomplished through ennobling, enabling, empowering, and encouraging ourselves and others. We must relentlessly pursue the release of authority and control."

7. *Let the magic happen.* "The final principle of leadership is to let go of the demands of our ego. We must become a member of the team and utilize our abilities—joining in the shared purpose—to help achieve its maximum potential. There are always three choices: lead, follow, or get out of the way. The wisdom of leadership in the Age of Interaction is to know which action to choose for each situation."

For some nursing organization leaders this kind of leadership will be easy and for others it will be more difficult. Clearly such leadership is necessary and will occur in the preferred future if nursing organizations are to do meaningful work and make a difference in nursing and health care. The value and effectiveness of nursing organizations is directly related to the quality of the nursing leadership. Like our predecessors—nurse leaders who had courage, insight, and a will to complete their objective—the women and men leading nursing organization will accomplish the preferred future laid out in this chapter.

## Preferable Futures Thinking

Nursing organizations have a proud legacy. Recently they have been very busy reacting and adjusting to the many changes in health care that have occurred in a very short time. That reaction has become the "modus operandi." In this new age of interaction, nursing organizations must do more. They must set the future.

Pesut (1997) makes the point that nursing takes a "wait and see" approach to change. Rather than moving forward, nursing is "associated with the past or the 'here and now' and not looking forward to the future." Pesut also questions the degree to which nurses engage in futures thinking. He urges nursing to do a better job of inventing and projecting preferred nursing futures. Nurses will use "future-think" because it will be necessary and because the leadership of nursing organizations will help it happen. The time also will be right.

The nurse leaders of the late 1800s moved the profession forward with their development of nursing organizations. It is now time for the leaders of the current nursing organizations to take the profession even further. They will do that by purposing a preferable future and helping nurses and other health care providers create that future. More involvement in futures work can make this happen.

# CONCLUSION

The preferable future requires a different way for nursing organizations to function. Both the leadership style and the functions of the organizations must change. Nursing organizations must work together; help their constituencies address the needs of the changing health care scene; and provide data for legislatures, reimbursers, and consumers about the value and activities of all kinds of nurses. Nursing organizations must speak with one strong voice. This means team work, collaboration, and targeting system issues.

Nursing education for all levels of nurses must change dramatically, and that means those nursing organizations that accredit programs must promote new directions that are workforce oriented. Those organizations that represent specialty areas of nursing must come together and address issues that are common to them all. They must also promote activities that are sensitive to what could be the world of tomorrow. "Future think" is imperative. Nurse practitioner organizations also must work together and with other health care worker groups, particularly physicians, if the needs of tomorrow's consumers are to be met. Again, "future think" is needed.

Whatever nursing organizations do, their activities must be consumer oriented and based on research data. Clearly the future of nursing depends on the reconstruction of how nurses function as caregivers and managers, how they are educated, how nursing research is conducted, and how nursing organizations provide leadership for these changes.

We again are faced with a need for the emancipation. Where early nursing organizations were forceful and successful in emancipating nurses, emancipation of the profession is now necessary. Nursing organizations must seize the opportunity, take advantage of the changes occurring, and shape the preferred future for nursing and health care. Our patients depend on it.

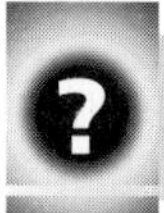

## *Discussion Exercises*

1. You are president of a major nursing organization. Select your organization and answer the following:
   a. What is your major goal for your term of office? Why?
   b. What issue causes you the most concern?
   c. What strategies will you use to meet your goal?
   d. How will you encourage collaboration with other organizations both in nursing and outside of nursing?
2. Do you belong to any nursing organization (e.g., student nurses, ANA, Sigma Theta Tau International)? Name them. Why do you belong? If not, why not?
3. After reading this chapter, have you changed your mind about the importance of belonging to nursing organizations? Explain.

## References


Bullough B, Bullough VL: *Nursing issues for the nineties and beyond,* New York, 1994, Springer.

Hancock T, Bezold C: Possible futures, preferable futures, *Healthcare Forum J,* 37(2):23, 1994.

Hegyvary ST: A guide to nursing organizations. In McCloskey JC, Grace HK: *Current issues in nursing,* St. Louis, 1994, Mosby.

Lewenson SB: *Taking charge,* New York, 1996, National League for Nursing Press.

Palmer S: *First and second annual conventions of ASSTSN,* Harrisburg, Penn, 1897, Harrisburg.

Pesut D: Future think, *Nurs Outlook,* 45(3):107, 1997.

Pew Health Professions Commission: *Critical challenges: revitalizing the health professions for the twenty-first century.* San Francisco, 1995, UCSF Center for the Health Professions.

Prestwood DL, Schumann PA: Seven new principles of leadership, *Futurist,* p. 68, January-February, 1997.

Senge P: *The fifth discipline,* New York, 1995, Doubleday/Currency.

Sigma Theta Tau International: *Mission statement,* Indianapolis, Ind, 1997, Sigma Theta Tau International Center Nursing Press.

Sigma Theta Tau International: *Nursing leadership in the 21st century: a report of ARISTA II,* Indianapolis, Ind, 1996, Sigma Theta Tau International Center Nursing Press.

Sponselli C: Newsmaker interview: managed care worries nurse leader, *NurseWeek* 1:27, 1997.

U.S. Department of Health and Human Services, Division of Nursing, Bureau of Health Professions, Health Resources and Services Administration: *National Sample Survey of Registered Nurses,* 1996, *http://www.hrsa.dhhs.gov/bhpr/dn/sample.htm.*

# 37 Scenarios for the Future

**Clement Bezold**
**Eleanor J. Sullivan**

*What lies behind us and what lies before us are tiny matters compared to what lies within us.*

**Oliver Wendell Holmes**

The future of society, of health care, and of nursing cannot be predicted with certainty, but there are patterns of change that can be anticipated. We know with some certainty, for instance, that there will be about 5 million people in the United States who are over age 85 by the year 2010, but we are less certain about how healthy they will be or what disabilities they may have.

We can anticipate scientific breakthroughs in such areas as mapping the human genome and understanding healthy aging. It is much harder to predict the specific timing of scientific discoveries or exactly when they will be reflected in practice.

Changes in societal values, public policy, and individual behavior are even more uncertain. However, these changes are often more important to the future of health than scientific breakthroughs. For instance, society may or may not adequately deal with poverty, the single biggest cause of ill health. Consumers may or may not become increasingly interested in health. Health care policy and financing may evolve in ways that directly affect people's health in the future.

The following alternative scenarios for U.S. health care in the year 2010 allow us to explore various answers to these and other issues.

## FOUR SCENARIOS OF THE FUTURE

### Business as Usual

Economic growth is irregular but persistent, and the United States holds its own in global competition. The majority of people in the United States are better off, but the percentage of poor continues to rise beyond the 15% it was in the mid 1990s.

Health care reform is left to the states, which in turn leave it to the marketplace.

As the percentage of poor rises and states have to carry the Medicaid burden, more states limit individual patients' access to expensive, radical care. Most states and health care providers have their residents share in the decisions over what is made available in the state-funded health plans.

Advances in biomedical knowledge and technology make it possible to forecast and increasingly manage people's health, profoundly altering health care delivery for those who are insured. As a result, health care providers no longer allow a patient's symptoms to grow acute and then rush to the rescue, guns blazing against symptoms of disease.

High-tech interventions become common, such as vaccines for cancers and medications that prevent plaque buildup in the arteries. The affluent or well insured also have access to such advanced therapies as biosensors, organ transplants, organoids (a new organ or organ part grown outside the body and then implanted in it), and performance-enhancing bionic implants (devices that enhance functions such as vision, hearing, mobility, and mental capacity).

Health care delivery becomes more effective and efficient. Multispecialty physician groups direct most care, aided by other health care providers and supported by expert systems. These expert systems constrain the decisions that physicians make but improve their outcomes.

The number of hospital beds is cut by two thirds in just over two decades, from more than 900,000 in 1989 to 300,000 by the year 2010. Hospitals become smaller, and their numbers decline. Those with a large share of insured or private payers can take advantage of new technologies and are able to move faster toward delivering more ambulatory care walk-in/walk-out treatment. Even poorer patients on Medicaid receive consistent care and are able to have their major illnesses forecast, prevented, or cured, including heart disease, cancer, arthritis, and Alzheimer's disease.

By the year 2010 health care's percentage of GNP stabilizes at 15%, and economists argue that it could be reduced further if the country did not spend so much on life extension and performance enhancement.

Bottom line: Most individuals have very effective care that prevents or cures most diseases. However, bionics and replacement hearts, for example, are limited to those who can afford them.

## Hard Times

Times are tough for the economy as a whole and for health care. The depression of 2001 is preceded and followed by recessions. Innovations in health care and throughout society move far more slowly than had been promised in the 1990s.

The relative affluence of physicians irks some consumers. Scandals regain attention involving doctors, hospitals, and insurers. Health care expenditures are at 15% of the GNP yet cover only 80% of the population when the recession begins. As unemployment grows so do the costs to the states for Medicaid. Sentiment shifts, encouraging the federal government to take back health care and to create universal access to a frugal basic package of care.

The federal government as the single payer sets prices and keeps them low but gives states discretion over what types of care are eligible for payment and what are the priorities among these. The "Oregon approach"—involving the public in consciously setting priorities for the services available—is taken not only for the poor but also now for the vast bulk of the population.

Health care innovation slows dramatically. The system favors paying only for what has the greatest return on limited funds. To become widely available, an innovation has to have a low price tag and quickly lead to lower overall costs.

Certain cancer vaccines are widely available; ultrasound diagnostic devices and bionic enhancers develop more slowly and are available only if you can afford them or if you "buy up"—purchase directly or through extra insurance coverage.

Over time the government encourages providers to implement a "forecast, prevent, and manage" approach to primary care. Heroic measures to prolong life of those near death (including extremely premature babies) have been dramatically reduced. Rationing of scarce resources push health care providers to become more active in creating healthy communities.

Affluent consumers, the 30% who "buy up," are satisfied, though some grumble about the extra charges they pay. Some members of the middle class resent their lack of choice, yet most are satisfied. The formerly uninsured are better off because of the greater emphasis on services for all.

Bottom line: With hard times and increased poverty comes greater illness, yet this is somewhat offset by the movement toward the "forecast, prevent, and manage" paradigm. The affluent are able to purchase better care and technology and thus significantly improve their health and functioning. Others benefit as well, because hard times force the health care system to become more efficient.

## Buyer's Market

The growing cost and growing dissatisfaction with health care prompts a dramatic shift toward letting the market determine health services. The cost of health care reaches $1 trillion and nearly 15% of the GNP and a powerful coalition emerges. Policy makers, employers, and consumer groups become convinced that modest changes will not work; responsibility for health and health care expenditures are returned to the consumer.

National health policy makes all individuals and families who are not poor or "near poor" responsible for their health expenditures up to 8% to 10% of their income. People can buy insurance, but the insurance has to meet certain criteria and includes administrative costs and profit of the insurer and a tax to help pay for the care given to the poor. Medicare and Medicaid coverage is adjusted to ensure that all poor and near-poor individuals have basic health care.

States now ensure that health care providers are effective in their work. They are certified on the basis of their knowledge and competence, not their profession. They are recertified on the basis of the outcomes of the care they provide. Ineffective physicians, nurses, and other providers lose their certificates of practice.

Nurses, other conventional health care providers, and alternative providers quickly seek to practice more independently. A diverse and active market for various types of providers and treatments emerges. Even managed-care plans begin providing both conventional and alternative therapies. Cost-effective innovation is rapid because the resulting outcomes are quickly known.

In-home information systems let patients compare how well their health care provider is doing in relation to others. People can even manage their own diagnosis and treatment for most nonacute conditions. Individuals can now forecast their health conditions, and they have better tools for changing their lifestyles and for adopting medical strategies to prevent or manage disease. The result: People have greater freedom from health care providers. Home information systems can now tap into the expertise of the best specialists in any field.

Individuals and families are now rewarded for good health and prudent buying, either by not having to pay out of pocket or by yearly rebates from their insurance company or managed-care provider.

Some people still make poor decisions regarding their health and assume that catastrophic coverage will take care of them. However, most people have learned to improve their health conditions and better manage their health care needs. This awareness includes a greater sophistication about which, if any, treatments make sense in the very late stages of life. Combined with greater acceptance of death throughout society, this has lowered expenditures in the days and months before death.

In this scenario health care's portion of the GNP is reduced from its high of 15% to 10% by the year 2010. These savings result from lower disease rates, better and cheaper diagnostics and therapeutics, the acceptance of dying (which cuts down on expensive and needless life-prolonging procedures), and other factors. The percentage might have dropped lower, except for the fact that the services of alternative providers (such as acupuncturists and various physical therapists) are now often sought by consumers on a recurring preventive basis.

Bottom line: People are smarter, savvier consumers of health care services and receive care from the good doctors, nurses, and other health care providers, as well as software/expert systems, and shun the ones who perform poorly. Giving individuals responsibility for their own health and managing their health care expenditures leads to better and more cost-effective care in this scenario.

## Healthy, Healing Communities

Healing the body, mind, and spirit of individuals and communities becomes health care's focus. The specific paths taken are as diverse as communities, but together they help to reinvent a twenty-first century U.S. democracy that is sustainable and healthy in communities throughout the country.

Most of the health care players who have long-term loyalty in communities also give people more control over the system's priorities and management. Health systems and the communities they serve realize that they can work together to eliminate problems such as drugs, teenage pregnancy, and the effects of poverty.

Health care's focus on healthy communities is important in overcoming problems with both the environment and unemployment. As the Information Revolution makes most workers more productive—or replaces many workers altogether—unemployment grows to 25% by the year 2005. Volunteering for various personal and community health-enhancing activities becomes an important source of personal identity and satisfaction. Making communities sustainable—environmentally and economically viable places for families—in the face of declining "paid work" becomes the goal that health care organizations help achieve.

Members of health care organizations are polled on the design and operation and priorities for care; this sophisticated polling becomes a significant model for other dialogues that enhance the nature of democracy. The discussions generally reinforce the commitments that most health care organizations make to building communities and a world that works for everyone—humans, other species, and nature as well.

In some communities where much community development is now done through health organizations, expenditures rise. Generally, the expenditures for what was thought of as medical-care expenditures and which accounted for roughly 15% of the GNP in 1995, now account for less than 10%, with higher health gains.

Older people now face fewer years of disability because of better nutrition, exercise, social interaction, mental stimulation, personal and spiritual growth, and the opportunity to contribute in rewarding ways in the community. As a result people spend much less time in long-term-care institutions. When loss of mental or physical capacity does occur, bionics, robotics, smarter homes, and more caring neighborhoods do much to allow the disabled elderly to remain at home.

Bottom line: People are healthier because their community is healthier and offers a secure and nurturing environment where neighbors look out for one another. Per capita health care spending is down one third from the mid 1990s and is viewed as an important long-term investment in a healthier society.

# WILD CARDS

What are some of the possible breakthroughs in health care that could dramatically alter our health in the future? And what could go wrong? Box 37-1 suggests some possibilities.

### Box 37-1
### *Wild Cards*

**Health Breakthroughs**

Microrobots or nanodevices circulate in the body and act as a general repair device for a disease that the immune system cannot handle. These devices also help slow the aging process.

Dream therapy comes into wide use by health care providers. The use of virtual reality and lucid dreaming techniques create out-of-body experiences that transcend our physical limitations. We "feel" healthier even if our bodies are ravaged by disease or disability.

Cyberspace is used again as a way to overcome our physical limitations. Our minds and our cyber-personae are physically fit, perhaps even superhuman.

There is a technology of consciousness that enhances health.

Electronics and human consciousness merge to form "psychotechnology." We can communicate with all the body's cells, telling them to "shape up."

Telepathic communication replaces electronic communication. We are all connected mentally. Mind-to-mind replaces computer-to-computer as the quickest and most preferred method of transmitting information.

Alternative medicine ranging from acupuncture to aromatherapy, which have been demonstrated effective, are fully integrated into the new health care system.

**Health Nightmares**

New diseases emerge, such as a successor to Ebola or a form of AIDS, that can be transmitted via sneezing or coughing.

A major portion of the planet experiences an ecologic collapse, for example, global warming might cause harsh weather patterns and severe crop losses, thus triggering widespread malnutrition.

Information technologies are flagrantly abused. Medical records are manipulated, causing erroneous treatment. Information on DNA profiles, health and psychological conditions, and economic patterns becomes available to computer hackers, criminals, and others who can threaten our health and well-being.

---

Modified from *Institute for Alternative Futures.*

# IMPLICATIONS FOR NURSING

So what does all of this mean for nursing? What are the opportunities and challenges in these predictions of the future? Can nursing take advantage of the changes in health care and thrive? Will nurses retreat from full participation in the health care system of the future?

What has nursing traditionally done when faced with new circumstances? We have responded with remarkable courage and determination in times of need, such as war or extreme poverty or other dire conditions. We have shown exceptional courage in disaster situations. Examples include the Hyatt Hotel disaster in Kansas City when the balcony fell and nurses on the staff of ANA headquarters rushed to the aid of the wounded and dying; the Sioux City plane crash; the Oklahoma City bombing; and the Vietnam War. Nurses' abilities, compassion, and cool headedness have cared and comforted many in those terrible situations.

Sometimes we have exhibited extraordinary ability to collaborate. Establishing the nursing institute at the National Institutes of Health was a remarkable achievement because Congress had to override President Reagan's veto. It resulted from coordinated efforts from all of organized nursing and thousands of individual nurses who convinced their senators and representatives that nursing research would improve health care. And it has. At other times we have either been inert or divisive and, as a result, ineffective or we have been as inappropriately self-protecting as other health care providers also can be.

## What Are Our Strengths?

- We have a commitment to our patients.
- We are willing to do the work.
- We have the skills and the knowledge.
- We can communicate and coordinate nursing care, the work of other professions, and family members and patients, which is needed today to provide care across the continuum of an episode of care or a life span.
- We are good leaders and team members.

## Why Might We Not Succeed?

- We might retain a parochial, narrow, rigid view of nursing.
- Nurses might be unwilling to collaborate with each other and with other professions, both individually and collectively.
- The health care system might be unwilling to accept nursing's input or recognize nursing's contribution to health care.
- Organized nursing may concentrate on increasing its status, preserving its image, and enhancing its power.
- In the face of a potential surplus our schools may continue overproducing graduates and current nurses may not be able to shift into other areas.

## CONCLUSION

Whatever forecast comes to pass, a multitude of opportunities awaits the creative visionaries in nursing, both individually and collectively. Nursing has overcome tremendous adversity in its brief history and persevered, putting patients first. The same tenacity and dedication to patients coupled with openness, flexibility, energy, enthusiasm, and willingness to take chances can ensure that people have continued access to expert nursing care, as well as provide nursing with a viable future in health care.

We are all creating the future by what we do today. Or don't do. Let's not miss the opportunity to create the best future for nursing that we can. Future generations of nurses and their patients depend on it.

## *Discussion Exercises*

1. The chapter suggests four scenarios for the future of health care. Which one do you think is most likely? Why? Explain.
2. The first chapter of the book explains that "wild cards," though unexpected, do occur. Select one of the wild cards listed in Box 37-1, and describe what changes might follow if it came true.
3. This book has been designed to help you participate in creating nursing's future. What is the most important lesson you have learned about influencing the future?

## References

This chapter was adapted from an article compiled by Clement Bezold from the writings and discussions of six leading North American health futurists: Clement Bezold, Roy Amara, Trevor Hancock, Lee Kaiser, Jeff Goldsmith, and Russell Coile and the forecasts of the Institute for Alternative Futures. The article, "Your Health in 2010: Four Scenarios," was published in *The Futurist,* March/April, 1997 and is used with permission from the World Futures Society.

**RN 4 EVR**

*Missouri license plate*

# Appendix A
# International Resources

## Welsh Health Planning Forum Portland House

22 Newport Road
Cardiff CF21DB
Wales
Phone: 0222-460015

Part of the National Health Service Directorate of the Welsh office, the forum has been developing a strategic direction for the NHS in Wales, serving a population of 2.8 million people since 1989. The forum "endeavors to operate at the interface between the leading edge of strategy development and the trailing edge of health futures."

## PAHO/World Health Organization Health Policies Development Program

525 23rd Street NW
Washington, DC 20037
USA
Phone: (202)861-3218
Fax: (202)861-2647
Contact: Christine Puentes-Markides

The Pan American Health Organization (PAHO) has an ongoing program to make health futures tools and forecasts available to their member states. See "On Futures for Health and Health Care in Latin America and the Caribbean: Trends, Scenarios, Visions, and Strategies" (Technical Reports series No. 12), October 1992.

## WHO/Euro Strategic Planning and Evaluation

Copenhagen, Denmark
Phone: +45 39 17 17 17

Fax: +45 39 17 18 18
Contact: Herbert Zollner

WHO/Euro has held a series of meetings on health futures in its region. See "Future Trends in Society and the European Health for All Strategy: A Report on the Second Consultation," Prague, July 2, 1992.

### OECD Futures Studies Information Base

2 Rue Andre Pascal
75775 Paris CEDEX 16
France
Phone: 45 24 82 00
Fax: (33-1)45 24 85 00
Contact: W. Michalski, Head, Advisory Unit to the Secretary General

OECD Supports dissemination of futures tools to a wider audience.

### World Health Futures Studies Federation c/o Turku School of Economics

Fehtorinpellonkatu 3
sf-20500
Turku, Finland
Phone: 358-21-638 3310
Fax: 358-21-330 755
Contact: Professor Pentti Malaska, Secretary General

This association of professional and academic futurists provides networks and publications.

### The World Futures Society

7910 Woodmont Avenue, Suite 450
Bethesda, MD 20814 USA
Phone: (301)656-8274
Fax: (301)951-0394

A group with both professional and lay members, this society publishes a popular magazine, *The Futurist,* a refereed journal, *Futures Research Quarterly,* and the most cost-effective environmental scanning of English language periodicals. "Futures Survey."

### Futuribles International

55 Rue De Varenne
75007 Paris, France
Phone: 011-33-1-42-22-63-10
Fax: 011-33-1-42-22-65-54
Contact: Hugues de Jouvenel

This organization has developed a network for the French-speaking community.

### Swiss Society for Futures Research

Haldenweg 10A
CH-3074 Mrui, Switzerland
Phone: 41 31 33 65 55
Fax: 41 31 33 68 00
Contact: Dr. Gerhard Kocher

For German speakers, this society compiles futures material from German and English sources.

### International Health Futures Network (IHFN) for Americas or Asia:

The Healthcare Forum
830 Market Street, 8th floor
San Francisco, CA 94102 USA
Phone: (415)421-8810
Fax: (415)421-8837
Contact: David Zimmerman

### Foundation for Strategic Health Policy Development

PO Box 7100
2701 AC Zoetermeer
The Netherlands
Phone: 079-710311
Fax: 079-510881
Contact: Ronald F. Schreuder

A coalition of a large number of futures groups, the IHFN has published a reader on health futures and has an ongoing newsletter. Projects are emerging that will catalogue efforts worldwide to invent twenty-first-century health systems and to explore the future of public health.

### Institute for Alternative Futures

100 North Pitt Street, Suite 235
Alexandria, VA 22314
Phone: (703)684-5880
Fax: (703)664-0640
The Institute for Alternative Futures works extensively on health futures efforts around the world. For the United States, former U.S. Sur-

geon General C. Everett Koop and other Americans developed "Healthy People in a Healthy World: The Belmont Vision for Health Care in America," which describes a preferable future for health. It is used by individual hospitals and health care systems around the country as a touchstone for developing or comparing their visions. Available materials include a newsletter, "Health Care Visions," as well as "Creating Community Health Visions: A Guide for Local Leaders."

---

Data from *Healthcare Forum J* March/April 1994.

Appendix B

# Doctoral Programs in the United States

## SCHOOLS OF NURSING THAT OFFER DOCTORAL PROGRAMS IN NURSING

University of Alabama at Birmingham
Birmingham, Alabama

University of Arkansas for Medical Sciences
Little Rock, Arkansas

University of Arizona
Tucson, Arizona

University of California–Los Angeles
Los Angeles, California

University of California–San Francisco
San Francisco, California

University of San Diego
San Diego, California

University of Colorado Health Science Center
Denver, Colorado

University of Connecticut
Storrs, Connecticut

Yale University
New Haven, Connecticut

The Catholic University of America
Washington, D.C.

Barry University
Miami Shores, Florida

University of Florida
Gainesville, Florida

University of Miami
Coral Gables, Florida

University of South Florida
Tampa, Florida

Georgia State University
Atlanta, Georgia

Medical College of Georgia
Augusta, Georgia

Loyola University of Chicago
Chicago, Illinois

Rush University
Chicago, Illinois

University of Illinois at Chicago
Chicago, Illinois

Indiana University
Indianapolis, Indiana

University of Iowa
Iowa City, Iowa

University of Kansas
Kansas City, Kansas

University of Kentucky
Lexington, Kentucky

Louisiana State University Medical Center
New Orleans, Louisiana

The Johns Hopkins University
Baltimore, Maryland

University of Maryland
Baltimore, Maryland

Boston College
Chestnut Hill, Massachusetts

University of Massachusetts–Amherst
Amherst, Massachusetts

University of Massachusetts–Worcester
Worcester, Massachusetts

University of Massachusetts–Boston
Boston, Massachusetts

University of Massachusetts–Lowell
Lowell, Massachusetts

University of Michigan
Ann Arbor, Michigan

Wayne State University
Detroit, Michigan

University of Minnesota
Minneapolis, Minnesota

Saint Louis University
St. Louis, Missouri

University of Missouri–Columbia
Columbia, Missouri

University of Missouri–Kansas City
Kansas City, Missouri

University of Missouri–St. Louis
St. Louis, Missouri

University of Nebraska Medical Center
Omaha, Nebraska

Rutgers, The State University of New Jersey
Newark, New Jersey

Adelphi University
Garden City, New York

Columbia University
New York, New York

New York University
New York, New York

State University of New York–Buffalo
Buffalo, New York

Teachers College, Columbia University
New York, New York

University of Rochester
Rochester, New York

University of North Carolina–Chapel Hill
Chapel Hill, North Carolina

Case Western Reserve University
Cleveland, Ohio

The Ohio State University
Columbus, Ohio

University of Cincinnati
Cincinnati, Ohio

Oregon Health Sciences University
Portland, Oregon

Duquesne University
Pittsburgh, Pennsylvania

University of Pennsylvania
Philadelphia, Pennsylvania

University of Pittsburgh
Pittsburgh, Pennsylvania

Widener University
Chester, Pennsylvania

University of Rhode Island
Kingston, Rhode Island

University of South Carolina
Columbia, South Carolina

Medical University of South Carolina
Charleston, South Carolina

University of Tennessee–Knoxville
Knoxville, Tennessee

University of Tennessee–Memphis
Memphis, Tennessee

Vanderbilt University
Nashville, Tennessee

University of Texas Health Science Center–San Antonio
San Antonio, Texas

Texas Tech University Health Sciences Center
Lubbock, Texas

Texas Woman's University
Denton, Texas

University of Texas Health Science Center
Houston, Texas

University of Texas–Austin
Austin, Texas

University of Texas–Galveston
Galveston, Texas

University of Utah
Salt Lake City, Utah

George Mason University
Fairfax, Virginia

University of Virginia
Charlottesville, Virginia

Virginia Commonwealth University
Richmond, Virginia

University of Washington
Seattle, Washington

University of Wisconsin–Madison
Madison, Wisconsin

University of Wisconsin–Milwaukee
Milwaukee, Wisconsin

## SCHOOLS OF NURSING THAT PLAN TO OFFER DOCTORAL PROGRAMS

Azusa Pacific University
Azusa, California

University of Southern California
Los Angeles, California

Emory University
Atlanta, Georgia

University of Hawaii at Manoa
Honolulu, Hawaii

Southern University and A&M College
Baton Rouge, Louisiana

Grand Valley State University
Allendale, Michigan

Michigan State University
East Lansing, Michigan

University of Southern Mississippi
Hattiesburg, Mississippi

University of Medicine & Dentistry of New Jersey
Newark, New Jersey

Binghamton University
Binghamton, New York

University of Texas–El Paso
El Paso, Texas

Old Dominion University
Norfolk, Virginia

West Virginia University
Morgantown, West Virginia

# Appendix C
# Directory of Nursing Organizations

Academy of Medical-Surgical Nurses
American Academy of Ambulatory Care Nursing
American Academy of Nursing
American Assembly for Men in Nursing
American Association for Continuity of Care
American Association of Colleges of Nursing
American Association of Critical-Care Nurses
American Association of Diabetes Educators
American Association of Neuroscience Nurses
American Association of Nurse Anesthesists
American Association of Occupational Health Nurses
American Association of Spinal Cord Injury Nurses
American College of Nurse Practitioners
American Heart Association Council on Cardiovascular Nursing
American Holistic Nurses Association
American Medical Informatics Association
American Nephrology Nurses' Association
American Nurses Association
American Nurses Foundation
American Psychiatric Nurses Association
American Public Health Association
American Radiological Nurses Association
American Society for Parenteral and Entéral Nutrition
American Society of Ophthalmic Registered Nurses
American Society of Pain Management Nursing
American Society of PeriAnesthesia Nurses
American Society of Plastic and Reconstructive Surgical Nurses, Inc.
American Thoracic Society
Association of Black Nursing Faculty in Higher Education, Inc.
Association of Community Health Nursing Educators

Association of Nurses in AIDS Care
Association of Occupational Health Professionals
Association of Operating Room Nurses, Inc.
Association of Pediatric Onocology Nurses
Association of Rehabilitation Nurses
Association of State and Territorial Directors of Nursing
Association of Women's Health, Obstetric, and Neonatal Nurses
Chi Eta Phi Sorority, Inc.
Consolidated Association of Nurses in Substance Abuse International
Council for Acute Care Nursing Practice
Council for Advanced Practice Nursing
Council for Community, Primary, and Long Term Nursing Practice
Council for Nursing Research
Council for Nursing Systems and Administration
Council for Professional Nursing Education and Development
Council on Graduate Education for Administration in Nursing
Dermatology Nurses Association
Developmental Disabilities Nurses Association
Drug and Alcohol Nursing Association
Emergency Nurses Association
Home Healthcare Nurses Association
Hospice and Palliative Nurses Association
International Society of Nurses in Genetics
International Society of Psychiatric Consultation Liaison Nurses
Intravenous Nurses Society
National Association of Directors of Nursing Administration in Long Term Care
National Association of Hispanic Nurses
National Association of Neonatal Nurses
National Association of Nurse Massage Therapists
National Association of Nurse Practitioners in Reproductive Health
National Association of Orthopaedic Nurses
National Association of Pediatric Nurse Associates and Practitioners
National Association of School Nurses, Inc.
National Association of State School Nurse Consultants, Inc.
National Black Nurses Association, Inc.
National Flight Nurses Association
National Gerontological Nursing Association
National League for Nursing
National Nurses Society on Addictions
National Nursing Staff Development Organization
National Organization of Nurse Practitioner Faculties
National Student Nurses Association
North American Nursing Diagnosis Association
Nurses Organization of Veterans Affairs
Nursing Division of the American Association on Mental Retardation
Oncology Nursing Society
Philippine Nurses Association of America, Inc.
Respiratory Nursing Society
Sigma Theta Tau International
Society for Education & Research in Psychiatric-Mental Health Nursing
Society for Vascular Nursing
Society of Gastroenterology Nurses and Associates, Inc.
Society of Otorhinolaryngology and Head-Neck Nurses, Inc.
Society of Pediatric Nurses
Society of Urologic Nurses & Associates, Inc.
Southern Nursing Research Society
The American Association of Legal Nurse Consultants
The American Association of Nurse Attorneys
Wound, Ostomy & Continence Nurses Society

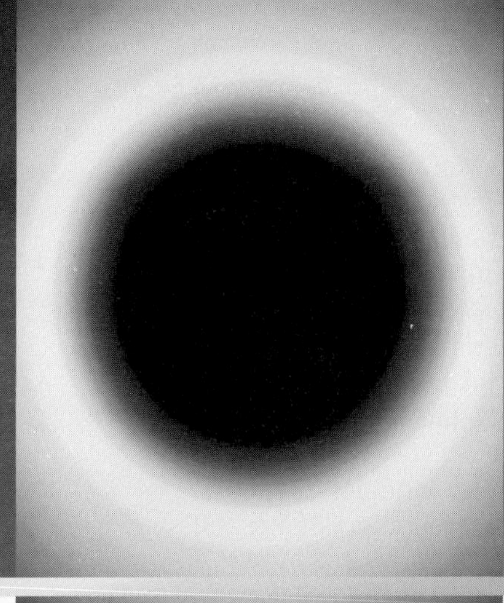

# Index

**E**